P9-ARE-983

Road
El Dorado, Kansas 67042-3280

LIBRARY IN A BOOK

THREATS TO FOOD SAFETY

Fred C. Pampel

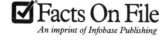

Facts On File
An imprint of Infobase Publishing

THREATS TO FOOD SAFETY

Facts On File, Inc.
An imprint of Infobase Publishing
132 West 31st Street
New York NY 10001

Library of Congress Cataloging-in-Publication Data

Pampel, Fred C.
  Threats to food safety / Fred C. Pampel.
    p. cm.—(Library in a book)
  Includes bibliographical references and index.
  ISBN 0-8160-6281-1
  1. Food adulteration and inspection. 2. Food—Quality. 3. Food—Safety measures. I. Title. II. Series.
  TX531.P26 2006
  363.19′264—dc22   2005031606

Facts On File books are available at special discounts when purchased in bulk quantities for businesses, associations, institutions, or sales promotions. Please call our Special Sales Department in New York at (212) 967-8800 or (800) 322-8755.

You can find Facts On File on the World Wide Web at http://www.factsonfile.com

Text design by Ron Monteleone

Printed in the United States of America

MP Hermitage 10 9 8 7 6 5 4 3 2 1

363.19 PAM 2006

Pampel, Fred C.
Threats to food safety.

CONTENTS

PART III
APPENDICES

PART I

OVERVIEW OF THE TOPIC

CHAPTER 1

INTRODUCTION TO THREATS TO FOOD SAFETY

Most Americans take the safety of their food for granted. The food supply seems so varied, plentiful, and satisfying that overeating and obesity rather than lack of safe foods occupies people's attention. Consumers often take simple precautions to ensure food safety, such as washing fruits and vegetables, refrigerating leftovers, and fully cooking meat, and some buy organic foods to minimize exposure to artificial chemicals. Otherwise, they give little attention to the issue. After all, government officials and politicians call the American food supply the safest in the world.

That attitude could change quickly, however. Food safety remains vulnerable to several threats that have become more worrisome in recent years. Experts disagree on the extent of the threats and on the ability of the government to protect the population from them, but warnings of serious problems in the future are unmistakable:

- New and deadly antibiotic-resistant strains of bacteria spread by food have emerged in the last several decades.
- A frightening new disease called mad cow disease that affects the nervous systems of its victims is spread by eating infected tissue in beef.
- Terrorists threaten to contaminate food with deadly poisons.
- Modern farming, production methods, and preferences for convenience foods have increased the use of chemical additives, pesticides, and hormones in food, which may cause cancer and other health problems.
- Techniques of passing meat through radiation and genetically modifying crops may present new food hazards.

Are these claims unnecessarily alarmist? Should Americans worry about food safety? Can the government protect consumers from the risks of

3

food-based disease? Determining the safety of food and the seriousness of the threats proves surprisingly difficult. It often involves more philosophical and moral judgments than scientific facts. Still, the questions remain critically important—and could become even more so in the near future. This chapter provides an overview of the threats to food safety and the controversies they generate. It begins with discussion of foodborne illness and mad cow disease and then considers terrorist actions, food additives, chemical and natural toxins, food allergens, and new food technologies.

FOODBORNE ILLNESS

The statistics on foodborne illnesses or food poisoning—diseases caused by ingesting food with bacteria, viruses, parasites, or toxins—are staggering: 76 million persons become sick each year, with 325,000 requiring hospitalization and 5,000 dying.[1] That translates into 890 hospitalizations and 14 deaths each day. Worse, some disease agents have become more resistant to treatment and more likely to cause serious illness or death. Even the currently accepted figures may understate the problem, as many infections of unknown cause may be transmitted by food. Simple precautions such as thoroughly cooking and refrigerating food can help but not eliminate the problem.

Most often the illnesses cause vomiting and diarrhea—more an inconvenience than a life-threatening condition. Yet the hospitalizations and deaths make the disease a serious threat, particularly when the victims are young children. For example, on July 18, 1993, six-year-old Alex Donley died of an infection he picked up from eating an undercooked hamburger that contained bacteria-laden cattle feces. His mother, Nancy Donley, wrote of his death over a four-day period:

> *I watched in horror his life hemorrhaging away in the hospital bathroom; bowl after bowl of blood and mucus gushed from his little body. Later, I helped change blood-soaked diapers that he had to wear after he could no longer stand or walk. Alex's screams were followed by silence as the evil toxins attacked his brain causing him to lose neurological control. His eyes crossed and he suffered tremors and delusions. He no longer knew who I was.[2]*

A small portion of those who survive foodborne illness, about 2 to 3 percent, suffer long-term health problems such as kidney failure, nerve damage, and arthritis. For example, Linda Deasley's young son Jimmy survived in 1987 the same infection that killed Alex Donley. In describing Jimmy's long-term health consequences, she says

Introduction to Threats to Food Safety

Today, you can tell by looking at him that something happened to him. He walks with a bit of a limp and he never regained the use of his left arm. His IQ will never be more than that of a 12 to 13 year old . . . For a while, Jimmy thought he would eventually get back to normal. It was hard for him to realize that this was not going to go away.[3]

These outcomes make foodborne illness more than an inconvenience. Despite their small numbers compared to heart disease, cancers, strokes, and accidents, disabilities and deaths from foodborne illness are undeniably tragic.

The problem will not disappear soon. Food-based forms of infectious disease have persisted in spite of modern technology, advanced medicine, and improved human health. Indeed, new strains have become more lethal and immune to antibiotics. The annual costs of foodborne illness likewise remain high, with related medical expenses, lost work, and premature death reaching $6.9 billion a year.[4] The public seems more concerned about the problem than ever before, and controversy exists over whether the government does enough to protect the public from foodborne illness.

FROM MOSES TO JACK IN THE BOX

Over time, humans discovered that salting, drying, or cooking and curing food with smoke did much to reduce the risk of foodborne illness, though it did not eliminate the problem. The Old Testament lists a variety of dietary practices designed to keep food safe: By the Law of Moses, Israelites were not permitted to eat pork, shellfish, rats, lizards, and other unclean foods. These and other dietary rules concerned with cleanliness in meal preparation helped protect them from unsafe food. Writers in Roman times and the Middle Ages also recognized the link between certain foods and sickness, even if they did not know about the microbes that cause the disease.

Modern science identified the sources of foodborne illness. John Snow demonstrated in 1851 that drinking water could spread the deadly disease cholera, and William Budd in the late 1850s demonstrated that typhoid fever could be spread by milk. Although bacteria had been seen through primitive microscopes dating back to 1676, Robert Koch and Louis Pasteur founded the science of microbiology in the late 1800s, and others led scientists to identify foodborne agents. In 1888, August Gaertner isolated a *Salmonella* bacterium from both the meat of a cow slaughtered while sick with diarrhea and the body of a man who died from food poisoning after eating that meat (59 other people became sick as well from the same cow). Around this same time, other scientists isolated bacteria such as *E. coli* and *Shigella* that could be transmitted to humans via food.

5

Threats to Food Safety

The public in the United States became more aware of the risks of unclean food with the publication of a best-selling exposé in 1906. *The Jungle* by Upton Sinclair described the filthy conditions in the Chicago stockyards. The novel was based on Sinclair's observations of activities in a slaughterhouse and meatpacking plant. Readers were sickened by his descriptions of the blood, feces, and filth on the plant floor; the use of diseased cattle and pregnant cows for meat; and the way workers scooped up dirt, rats, and poison from the floor in making sausages. The scandal created by the book led to investigations and, with the support of President Theodore Roosevelt, to passage by Congress of the Pure Food and Drug Act and the Meat Inspection Act in 1906.

Around the same time, "Typhoid Mary" Mallon created headlines about the danger of foodborne illness.[5] Mallon, an Irish immigrant who worked as a cook, carried typhoid bacteria but did not get sick from it. However, she passed the disease from her hands to the food she prepared. When several people came down with the disease at a well-to-do summer home, she was identified as the culprit. After refusing to stop cooking and revealing mental instability, she was arrested and quarantined in 1907. Called the most dangerous women in America, she was detained until 1910 and then released on the condition that she not cook for the public again. However, she continued to do so, spreading typhoid fever wherever she went.

Improvements in public health lessened concern about foodborne illness in the first half of the 20th century. Stories about Typhoid Mary, new clean-food laws applied to meatpacking, the widespread pasteurization (or heating) of milk to kill microbes, and the use of safe canning methods all helped address the problem. People instead worried more about diseases spread through human contact. In 1918–19, 675,000 Americans died from an influenza epidemic, and diseases such as scarlet fever, tuberculosis, and pneumonia still killed many people. Later, concern about rising rates of deaths from heart disease, cancers, and smoking-related diseases overshadowed problems of foodborne illnesses.

In the second half of the century, attitudes began to shift again. In 1971, the American Public Health Association (APHA) took the U.S. Department of Agriculture (USDA) and its secretary, Earl Butz, to court over inspection procedures.[6] Based on the 1906 Meat Inspection Act and later revisions in the laws, the USDA inspected meat largely by looking, poking, and smelling the product. Inspectors could identify obviously spoiled products but, without microscopic exams, could not really certify that meat was safe. The APHA demanded that labels be placed on raw meat packages that warned of the risks of bacterial infection and the need for thorough cooking.

In the 1980s, other groups expressed alarm about the safety of meat. The General Accounting Office (GAO) offered a critical report on meat exami-

6

nation procedures, claiming that inspectors could no longer keep up with the increased speed of meatpacking. A 1985 report from the National Research Council (NRC) recommended that the USDA improve its food inspection system, echoing other claims that the sight, touch, and smell methods were inadequate and unscientific.

The government responded grudgingly to concerns about foodborne illness. In reaction to a 1971 suit, the USDA argued that because many foods contain bacteria, it made more sense to educate consumers about the broad risk of foodborne illness rather than single out meat as hazardous. In *APHA v. Butz*, an appeals court ruled in 1974 that the USDA could choose education over warnings and leave its approval and inspection labels unchanged. In the 1980s, Congress refused as well to respond directly to concerns expressed by the GAO and NRC about meat inspection and foodborne illness. To the contrary, they passed a 1986 law that gave new inspection responsibilities to meat companies and gave government inspectors more choice in deciding how often plants had to be inspected.

Recent Outbreaks Raise Concerns

Highly publicized and deadly outbreaks of foodborne disease in the 1990s led to new action and widespread recognition of the problem. In January 1993, doctors in a pediatric hospital in Seattle, Washington, reported an unusually large number of children with *E. coli* infections. Several had to undergo dialysis when the infections caused their kidneys to stop working properly. One two-year-old boy soon died. State inspectors discovered that the outbreak resulted from eating hamburgers from area Jack in the Box restaurants. The restaurant chain accused its meat supplier of providing hamburger that had been contaminated with fecal matter in the slaughterhouse, but state officials held the restaurants responsible for not fully cooking the hamburger and killing the bacteria. In the end, the incident led to 501 reported incidents, 151 hospitalizations, three deaths, and untold negative publicity for Jack in the Box hamburgers.[7]

In 1996, the makers of Odwalla fruit juice recalled 13 types of juice after an outbreak of *E. coli* was linked to their product. Although previous outbreaks had come from undercooked hamburgers, these cases stemmed from contaminated apples that the company had used in its unpasteurized apple juice. Perhaps the apples had become contaminated with the fecal matter of cows grazing nearby. In any case, one 16-month-old girl died, 14 children developed life-threatening kidney ailments, and 70 persons became sick.[8]

In 2000, more than 60 people contracted *E. coli* from eating watermelon in a salad bar at a Milwaukee Sizzler steakhouse. Fifteen of the victims were children, with three developing severe kidney failure and one three-year-old girl dying.[9] Restaurant employees had used the same knives to cut watermelon that they had used earlier to slice some tainted beef. The beef was cooked enough to kill the bacteria, but the raw watermelon in the salad bar allowed the bacteria to pass directly to the customers. Worse, older fruit was not discarded as new fruit was added, which allowed the bacteria to grow and spread.

Of special concern, these outbreaks involved a dangerous form of the normally harmless *E. coli* bacteria. This new strain, called *E. coli* O157:H7, seemed to have picked up genes from other deadly bacteria and caused the release of dangerous toxins into the body of its human hosts. Antibiotics do little to kill this strain and may even increase the risk of death (the bacteria respond to the antibiotic with increased output of toxins).[10] The toxins poison the blood supply and organs, often overcoming the underdeveloped defense system of young children.

These incidents raised the awareness of the public about foodborne illnesses. Government agencies began to take more seriously the need to prevent contamination of food in food plants, better inspect meat and other products, remove tainted items before they could be sold and eaten, and educate consumers about food safety practices. In recent years, the Centers for Disease Control and Prevention has begun to track the most common and dangerous types of foodborne disease.

AGENTS OF FOODBORNE DISEASE

Understanding issues of food safety does not require a course in microbiology, but it helps to know something about the bacteria, viruses, and parasites most often spread by food (and the dangerous toxins sometimes produced by the microbes). Although there are more than 250 foodborne pathogens (a term used to describe microbes such as bacteria, viruses, and parasites that cause illness), the Foodborne Disease Active Surveillance Network (FoodNet) has identified several of most concern.[11] The unfamiliar names of bacteria and viruses in the selective list that follows should not hide their common presence in the food people enjoy.

Bacterial Agents

Campylobacter jejuni: This germ is the leading cause of bacterial diarrhea, affecting more than a million persons each year. Although responsible for more food poisoning than any other organism, it remains unknown to the public. The lack of publicity may stem from the relatively mild symptoms of the diseases, which typically last about a week. However, in rare cases it can lead to life-threatening infections and Guillain-Barré syndrome, a neurological disease causing paralysis that can last several weeks. *Campylobacter jejuni* is spread most often from raw poultry and less often from unpasteurized milk. Most chicken flocks carry the bacteria in their intestines but are not harmed by it. When slaughtering the chickens, material from the intestines can transfer to the meat. The bacteria show up in more than half of raw chicken products, which require careful handling and full cooking. Cows can also become infected and pass the bacteria into milk, which can infect humans if not pasteurized. Efforts in the last few years of the USDA to improve its inspections have reduced but not eliminated the presence of this disease on chicken meat and in milk.

Clostridium botulinum: These bacteria produce a nerve toxin that causes botulism, a disease causing paralysis, breathing failure, and death. An antidote exists for the disease but must be given quickly to be effective.[12] The bacteria are found in soil but remain dormant until they find low oxygen and low acid conditions—the environment of canned products. Improvements in home canning procedures have done much to eliminate the disease, but shoppers should beware of swollen cans at grocery stores. On rare occasions, outbreaks have occurred from eating cooked onions and chopped garlic that had been placed in conditions where low oxygen and acidity allowed the bacteria to grow and produce dangerous toxins.

Escherichia coli (E. coli) O157:H7: This strain of the generally harmless bacteria present in the intestines of healthy animals and humans has the trait of producing dangerous toxins. The genus name *Escherichia* comes from the scientist who discovered it, Theodor Escherich; the species name *coli* comes from its presence in the colon; and the number O157:H7 comes from markers found on the cell surface that define this particular strain. An estimated 73,000 cases of infection and 61 deaths occur each year. The usual symptoms of diarrhea, nausea, and low-grade fever usually disappear in a week, but in some cases the toxins released by the bacteria can cause hemolytic uremic syndrome that can lead to kidney failure in children. Cattle, deer, and other grazing animals carry the organism in their intestines, so contact with intestinal material and feces will infect meat. Although it can spread through water, unpasteurized apple juice and milk, and fruit and vegetables, it most often affects humans who eat undercooked hamburger. The lethal threat of the bacterium led the USDA to target it for its first microscopic testing program.

Listeria monocytogenes: Although most healthy adults are not affected by the bacterium, it has a high mortality rate among those who are vulnerable. It causes fever and muscle aches along with nausea and vomiting that, among vulnerable groups such as pregnant women, newborns, and the elderly, leads to serious illness and death. Of the 2,500 persons who become seriously ill each year from *Listeria monocytogenes,* about 500 die—an extremely high number for infected persons. It is more difficult to eliminate than other foodborne diseases because it is so common in the environment and can continue to grow even in the cool temperatures of a refrigerator. Its presence in soil and water contaminates raw vegetables, and it also appears in meat, cold cuts, and unpasteurized liquids. One outbreak that led to 48 deaths came from eating Mexican-style soft cheese, and another outbreak came from eating contaminated hotdogs.

Salmonella: This group of bacteria, first discovered by E. E. Salmon, causes the most deaths from foodborne illness in the United States. It usually leads to diarrhea that lasts four to seven days and requires victims to rest and replace lost liquid. In some cases, it can spread to the bloodstream and organs, where, without antibiotic treatment, severe illness can result. Humans can contract the illness by eating food contaminated with animal feces, but hens infected with the bacteria can pass it directly to their eggs. Eating raw or inadequately cooked eggs has become a major source of the disease. For example, 71 illnesses and 17 hospitalizations resulted from eating undercooked scrambled eggs from a breakfast bar in a Maryland restaurant.[13] Overall, 40,000 cases of *Salmonella* poisoning are reported each year, and 2–4 million other unreported cases likely occur. Of special concern, some scientists believe that antibiotic-resistant strains of *Salmonella* have emerged. If so, it is all the more important to thoroughly cook eggs and other products; avoid raw eggs in homemade Caesar salad dressing, ice cream, mayonnaise, and cookie dough; and take care in eating other uncooked food.

Shigella: A group of bacteria discovered by Japanese scientist Kiyoshi Shiga, *Shigella* is most closely associated with poor sanitation and hygiene. It causes diarrhea and stomach cramps in most people it infects but can more seriously harm young children, the elderly, and those with weak immune systems. Antibiotics can help with the illness, but some of the bacteria have become resistant to the usual medicines. A small portion of victims later develop a condition called Reiter's syndrome that involves joint pain, eye irritation, and painful urination and eventually can lead to chronic arthritis. The disease passes through the stools of infected persons, who may spread it to food by not washing properly. Raw sewage leaking into cropland or water can also infect humans; for example, a 1998 outbreak was traced to imported parsley grown and harvested in unsanitary conditions. About 18,000 cases are reported each year, but the number of unreported cases may reach 360,000.

Vibrio parahaemolyticus: This bacterium resides in coastal waters and infects shellfish that inhabit those waters. Outbreaks usually occur during the summer months from eating raw oysters and clams. In 1998, for example, 368 persons became ill from eating raw oysters harvested from Galveston Bay on the Texas Gulf Coast. Severe disease occurs rarely, with illness usually striking within 24 hours and lasting no more than three days. The illness is relatively rare, with 30–40 cases a year found in the Gulf Coast area. The government makes special efforts to monitor the presence of the bacterium during periods of oyster and clam harvest.

Yersinia enterocolitica: This bacterium is spread to humans most often from pigs and undercooked pork but can also be spread to other food from the unwashed hands of cooks handling pork products. It can also infect unpasteurized milk. About 17,000 cases occur each year.

Viral Agents

Hepatitis A: This viral disease can pass directly from contaminated food to uninfected persons and indirectly from an infected person to food and then to uninfected persons. In 1997, contaminated frozen strawberries transmitted the virus to 262 persons in five states; in 2001, an infected food handler passed the disease to 43 patrons who ate restaurant sandwiches.[14] Once it infects a host, the disease can take several weeks to develop, beginning with symptoms of diarrhea, nausea, and fever and later inflaming the liver and producing jaundice. Most people recover in a few weeks, but some can have symptoms for six to nine months. No effective treatments exist at present.

Norwalk Virus: Named after a small Ohio town where an outbreak occurred, this virus belongs to a family of similar diseases called noroviruses. It causes vomiting, nausea, abdominal pain, and diarrhea for a period of one or two days. The illness is spread through eating raw clams and oysters, but outbreaks have also been linked to eating fresh salads, coleslaw, fruit, and eggs. In the case of oysters, the disease was probably present in fishermen stools that were dumped into the sea and subsequently absorbed by oysters that later infected diners who ate them. The Norwalk virus is spread in other ways besides eating contaminated food. Several well-publicized instances of passengers on cruise ships contracting the virus likely resulted from contact with infected persons or contaminated parts of the ship.

Parasites

Cryptosporidium: This microscopic parasite lives in the intestines of animals and humans but has the ability to survive outside its hosts for long periods of time. It is typically found in water, soil, feces, and sewage and can affect people through drinking water and eating contaminated food. The parasite produces diarrhea in about a week and the symptoms can last one to two weeks.

Cyclospora cayetanensis: This single cell parasite has been found to infect water and fresh produce, particularly in developing countries. Besides diarrhea, it can cause cramps, bloating, weight loss, and persistent fatigue and, in some cases, last for up to a month.

Toxoplasma gondii: A parasite that proliferates in cats, the microorganism causes toxoplasmosis in humans. Cats are often the direct source of infection, but foods can spread the parasite as well. The parasite can be found in undercooked pork and lamb, in raw beef (such as steak tartar), and wild game. The parasite has little effect on most persons with a healthy immune system but can cause flu-like symptoms in some and severe damage to the brain and eyes of those with weak immune systems. Newborns, HIV/AIDS patients, and those undergoing chemotherapy are most at risk of damage and death.

EXTENT OF THE PROBLEM

Even this partial list of foodborne disease agents makes regular eating sound dangerous—most foods are vulnerable to one type or another of foodborne diseases. In fact, people continually come in contact with pathogens but show no symptoms or only mild symptoms. How then do experts determine the incidence of the diseases? The reported cases include only the most serious incidents, particularly when a group of people who ate the same food become sick, but miss illnesses left unreported by victims or assumed to be flu. The numbers instead come from calculations.

One method sums reported incidents and estimates of unreported incidents to obtain the total figures cited earlier: 76 million illnesses, 325,000 hospitalizations, and 5,000 deaths. Figures of known foodborne diseases account for 14 million illnesses, 60,000 hospitalizations, and 1,800 deaths.[15] Using other figures from smaller studies that determine the incidence of unreported foodborne disease and some complex mathematics produces the total estimates. Another method suggests even higher figures. Given estimates that each person on average has diarrhea 1.4 times each year and that 25 percent of diarrheal episodes are caused by foodborne diseases, the method suggests that there are 91 million incidents of foodborne disease in the country each year.[16] Still others suggest that foodborne diseases not associated with diarrhea are understated with these methods and produce even more incidents and deaths from foodborne disease.[17]

Some 1999 figures on the distribution of reported diseases can contrast the harm of most common foodborne illnesses.[18] The figures do not include unreported or undiagnosed incidents but for the most serious outcomes—death and hospitalization—highlight the main threats to the public. *Salmonella* causes the most deaths (556), followed by *Listeria monocytogenes* (499), *Toxoplasma gondii* (375), Norwalk-like viruses (120), *Campylobacter* (99), and *E. coli* O157:H7 (52). The ranking differs for incidents of hospitalization, where Norwalk-like viruses (20,000), *Salmonella* (16,000), and *Campylobacter* (10,500) lead to the most incidents.

Introduction to Threats to Food Safety

A study of the trends in the reported illnesses between 1996 and 2002 shows a decline for several diseases.[19] Reported incidents of *Campylobacter, Yersinia,* and *Listeria* have declined steadily, but no sustained decline appears for other major foodborne infections such as *Escherichia coli* O157:H7, *Vibrio,* and *Salmonella.* These findings are limited to reported incidents in areas within the FoodNet surveillance system and do not allow inferences about unreported incidents outside the system. Still, they give some possibly reassuring evidence that the problem has not worsened in recent years.

SOURCES OF INFECTION

Microbes are everywhere. They exist in the soil where food is grown, in the water where fish live, and in the bodes of healthy animals and humans. In one sense, it is no surprise that food comes in contact with many microbes that can cause sickness—it is surprising that people do not get sick more often than they do. The immune system generally deals well with foodborne infections and protects people from serious illness. In another sense, however, certain practices increase the risk of getting infections through food and suffering serious illness as a result.

The source of most foodborne illness is contact of food with fecal matter. Distasteful in any circumstances, such contact allows microorganisms to spread from the bowels of healthy animals and humans to food. If the animals or humans are sick from a potent bacterial or viral strain, the risk of spreading a more serious illness increases. Most commonly, contact between food and fecal matter occurs in slaughterhouses and meatpacking plants. Without careful butchering, material from the intestines can contaminate other parts of the animal carcass and the meat sold to consumers. Less commonly, fruit and vegetables can come in contact with the manure of grazing animals or with irrigation water that has been contaminated by sewage, and oysters and clams can come in contact with human sewage dumped into the sea.

Microbes can infect food in other ways besides contact with fecal matter. A hen with *Salmonella* can directly pass the bacteria to the eggs it lays. A sick cow can similarly pass *Salmonella* and other disease organisms into milk and, without pasteurization, into milk products such as cheese and ice cream. These hens and cows do not always appear sick but nonetheless transmit disease.

Modern Food Production

Tracing the sources of contamination backward ultimately leads to modern agricultural and food production methods. In the past, meat came from local ranches and farms that produced small amounts of food and allowed animals to graze in open fields. In contrast, modern agriculture has increased

13

its efficiency and productivity by crowding thousands of cattle, hogs, and hens together. Animals kept in these conditions inevitably come in contact with the feces of other animals, and diseases spread quickly and easily.

Shipping animals in crowded trucks and trains to distant locations for slaughtering also increases the risks of coming in contact with disease. Packing plants then mix meat from numerous animals to make hamburgers and sausages so that one infected carcass may contaminate other uninfected meat.

A description of poultry processing illustrates the risks of modern techniques compared to old-fashioned butchering.[20] After birds are killed by severing the major neck artery and the blood drains, they are scalded in hot (though not boiling) water to ease removal of the feathers. Then a machine with fingerlike rubber attachments removes the feathers. When *Salmonella* become attached to the skin of the birds, the scalding does not kill the pathogen, and the feather remover spreads it from those with infected skin to uninfected skin. A vacuum machine designed to remove the intestines without allowing any of the contents to spill nonetheless cannot reach 100 percent effectiveness and can allow fecal matter to come in contact with meaty parts of the bird. Cutting the carcass into parts can further spread pathogens via cutting tables and knives.

These production techniques do not cause the disease but allow it to spread. As a result, "Salmonella bacteria are found in 15 to 70 percent of poultry. High rates of contamination with campylobacter and *Listeria* bacteria have also been reported. If you consider all types of pathogens, the majority of chickens currently on sale are very likely contaminated with one form or another."[21] More expensive production techniques and higher paid employees in meatpacking plants would help minimize the problem but would also raise the cost of poultry. Businesses have focused on improving efficiency and lowering cost.

The mass production of eggs and milk has many of the same characteristics as the production of meat. Hens and cows are kept inside buildings and pens to produce their products. The crowding makes it easier for disease to spread and harder to identify sick hens and cows that may contaminate products. Thus, efficient production can increase the risk of *Salmonella* infection in eggs and milk.

Low-Dose Antibiotics in Animals

Ironically, using antibiotics to kill bacteria in animals may actually worsen the safety of food among humans. For nearly 50 years, antibiotics in low doses have been routinely mixed with feed to promote fast growth of animals. When given to animals without serious infection, the antibiotics allow

14

the animals to digest feed more efficiently, reach the size for slaughtering sooner, and reduce production costs. Low-dose antibiotics, received by roughly 60 to 80 percent of all cattle, sheep, swine, and poultry in the United States,[22] may also prevent the spread of infections among large numbers of animals kept in close confines—further helping to keep costs down.

It might seem that preventive antibiotics would reduce the bacteria in animals going to slaughter and the risk of infected meat getting to humans. In practice, something different occurs. Antibiotics similar to those used in humans kill normal bacteria but indirectly allow resistant bacteria to multiply. These resistant bacteria represent a serious threat when they make their way into meat consumed by humans. Because normal antibiotic treatments are ineffective against resistant strains, doctors can do little to treat the infection. The problem stems not from the occasional use of these drugs to treat sick animals but from regular nontherapeutic use to promote fast growth. In other words, overuse of antibiotics in animals contributes to the ineffectiveness of antibiotics in humans and increased risk of serious illness or death from foodborne pathogens.

The routine feeding of antibiotics to animals has encountered major opposition in recent years. In 1999, the American Public Health Association urged the Food and Drug Administration (FDA) to ban their use for nonmedical purposes. In 2001, an editorial in the *New England Journal of Medicine* noted that several studies had demonstrated the presence of drug-resistant bacteria in food. It concluded that the presence resulted from the use of antibiotics in feed, and called for an end to the practice.[23] The World Health Organization and the European Union have likewise supported this goal. Denmark has already ended nonprescription use of antibiotics in its animal production. Even McDonalds requires its meat producers to minimize use of antibiotics.

The practice continues in the United States, however. The FDA remains open to banning particular antibiotics that might need to be reserved for humans but has taken no action in general against the use of antibiotics for fattening animals. The Animal Health Institute, which represents manufacturers of pharmaceutical products for animals, fully supports the FDA. It argues that there is little evidence of the transfer of antibiotic-resistant bacteria to humans and that banning antibiotics would certainly raise meat prices and increase the incidence of animal health problems.

Food and Diet Trends

Although thorough cooking kills most dangerous microbes found on fresh food, trends in diet make this custom less common than in the past. The

15

public eats more fresh fruits and vegetables than it once did, in part because of recommendations from health experts and the government. The demand for off-season fresh fruits and vegetables requires importers to ship them from countries that have different climates but also may lack the sanitation regulations of the United States. The popularity of uncooked fish in sushi, raw oyster bars, and rare tuna steak raises the risk of contracting foodborne disease. With less free time than in the past, cooks are less likely to serve well-cooked roasts and more likely to quickly grill or sauté meat and reheat leftovers and fast food.

Given trends in eating out, restaurants and catered events have become a major source of foodborne illnesses. The threat of failing a health inspection or suffering the negative publicity of food poisoning heightens the concerns of restaurants for food safety. Still, the sheer amount of food served in popular restaurants increases the risk of an outbreak. Employees that do not follow rules concerning cleanliness and cooking procedures can inadvertently serve contaminated food. Cooks may avoid fully cooking meat to preserve taste and texture and may not fully refrigerate products in order to keep ingredients close. Transportation of food to catered events similarly increases the risk of improper refrigeration and spoilage.

Even under the best of efforts, salad bars pose special risks to restaurant patrons. The popularity of fresh fruit and vegetables has led grocery stores and fast-food outlets to offer this option to customers. Yet uncooked items in salad bars contain bacteria and the difficulty of keeping all the food properly chilled allows bacteria to grow. Many of the salads containing egg products such as mayonnaise pose a special risk for food poisoning. Other foods have likely been touched by food preparers during chopping and cutting. Germs from customers may spread to the open bar despite sneeze guards and utensils to prevent direct contact. Once infected, an item in a salad bar will sicken the tens or even hundreds of customers who share the item.

Because they produce so much food so quickly, fast-food restaurants also face special food safety problems. The television show *Dateline NBC* recently gathered information on critical health violations in 100 fast-food restaurants in each of 10 chains.[24] Researchers then called state, county, and local health departments to obtain inspection reports and counted the number of reported critical violations. Critical health violations include the presence of insects or rodents, lack of cleanliness, improper food temperatures, and failure of employees to wash hands. The study found that Jack in the Box had the fewest critical violations—45 per 100 inspections. Taco Bell restaurants had the next fewest, with 65 critical violations, and Wendy's restaurants followed with 84 critical violations. Seven other restaurant chains—Subway, Dairy Queen, KFC, Burger King, Arby's, Hardee's, and McDonald's—had critical violations ranging from 98 to 126 violations per

100 inspections. Despite efforts of the food companies to improve food safety, the nature of food service makes full compliance difficult.

WHAT CONSUMERS CAN DO

Although consumers have little control over food production, meat processing, and restaurant practices, they can take actions to protect themselves from foodborne illnesses at home. Vegetarians eliminate meat and perhaps egg and milk products from their diet but then cannot stop eating fresh fruit and produce. Vegetarians and nonvegetarians alike can select food carefully to avoid expired products but cannot check for the presence of microbes. At home, they can follow the four steps recommended by the government to protect consumers from foodborne illness.

- Cook meat and eggs thoroughly.
- Separate foods, knives, and cutting boards so that raw meat does not contaminate fresh produce.
- Chill leftover foods and open containers of food quickly in the refrigerator to prevent bacteria from growing.
- Clean food with water and clean knives, cutting boards, and hands with soap and water.

Sometimes following these rules proves unexpectedly hard. A leaky package of meat can accidentally contaminate fresh produce in grocery bags or the refrigerator; a cook checking the recipe by tasting food before it is fully cooked can ingest active pathogens; microwave ovens can leave parts of a reheated dish cold and fail to kill all bacteria; and adding a raw hamburger to a grill with nearly done hamburgers can newly contaminate the cooked meat. In short, consumers should assume that any food they plan to eat could contain foodborne disease and should do whatever they can to minimize the risk.

Consumers wanting to know about food safety will find no shortage of other sources of information. In 1997, the USDA, Department of Health and Human Services (DHHS), and Department of Education joined with food industry groups to form the Partnership for Food Safety Education (PFSE). Aiming to educate the public about safe food handling and to reduce foodborne illness, the partnership sponsors a program called Fight BAC! (a name based on the first three letters of both "back" and "bacteria").[25] As part of the program, McDonald's has distributed a brochure called "A Parent's Guide to Playing It Safe at Home" with its Happy Meals for children.

The Food Safety Inspection Service of the USDA sponsors a bus that travels across the country with food safety resources and distributes guidelines that, among many other things, recommends greater use of thermometers to ensure foods are fully cooked. The USDA and the FDA have collaborated as well to create the Food Illness Education Center that provides special information for food service workers, child-care providers, and children. The Food Safety web page (http://www.foodsafety.gov) lists links to hundreds of food safety sources.

Few oppose efforts to make the public more aware of food safety practices, but critics can rightly point out that educational efforts alone are inadequate. The need for consumers to take care about foodborne illness might be viewed as a failure of the government and food industry to produce food in a way that eliminates or minimizes the presence of dangerous microbes. The educational strategy focuses on the end of the food chain—when people eat the food—rather than on the beginning. Critics believe the government can do much more in the first place to prevent the bacteria, viruses, and parasites from getting into food sold to restaurants and consumers.

WHAT THE GOVERNMENT HAS DONE

Government food agencies, primarily the Food Safety Inspection Services (FSIS) of the USDA and the FDA of the Department of Health and Human Services, have the goal of ensuring safe food. However, until the 1990s, the USDA argued that because bacteria were a natural part of all raw food, they could not guarantee its absence from products consumers bought. With support of the industry, they would approve meat as safe even if it contained foodborne illness, assuming that proper food handling would kill the germs later.

Government agencies began to change their approach after the serious food outbreaks in the early and mid-1990s, especially the one involving the deaths of three children from the dangerous *E. coli* O157:H7 bacteria contained in Jack in the Box hamburgers. In regard to meat, the FDA changed the recommended temperature for cooking hamburger from 140 degrees to 155 degrees and then 160 degrees. The FSIS announced in 1994 a new policy to test for *E. coli* O157:H7 in ground meat. The policy requires testing only of randomly sampled producers and outlets of ground meat, but the FSIS expects companies—if they want to prevent a recall of meat—to do their own testing as well.[26]

The meat industry vigorously opposed the new regulation, but public opinion and ultimately a 1994 court decision in *Texas Food Industry Association, et al. v. Mike Espy, et al.* favored the plans of the government. Victims of the Jack in the Box *E. coli* O157:H7 outbreak, including family members of those who died, formed an organization called Safe Tables Our Priority (S.T.O.P.) that proved effective in advocating for reform. However, efforts to extend testing to all meat or to microbes other than the *E. coli* strain failed. In a 2001 case, *Supreme Beef v. USDA*, the Fifth Circuit Court of Appeals ruled that the USDA had overstepped its authority in threatening to shut down a Texas beef plant after tests revealed high levels of *Salmonella* in its meat.

Absent the microscopic examination of all meat, government agencies advocated a comprehensive approach to food safety named Hazard Analysis and Critical Control Point (HACCP, pronounced "hassip"). Originally developed to ensure that astronauts did not get sick from contaminated food while in space, HACCP provided a more general model for improving food safety. The Food and Drug Administration first applied HACCP to seafood in 1994, then later to juices, and now to dairy products. The USDA implemented the program for meats with new regulations approved in 1996 by President Bill Clinton, who later increased funding for the program. The implementation plan began with compliance among large companies before extending it to smaller companies. Ultimately, the plan aimed to bring all meat-processing plants under the system.

What is HACCP? In brief, it specifies a seven-step process of controlling contamination from the start to the end of food production.[27] According to the steps, establishments should first analyze the hazards of food contamination and second identify critical control points where they can eliminate or minimize the hazard. For each identified critical control point, they should establish control procedures (step 3), monitor the effectiveness of the procedures (step 4), and correct problems as they occur (step 5). The last two steps involve verifying continually that the procedures work properly and keeping effective records to document the system.

For example, a plant that sells cooked meat would

- specify the temperature needed to kill germs;
- measure the meat temperature to make sure it reaches desired degrees during cooking;
- specify the time needed to chill the meat to a temperature cool enough to keep germs from growing;
- measure the time taken to reach that temperature;
- check the temperature during packaging to make sure the meat remains appropriately chilled; and
- check to ensure the package is correctly labeled.

The process shifts responsibilities for safe food to the establishments but continues to involve the government. Companies are expected to anticipate and prevent problems rather than react to them after they occur. Systematic measurement plays an important role in the process, as does the reliance on careful records that government inspectors can check. Done carefully and with effort, the HACCP system appears to work well. Independent scientific organizations have favorably evaluated the system, and some tests have demonstrated its ability to reduce the presence of foodborne disease agents. It cannot eliminate all disease agents and does not require testing of all meat for the presence of pathogens—goals that would be enormously expensive. Instead, it aims to minimize the extent of contamination.

Industry groups and government agencies laud the efforts they have made to make meat the most regulated food in the United States and among the safest in the world. Defenders of the food inspection system note that inspectors are present in meat plants, examine animals before and after slaughtering, and check the processing of meat products. The meat industry willingly cooperates with these inspections according to Patrick Boyle of the American Meat Institute:

> *We have federal inspectors in our plants everyday. . . And in some of the larger plants, it's not one or two inspectors; there are literally dozens of USDA inspectors on site everyday in all parts of our operations, ensuring that we are fulfilling our primary responsibility for maintaining the safety and the integrity of our nation's meat supply.*[28]

Despite improvements in the safety of food, the government aims for continued progress. The Healthy People 2010 initiative lists goals of reducing foodborne infections from *Campylobacter* species, *E. coli* O157:H7, *Listeria monocytogenes*, and *Salmonella* species by 50 percent. Along with these efforts, the Centers for Disease Control and Prevention (CDC) has improved its surveillance and tracking programs. By collaborating with state health agencies to track the emergence of reported foodborne illnesses, the CDC can coordinate better the response to outbreaks and eliminate the source of the problem.

The Critics Weigh In

If HACCP works well in principle, the question remains as to whether it works well in practice. Employers who cut corners, workers who do not follow the rules diligently, and inspectors who are overwhelmed by the documents they review can compromise the HACCP system. Critics point to the continued need to recall meat and persistent outbreaks of foodborne disease as evidence of the limitations of the food safety system. For example, after the CDC identified multiple cases of illness, ConAgra Beef Company of Greeley, Colorado, voluntarily recalled 19 million pounds of beef in 2000 that were contaminated with *E. coli* O157:H7. If HACCP worked properly, companies would discover tainted meat before it is shipped and eaten. The flaws may indicate the need for microscopic testing for the most common and dangerous pathogens in all meat.

The problem of inadequate HACCP execution may stem from the nature of government regulation. Too often, federal regulatory agencies have close ties to the groups they regulate. The USDA, for example, both regulates and supports the meat industry—it must protect consumers from unsafe food at the same time it must promote the economic vitality of ranchers, farmers, and food producers. Such conflict shows in publicity about both the safety of food and the need for consumers to cook food carefully to avoid diseases. It likewise shows in agency efforts to enforce HACCP procedures at the same time it allows food plants to produce more food at lower cost by speeding up production lines. When conflicting goals exist, critics claim that economic interests of the industry override consumer interests for food safety. As evidence, they point to the substantial contributions made by the meat industry to the election funds of politicians from both parties.[29]

Even if government agencies had a more single-minded focus on food safety, the organization of the government agencies would limit their effectiveness. Right now, the FDA and the USDA share inspection duties, and both agencies lack the authority, except in the worst violations of the law, needed to force companies to recall food or close down a plant. Both agencies lack the power to require HACCP procedures in foreign meat plants and can inspect only a small portion of imported food. Many outbreaks of foodborne disease come from infected fruits and vegetables imported from other nations. These gaps in enforcement power limit the effectiveness of the government agencies.

A single food-enforcement agency with the authority to require recalls of food and fine offending agencies might overcome these problems. Yet calls for change have had little effect. Bills introduced in Congress to streamline the agencies and give them more power have made little headway. Critics worry that it will take another major outbreak and large death toll to bring about further change.

How can consumers make sense of competing claims? It is not easy given contrasting and plausible sides to these debates. First, reliable data that might settle the question are not available. Agencies can point to the downward trend in reported incidents of some foodborne illnesses, but critics can point to the rise of new and dangerous pathogens. The choice between contradictory and unreliable data makes it hard to settle the debate. Second, the standard for the presence of foodborne illnesses differs between defenders and critics of the system. Defenders argue that foodborne illness can never be eliminated in a large nation like the United States with modern agriculture and food-processing practices. With a more reasonable goal to control or reduce outbreaks, some foodborne illness will always be present. Critics prefer a more stringent standard, arguing that even if foodborne illness will always be present, it can be reduced to much lower levels than exist today. Third, economic interests distinguish sides in the debates. Defenders might claim that stricter regulations would raise the costs of food faced by all consumers but bring only limited benefit for food safety. Critics claim that companies exaggerate the cost of better procedures and that the loss would come primarily from the profits of companies rather than the pocketbooks of consumers.

Despite the disagreement, the debates might offer an insight all consumers can accept. Meat, vegetables, fruit, processed foods, and other edibles cannot be viewed as safe or unsafe. Rather, all food is safe or unsafe to a matter of degree. All else equal, it would be better to have more safe than less safe food, but people will differ in the degree of risk they are willing to tolerate and the cost for food they are willing to pay. Some will want to spend more on food to reduce the occasional but mild risk (or the rare but serious risk) while others will not. Most in the food industry will prefer a slightly higher risk for a lower cost, while most public health advocates will prefer the opposite. Without consensus on the degree of acceptable risk, substantial changes in policy are not likely. Unless a new and deadly outbreak of foodborne illness changes attitudes dramatically, consumers should recognize that all food carries a small but potentially serious risk.

MAD COW DISEASE

The most frightening threat to food safety is fortunately the least likely. For Americans, the risks of eating beef infected with mad cow disease or bovine spongiform encephalopathy (BSE) appear slim, as do the risks of getting the human version of the disease—variant Creutzfeldt-Jakob disease (vCJD). Yet the diseases have two particularly worrisome traits that make it different from other foodborne diseases. First, unlike bacteria and viruses, the agent in mad cow disease and vCJD cannot be killed by cooking, freezing, or boiling—it survives even in acids that kill human cells. This indestructibility makes traditional methods of food safety ineffective. Second, the disease leads to a debilitating and horrible death. It slowly destroys the brain and the nervous system, making its victims incapable of walking, talking, remembering, and caring for themselves.

Is the food supply safe from mad cow disease and are beef eaters safe from vCJD? The questions have been the subject of heated debates and one celebrated court case.

CREUTZFELDT-JAKOB DISEASE

Dr. Hans Creutzfeldt, a German neurologist who worked with Dr. Alois Alzheimer on brain disorders common in elderly people, first described the symptoms of the disease that would take his name (Creutzfeldt-Jakob disease). A young woman named Bertha Elschker was hospitalized in 1912 because her legs would jerk with spasms and she walked unsteadily. Over the next year, the symptoms worsened. She would fall over while standing, refuse to eat or bathe, scream that she was possessed of the devil, and appear dazed and confused. Falling into a deep coma, she died in 1913, and Creutzfeldt described the case in a 1920 article.[30]

About the same time, the head of a German psychiatric state hospital, Alfons Jakob, had several patients with many of the same symptoms as Bertha Elschker. The patients initially complained of weakness in their legs, later had difficulty walking, and still later exhibited dementia (the loss of mental capacity). Their thinking, memory, personality, and coordination seriously deteriorated, and they became depressed and apathetic. Although later analysis suggested that some of these patients likely suffered from mental illness, the symptoms of others rightly convinced Dr. Jakob that he had identified a new disease.

In examining the brains of the patients after they died, Creutzfeldt and Jakob discovered something unusual. The nerve cells appeared to be full of holes, resembling a sponge in texture. This observation appeared so unusual that neither scientist would report it in their publications.[31] Yet this sponge-like, or "spongiform," change in the brain would define a critical outcome of the disease.

Over the following decades, the neurological disease took the name of the first two physicians to identify it. Creutzfeldt-Jakob disease, or CJD, now occurs in only one person per million in the United States, is most common among persons over 50 years old, and is inherited in about 15 percent of cases.[32] Although rare, the disease turns up in some unusual groups. Cannibals in Papua New Guinea tribes, particularly women and children, have contracted a form of the disease. Children taking human growth hormone to deal with growth deficiency had unusually high instances of the disease. And some recipients of donor corneas for eye transplants and some brain surgery patients came down with the disease. For these groups and others, the disease has no known cure and remains fatal.

The discovery of the source of the disease took many decades and led to two Nobel Prizes. Even today, our knowledge of the causes remains limited. Scientists do not yet understand how the disease harms nerve cells and reproduces itself. It is so unusual that for a while scientists thought it violated basic laws of microbiology.

A breakthrough came from Dr. D. Carleton Gajdusek, the son of immigrants from Slovakia who was raised in New York City, studied at Harvard Medical School and the California Institute of Technology, and specialized in clinical pediatrics. In the 1950s, he began to investigate an unusual disease common in the Fore Tribe region of New Guinea called kuru, a word referring to trembling. The disease had similarities to CJD, but its source presented a puzzle. After visiting the region, living with the tribe, and performing autopsies on kuru victims, Gajdusek concluded that the disease was spread by eating the brains of deceased relatives. This practice, part of a funeral ritual rather than a form of nutrition, passed the disease from sick relatives to healthy relatives. After ending this cannibalistic tradition, the disease largely disappeared within a generation. Gajdusek won the Nobel Prize in medicine in 1976 for discovering how the disease was spread.

A second and more controversial breakthrough came from the work of Dr. Stanley B. Prusiner. After attending medical school at the University of Pennsylvania and beginning a residency at the University of California, San Francisco, in neurology, Dr. Prusiner admitted a woman patient who had steadily been losing her memory and ability to perform routine tasks. It turned out that she was suffering from CJD, a disease Dr. Prusiner found intriguing because it differed from diseases caused by other known infectious agents such as bacteria, viruses, and parasites. When hired as a professor at the school, he began to research what he called a "slow" virus. Unexpectedly, however, tests showed no evidence of the presence of a virus. Rather, they showed the presence of an unusual, deformed protein that Dr. Prusiner called a prion. The prion seemed to disrupt the normal operation of other proteins in the brain, ultimately destroying nerve cells and producing holes in infected brains. Although scientists viewed the initial claims about prions with skepticism and still do not understand fully how prions do their damage, they have come to accept the existence of a new type of infectious agent. For this discovery, Dr. Prusiner received the 1997 Nobel Prize in medicine.

The work of Dr. Gajdusek and Prusiner established that CJD was not transmitted through personal contact such as with a normal infection but, at least in the case of kuru, came from consuming affected body parts. It also established that the agent of the infection was not a virus. It did not lead to an immune system response, survived under extreme heat or cold, and was not affected by antibiotics, vaccines, and other medicines. The prion agent, in other words, could spread to new hosts through eating contaminated food despite cooking, and the body could do little to fight this kind of infection.

A NEW AND DEADLY FORM OF CATTLE INFECTION

The link between contaminated food and CJD began in England. Since at least the late 1700s, English shepherds and scientists had known of a disease in sheep call scrapie. The name came from the tendency of sheep with the disease to scratch themselves so intensely that their wool would be scraped off. As symptoms worsened, infected sheep would stagger, shake, go blind, and die. Although the disease spread to sheep throughout the country and other parts of Europe, it did not appear to affect humans. Despite their high consumption of lamb and mutton, the English population did not contract any similar kind of disease. Rather, the major harm came from the economic loss to sheep owners.

Scientists eventually came to realize that scrapie caused sponge-like holes in the brains of sheep. The symptoms of loss of coordination and tremors appeared similar to the symptoms of kuru found among New Guinea tribe members. Both diseases also produced the odd, sponge-like holes in the brain tissue.

Until 1984, nothing similar had emerged among cattle in Britain or any other country. On December 22 of that year, a farmer in Sussex in southern England reported to his veterinarian that one of his dairy cows had started to act oddly. Dairy cows are docile creatures, but this one had aggressively menaced other cows and staggered when walking.[33] Hostile cows soon emerged in other farms in southern England. A veterinarian described one of the sick cows this way:

> *When you approached her, she would shy away. She was previously a ° cow and started becoming aggressive, rather nervous, knocking other cows, bashing other cows and so on and becoming rather dangerous to handle. She would also at the same time become rather uncoordinated. If you shooed her, she would stumble, particularly on the back legs and go down.*[34]

Within a few years, the mysterious disease had spread to herds elsewhere in Britain. Yet veterinarians had been unable to either understand or treat the cause of the disease. Given the odd behavior of infected cows, the informal and misleading name of mad cow disease became common. Going beyond outward symptoms to study the brains of sick cows, scientists found that infected tissue resembled that of sheep with scrapie: They exhibited similar sponge-like holes. The first publication on the new disease in 1987 used the term *bovine spongiform encephalopathy* (BSE), with "bovine" referring to cows, "spongiform" to the sponge-like change in tissue, and "encephalopathy" to a disease of the brain.

Identifying the Source

Where had this new disease come from and how did it spread? Government officials quickly suggested one answer. It came from eating infected body parts of sheep with scrapie. The disease emerged in several parts of England at about the same time and did not appear to spread from one location to another, as would occur with a disease transmitted by contact between cows. Consistent with the emergence of the disease in multiple locations at the same time, all the cows with the disease had been fed a dietary supplement consisting of protein. Although cows are vegetarians, supplementing their diet with protein from otherwise unused meat and bone of dead animals led to rapid growth of young cows and greater milk production. If the meat and bone product contained body parts of sheep infected with scrapie, it could have caused a new form of the disease in cattle. If cows with infections were in turn used in the protein supplement, the disease would no longer have to cross species but could be transmitted from cow to cow. This cattle cannibalism might lead to transmission of BSE, much as human cannibalism in New Guinea led to the transmission of CJD.

By 1988, researchers had accumulated evidence that the disease had indeed emerged through contaminated feed.[35] The disease occurred only in places in England and in other nations that used meat and bone animal feed. The disease agent in scrapie could survive the process of creating the protein feed from dead animals (even though the process killed bacteria and viruses). And the feed used the tissue from the brain and spinal cord, where the infectious agent was concentrated. These facts plus evidence that infected animals had consumed animal products made the explanation of contaminated feed the most plausible one.

More worrisome, estimates suggested that the infections occurred some four to five years earlier. That the feed was used with young calves while symptoms first occurred in older cows indicated a long incubation period for the disease. This meant that calves given the feed in recent years might be infected, even if they did not show symptoms until many years later. In 1988, the British government banned the use of cattle and sheep-derived protein for cattle feed, yet that would not deal with the large number of animals that may have already been infected by the protein supplement. Many more cattle might die from the disease in years to come.

In responding to the potential for an epidemic, the British government was greatly concerned about the impact on the beef industry. It banned the selling of cattle with BSE and required that milk from BSE cows be destroyed, but it did not do the same for nonsymptomatic cattle in infected herds. Any more drastic action would have seriously harmed the industry. At the same time, the government was not willing to provide the resources to support farmers for the financial losses from a more drastic action. The government treasury offered half the market value of the sick animals to farmers but no more.

In the end, BSE severely damaged the cattle industry anyway. Estimates are varied, but recorded cases of BSE ended up affecting 182,552 cattle, with new cases still occurring; some suggest that unrecorded cases raise the figure to 2 million.[36] Since 1996, 6.5 million cattle over 30 months have been bought by the government and killed because of their higher risk of having BSE.[37] Once a link appeared between BSE and human disease, though, officials could do little to protect the industry.

CONTAMINATED BEEF PROVES FATAL FOR HUMANS

Responding to the BSE epidemic in their country, British experts noted that no evidence had yet indicated that the cow disease could be transmitted across species to humans. Scientists carefully qualified their language, noting that they did not fully understand the nature of the disease. Since scrapie in sheep did not affect humans and BSE had similarities to scrapie, it seemed reasonable to infer that humans might be immune from BSE. Still, some noted that the disease might cross species again, to jump from cattle to humans, as it jumped from sheep to cattle.

British Government Denials

Government officials continued to reassure the public that they were not at risk of contracting BSE. In 1990, the agriculture minister, John Grummer, hoped to dramatize the safety of British beef by eating a hamburger with his four-year-old daughter, Cordelia, in front of a television camera. In 1995, Prime Minister John Major told Parliament, "There is currently no scientific evidence that BSE can be transmitted to humans."[38] Although many did not believe them, government officials claimed for nearly a decade that British beef posed no health risk.

Economic issues again played a role in the government's actions. Accepting a risk for transmission of BSE to humans would have required the slaughter of all herds that had been given animal-based feed and were vulnerable to developing BSE. The cost would have reached £12–15 billion (or roughly $24 billion).[39] Widespread slaughter would in turn shake the confidence of the public in the safety of beef, milk, and dairy products. In claiming that BSE would not affect humans, the government tried to limit the short-term economic consequences of the disease for the food and cattle industry.

During the early 1990s, however, disconcerting evidence emerged that eating beef might cause disease. The death of a Siamese cat made national headlines in 1990.[40] The cat, named Max and later called Mad Max, had begun to stagger, would frantically lick and chew his hair and skin, and seemed unable to hold his head steady. Euthanized as symptoms worsened, Max presented a puzzle to veterinarians. When they examined the brain tissue under the microscope, they found the holes characteristic of spongiform encephalopathy. Several zoo animals also died from the disease, again indicating its ability to cross species.

The story about the cat created a near panic given the concern that eating cooked beef had caused Max's disease. Soon other cats reportedly contracted this new disease called feline spongiform encephalopathy. Having crossed species again, this time from cattle to cats, the disease might cross species to infect humans.

Confirming such fears, several young people in England appeared to contract a variant form of CJD around the same time.[41] Sixteen-year-old Vicky Rimmer was one of the first. As described by her grandmother, "She's blind. She can't move. She can't swallow. It's just living hell, seeing her everyday." Stephen Churchill, a young man, had begun to stagger in ways that reminded his parents of diseased cows shown in the news. He died in 1995, the first known human victim of the disease. Peter Hall, a 20-year-old student, died of the disease as well. His mother described the symptoms by saying it was like babyhood developing in reverse.

As described by a report from the Centers for Disease Control, the experience of one 22-year-old patient illustrates the horror of the disease.[42] The victim first visited her physician for help with depression and memory loss that recently had affected her job performance. She soon experienced trouble driving, receiving a ticket for failing to yield right of away. A little over a month after a visit to the doctor, she started to have trouble dressing and walking. Within two months, "the patient experienced falls with minor injuries, had difficulty taking a shower and dressing, and was unable to remember a home telephone number or to make accurate mathematical calculations. The patient subsequently became confused, hallucinated, and had speech abnormalities." Shortly before she died, "the patient had become bedridden, experienced considerable weight loss requiring surgical insertion of a feeding tube, and was no longer communicating with family members."

The disease in these cases resembled Creutzfeldt-Jakob disease but was not identical. The brain tissue of its victims revealed holes, but the pattern of damage to the nerve cells differed from that found in the tribe of New Guinea and in other classic cases. Scientists labeled the disease as variant Creutzfeldt-Jakob disease (vCJD). It belonged to the same family of brain diseases likely caused by the recently discovered prion proteins but had taken a new form. The variant form also differed from the classic form in another way: It attacked young people rather than older people. The classic form appeared most common in persons over age 50 and seldom among young people. The death of teenagers and young people indicated something new and terribly threatening.

The critical question in Britain was whether the deaths of the cats and young people came from eating infected beef. Despite government claims of the safety of its beef, sales had already declined substantially, with 1.4 million British households having stopped buying the meat.[43] Many schools, worried about the health of their students, had banned beef in their cafeterias. A climate of mistrust about food safety existed in Britain throughout the early 1990s.

British Government Reversal

Confirming the reasons for mistrust, the government reversed its position with an announcement to Parliament. On March 20, 1996, the secretary of state for health, Stephen Dorrell, stated that a variant form of Creutzfeldt-Jakob disease had been discovered among humans and that it most likely stemmed from the consumption of beef from cattle with BSE. With headlines announcing the threat to health, the market for British beef collapsed and the European Union banned exports from the country to its members. Even those who had no symptoms but had eaten British beef over the last decade worried about succumbing to this horrible disease.

The next year, the highly respected scientific journal *Nature* published an article written by a Scottish research team that provided stronger evidence for the link between BSE and vCJD.[44] After injecting one group of mice with BSE-infected tissue from cattle and another group with vCJD from human tissue, the researchers observed the outcomes. Both groups of mice died at similar rates and showed similar brain deformities. Other studies would further confirm the link, eliminating any doubt about the harm of infected beef for humans. Scrapie, BSE, and vCJD all appeared to represent different strains of the same disease that scientists had labeled as transmissible spongiform encephalopathy (TSE).

Deaths of others from vCJD in Britain followed the government announcement. According to the Centers for Disease Control and Prevention,

As of December 1, 2003, a total of 153 cases of vCJD had been reported in the world: 143 from the United Kingdom, six from France, and one each from Canada, Ireland, Italy, and the United States (note: the Canadian, Irish, and U.S. cases were reported in persons who resided in the United Kingdom during a key exposure period of the U.K. population to the BSE agent). Almost all the 153 vCJD patients had multiple-year exposures in the United Kingdom between 1980 and 1996 during the occurrence of a large U.K. outbreak of bovine spongiform encephalopathy.[45]

Although millions had been exposed to the BSE agent through eating contaminated beef, the death of 153 fell well below the expected number of deaths. As explained by Philip Yam,

With 1.6 million infected cattle having presumably entered the food chain, potentially 800 billion doses of BSE were consumed between 1980 and 1996. That would imply that virtually all of the 60 million people living in the UK before 1996, and any visitors, were exposed to a massive amount of infected material. Not all Englishmen have gone mad and died, meaning that several other factors must be at play in determining who succumbs to vCJD.[46]

Indeed, victims of vCJD shared the same food with other family members but were the only ones to die.

Scientists do not fully understand the nature of the vCJD disease and why it attacks some people—particularly those who are young—but not others. Nor can they predict with certainty the deaths from vCJD to come. Because strict regulations since 1996 have, as best as can be determined, prevented beef with BSE from being used for food, it should have eliminated new exposure to the disease in Britain. Yet a long development period for the disease could produce delayed deaths: Those having eaten infected beef in Britain nearly a decade ago might remain vulnerable.

CONTROVERSY IN THE UNITED STATES

During the late 1980s and early 1990s, the United States was spared the disaster that occurred in Britain. No identified cases of BSE appeared in U.S. cattle, and a ban on imported cattle, sheep, bison, and goats from countries known to have infected cattle—and from Britain in particular—minimized the risk of the disease emerging. The only person known to die from vCJD in the United States had been born and raised in Britain where she had contracted the disease before moving to Florida.[47]

Many groups opposed to beef consumption—vegetarians, animal rights activists, and health-food advocates—worried that what had occurred in Britain could also happen in the United States. Most Americans, however, seemed unworried. They had heard of the disease and the threat it presented to food safety elsewhere but for the most part continued to eat beef as they had in the past. A 1990 story in the *New York Times*, for example, reported the infection of British cattle with BSE and concerns that the death of cats from a related disease indicated its potential to spread to humans.[48] The same article reported that all cows with the disease had been destroyed and that British beef was safe to eat.

Not until the 1996 announcement from the British government that eating beef with BSE likely caused several deaths from vCJD did the U.S. public express serious concerns about the disease. On April 15, 1996, soon after the British announcement, talk show host Oprah Winfrey responded to the publicity by devoting one of her popular television shows to mad cow disease.[49] To debate whether the mad cow disease crisis could occur in the United States, Oprah invited three guests: Howard Lyman, the executive director of Humane Society's Eating with Conscience; Dr. Gary Weber, a representative of the National Cattlemen's Beef Association; and Dr. Will Hueston, from the USDA. The introductions contrasted Mr. Lyman's claim that mad cow disease could makes AIDS look like the common cold with the views of Drs. Weber and Hueston that beef was safe.

Mr. Lyman, a former rancher turned vegetarian, told Oprah that parts of dead cattle were still being fed to live cattle in the United States, a practice that could spread BSE much as it did in Britain. The other guests responded that 10 years of surveillance had revealed no BSE in the United States and that government and industry efforts to identify any cattle with the disease would safeguard the public in the future. Mr. Lyman countered that the denials of risk from U.S. officials echoed those made by British officials over the previous 10 years. Since inspection agencies did not have the personnel to check all cattle, the disease could enter into U.S. herds and the food supply before anyone could stop it.

Oprah and the audience expressed much concern over the risk of getting the disease. When told that cattle eat food made from other cattle, Oprah asked the audience if hearing that caused them some concern. After the audience clapped loudly and shouted yeah, Oprah said that hearing about the practice "Just stopped me cold from eating another burger." Later, Oprah told the audience that "we don't want to just alarm you all, but I have to tell you, I'm thinking about the cattle being fed to the cattle and that's pretty upsetting to me." When one audience member asked if all cows ground up for use in feed had first been tested for BSE, Dr. Weber admitted this could not be done.

The day after the program was broadcast, cattle prices dropped more than 10 percent, causing the industry to lose an estimated $36 million in two weeks.[50] Responding to the loss, a group of Texas cattlemen used a 1995 Texas statute to sue Oprah and Lyman for estimated losses of $12 million. The statute, which made anyone spreading false information about agricultural products liable to a civil suit, aimed to counter increasingly negative publicity about food safety. In this particular case, the plaintiffs believed that Oprah's show whipped up unfounded hysteria about the risks of beef, promoted false beliefs as fact, edited out reassuring comments from the experts about the safety of beef, and directly caused the decline in beef prices. Despite some concerns that the law violated free speech rights, the case went to trial in January 1998 in Amarillo, Texas, the center of a region that produces much of the nation's beef.

After a six-week trial, a jury ruled that Oprah and Howard Lyman had no liability for the drop in beef prices that occurred after her show. Oprah took pride in the victory for free speech rather than for her belief about the safety of U.S. beef; the cattlemen faced an embarrassing defeat but declared their belief that American beef was the safest in the world.[51] The trial gave much publicity to the debate over mad cow disease and may have acquainted the public with potential problems, but it did little to settle the issues debated on Oprah's show.

FIRST CASE OF BSE IN THE UNITED STATES

Given stories from Britain about new cases of vCJD and their efforts to prevent any further outbreaks of BSE, mad cow disease remained in the news after the Oprah trial. The Food and Drug Administration banned the use of protein from cows, sheep, and deer for use in animal feed in 1997, the USDA commissioned experts at Harvard University to evaluate their mad cow disease prevention measures in 1998, and the U.S. government banned the import of animal protein products in 2000. None of these changes, however, garnered the widespread public attention the Oprah trial had.

This lack of public attention changed on December 23, 2003. That day, the USDA announced that a cow in Washington State had contracted BSE—the first confirmed case in the United States. Tissue from a Holstein cow, which had been slaughtered nearly two weeks earlier near Yakima, Washington, had been sent for routine testing to Ames, Iowa. The lab there identified the presence of the disease and reported the results to government officials.[52] The USDA and its secretary, Ann Veneman, acted immediately. The agency set in motion a plan to determine where the infected cow had come from and where its meat went.

Investigators traced the origin of the cow to a dairy farm in Alberta, Canada. Perhaps other cows shipped to the United States from the farm had the disease. Of 25 cows in the herd with the infected cow, 14 were found and tested negative, while the other nine had likely already been slaughtered.[53] Investigators also found that the brain and spinal cord of the infected animal had not been used for food, and they were able to recall the meat that came out of the plant on the day the infected animal was processed. No further evidence surfaced that other U.S. cattle had BSE or that infected meat had entered the human food chain.

The discovery of the infected cow stemmed from a practice of testing tissue from samples of cows that fit a certain high-risk profile. Farmers refer to cows that, for a variety of reasons, cannot stand or walk as "downers." Since mad cow disease caused problems in movement and balance, downers have a higher risk of BSE infection than cows that can stand and walk normally. With the resources to test only a small portion of cattle, the Agriculture Department focuses its testing on this high-risk group. In this case, the infected cow was a downer.

Response to the News

Nearly all trading partners banned the import of U.S. beef after the December 23 announcement, causing a 15 to 20 percent decline in cattle prices.[54] Even if the U.S. beef supply appeared safe, efforts to do more to prevent similar events took on added urgency with the drop in cattle prices. The American cattle industry earns $56 billion in business each year and estimates suggest that a mad cow crisis similar to that in Britain would cost the nation $15 billion in lost sales and $12 billion in disposal costs.[55]

On December 30, Secretary Veneman announced new actions to further ensure the health of slaughtered cattle. The USDA immediately banned downers from the food system and tightened restrictions on the use of brain and spinal cord parts for food. Domestic producers and foreign farms supplying cattle and animal feed to the United States would now have to follow these rules. It also announced that it would move forward with a national system of animal identification. The system would make it easier to trace infected cattle, locate other cattle from infected herds, and recall contaminated meat.

The Food and Drug Administration, which takes responsibility for ensuring the safety of food, acted to ensure that animal-based food did not spread BSE. Since BSE is transmitted by infected animal feed rather than by contact between live cows, the purity of feed creates one safeguard against the disease. The agency had banned use of animal protein in feed for cattle and other grazing animals since 1997. In congressional testimony, one agency director stated that it had inspected all plants that render animal products or produced animal feed and had found 99 percent compliance.[56] For the 1 percent of firms not in compliance, the agency issued warning letters, obtained court injunctions, and required product recall. In response to the Washington BSE case, it intends to use increased funding from Congress to step up inspections.

Federal agencies have received praise for their efforts to prevent BSE in the United States and to respond to the first case of the disease in the nation. Senator Thad Cochrane, the chairman of the Committee on Agriculture, Nutrition, and Forestry, summarized his views in a hearing of the committee held on January 27, 2004:

> *The discovery of the BSE-positive cow has reaffirmed the effectiveness of the surveillance and food safety procedures in place by the Department of Agriculture and the Food and Drug Administration, and I commend them for having a good contingency plan in place to deal with this discovery. U.S. beef remains very safe, and consumer confidence in our nation's food supply remains strong.[57]*

Indeed, other senators at the hearing, concerned about the economic viability of the cattle industry in their states, urged the agencies not to overreact to the single case and thereby further harm the market for U.S. beef.

With beef prices, exports, and consumer purchases returning to normal levels nearly a year after the scare, the major outcome of the crisis has been the early steps to institute a national cattle identification system. The USDA has regulations in place that require a diseased animal or tainted beef to be traced within 48 hours. The way to meet this goal, instituting a national identification system, involves a massive and expensive undertaking. Ranchers in the northwestern United States have started a pilot program that involves recording the births, sales, and deaths of their cattle in a system that state and federal governments can access.

DEBATE OVER THE FUTURE SAFETY OF BEEF

The USDA has acted to ensure that consumers both in the United States and abroad can safely continue to eat U.S. beef. Although still focused on the more common bacteria and viruses that can affect beef, the agency has given special attention to protecting the meat from mad cow disease. Perhaps more important, the USDA surveillance program obtains tissue samples from high-risk adult cattle—those that cannot walk, have a central nervous system problem, or died from an unknown cause. The goal is to test nearly all such cattle and sample other healthy cattle for testing. With these numbers, the odds are high that the program would identify the presence of the disease even if it exists in only one in 10 million cattle. The sampling procedure avoids examining millions of cattle while focusing on those at highest risk.

After tests of 682,552 cattle by April 2006 and a few inconclusive tests that eventually proved negative, two other cases of BSE in American cows were confirmed.[58] As downers, the cows were blocked from use for human food, a fact noted by Secretary of Agriculture Mike Johanns. He argued that the disposal of the animals even before test results had determined they had mad cow disease demonstrated the effectiveness of the system.

Given prevention efforts and the rarity of the disease, Abigail Trafford, a health columnist for the *Washington Post*, called fears about getting mad cow disease from eating beef irrational. "Of all the things to worry about, getting mad cow disease from a nice juicy filet mignon is not one of them. Not yet, anyway."[59] With other foodborne illnesses much more common, the perception of risk of getting mad cow disease is wildly out of proportion. Trafford recognizes that the mysterious nature of the disease, its lethal consequences, and its unpredictable spread all tend to produce panic. Yet the risk is so slight that Americans should, she believes, worry about other more serious and immediate food safety problems.

Government officials would agree. A 2001 study by Harvard University determined that the chances of BSE entering the United States and posing a risk to consumers and the agricultural industry were "extremely low."[60] The study further concluded that, in the unlikely event that BSE would appear in U.S. cattle herds, the protection system in place would keep the disease from spreading so that it would eventually die out. Beef consumption has returned to the level found before the first BSE discovery and likely will change little with the second discovery.

Glaring Deficiencies in Regulation?

Other groups and individuals remain unconvinced. The Center for Food Safety, a nonprofit environmental food advocacy group that is critical of many modern food technologies, cites what it calls glaring deficiencies in regulation of U.S. meat production industry.[61] It notes that while only a small percentage of cows are tested in the United States, 70 percent of cows in Britain and 100 percent of cows in Japan are tested. The European Union has mandated since June 2001 that all cattle over 30 months of age be tested. Although the USDA has increased the inspection of cattle, it does not reach the inspection figures in other nations.

The disease could, according to government critics, spread in several ways. First, most food products imported into the United States cannot be tested. For example, dietary supplements from other countries sometimes contain ingredients from cow organs. Second, the FDA bans use of animal feed for ruminants—cows, sheep, goats, and other grazing animals—but not for pigs, fish, chicken and nonruminants that remain free of spongiform encephalopathy diseases. Despite safeguards, processing plants can accidentally mix the two types of feed. If cows get some of the feed intended for pigs, it could spread BSE. Third, regulations require separation of the brain and spinal cord for use in feed, but the slaughterhouses' process to do so is not precise. The usual way of killing cattle through injection of a bolt and compressed air into the head may force brain tissue into other parts of the body. Such stun devices may need to be banned as they are in Europe. Slaughtering practices should also remove the brain and spinal cord carefully before doing other butchering, but this is not always done.

A new threat to the safety of food has recently emerged from an unexpected source—deer and elk. Chronic wasting disease, a form of transmissible spongiform encephalopathy, has infected wild and captive deer and elk in several parts of the country. Because there is no evidence yet that this disease can spread to humans, food regulations do not prohibit use of animals with this disease for food. Should the disease change slightly, however, it could begin to infect cattle and humans.

The debate over the safety of beef from mad cow disease and humans from vCJD comes down to different emphasis on what has happened in the past and what could happen in the future. Since Americans have remained safe from these diseases so far, government agencies can reasonably claim that the procedures used in the past will continue to prove effective in the future. Others focus more on potential rather than past experience. Since the disease has shown it can change in unexpected ways, the government needs to do more than it has. Critics argue that agencies have been more concerned with protecting the financial interests of the beef industry than the health of the population. They point to the recently discovered second case as evidence of loopholes in the regulations.

Individuals concerned about the risk of mad cow disease could limit the chance of transmission by eating steaks and roasts cut from the muscle of cattle. It would be more dangerous but still safe, according to most experts, to eat meat in sausages, hotdogs, and other processed foods. Were BSE to spread, the tissue used in these foods are those most likely to contain the disease agent. Of course, avoiding beef altogether would prove safest, although most Americans do not view the risk as serious enough to make this change. If, as many suggest, regulations will prove unable to keep BSE out of American cattle and contaminated meat out of the human food chain, this, too, will likely change. In the meantime, it is impossible to say if beef is completely safe.

TERRORIST THREATS

On resigning in December 2004 after four years as the secretary of Health and Human Services, Tommy Thompson talked candidly about his worries over a possible terrorist attack on the food supply. "For the life of me," he said, "I cannot understand why the terrorists have not attacked our food supply because it is so easy to do. We are importing a lot of food from the Middle East and it would be easy to tamper with." Thompson notes that despite increased inspections, only "a very minute amount" of imported food is tested.[62]

Given the threat of foodborne illness to the public, the deliberate contamination of food offers an opportunity for those who want to harm the nation and its citizens. Natural or accidental outbreaks of foodborne illnesses alarm the public, but intentionally caused outbreaks would create even greater fear. While accidental contamination can generally be traced to a single plant or food shipment source, deliberate contamination can strike in multiple locations and infect a variety of foods. While the source of accidental contamination can be identified and corrected, deliberate contamination results from individuals doing all they can to avoid getting caught. The disease may be the same whether part of a natural or deliberate outbreak, but the potential for harm appears greater from a deliberate outbreak.

Motives for deliberate contamination might be many, but terrorism remains one of the most important. Terrorism involves the unlawful use or threatened use of force or violence with the intention of intimidating or coercing societies or governments, often for ideological or political reasons. It typically involves disenfranchised, small, and radical groups but sometimes has the sponsorship of nations and governments.

The public usually thinks of terrorist violence in terms of bullets, bombs, and more recently the use of airplanes as weapons. The September 11, 2001, attacks on the United States by al Qaeda and the suicide bombings in crowded areas of Jerusalem by Palestinians illustrate these types of attacks. In addition, the public recognizes that terrorists might use biological weapons— microorganisms or toxins derived from living organisms—to attack their enemies. For example, in 1995 Aum Shinriyko, a terrorist cult in Japan, killed 12 and injured thousands by releasing deadly sarin gas in a crowded subway. A week after the September 11 attacks, anthrax spores mailed in envelopes to a variety of locations infected 18 and killed five Americans.

Perhaps less well recognized, contaminating food can also serve the goals of terrorist groups. Contaminated food can kill and sicken the civilian population, create worry about the safety of citizens, disrupt the economy, and create general havoc. Such contamination represents one serious form of agroterrorism, or the use of biological weapons by terrorists against animals, crops, and food in order to harm societies or governments. As described in a government report,

> *The threat to the U.S. food supply is more than theoretical. When U.S. troops entered the caves and safe houses of members of the al Qaeda terrorist network in Afghanistan in the months following the September 11th attacks, they found hundreds of pages of U.S. agricultural documents that had been translated into Arabic. A significant part of the group's training manual is reportedly devoted to agricultural terrorism—specifically, the destruction of crops, livestock, and food processing operations.*[63]

Terrorist threats thus raise important concerns about the safety of the food supply.

DISRUPTION RATHER THAN DESTRUCTION

Consider a few instances of terrorist attacks on food sources.[64] In 1984, the followers of Bhagwan Shree Rajneesh, a leader of a religious commune in

37

Oregon, caused the illness of 751 people by poisoning a salad bar with *Salmonella*. Their goal, however illogical as it sounds, was to influence a local election in their favor. Fortunately, no one died from the poisoning, but the ability to make people sick by infecting the food supply illustrates the potential threat of the approach. The difficulty in determining that the effort was intentional rather than accidental made it even more effective. Attacks like this do not require a highly skilled organization and coordinated action but could come from the efforts of a few individuals.

In 1978, members of the Arab Revolutionary Council injected a poisonous liquid into oranges being exported from Israel to Europe. Although only 12 people were injured by eating the oranges, the publicity led to a 40 percent drop in sales of Israeli fruit and harmed the nation's farmers and exporters. In another scheme, Palestinians used counterfeit stamps to allow bacteria-laden eggs to be sold in Israel, leading to many incidents of food poisoning and perhaps two deaths. Still other efforts to harm the Israeli food supply were discovered and stopped by authorities. In one case, a plot to poison patrons at a Jerusalem café led to the arrest of the chef and two others.

In many cases, harm can come from threat alone.[65] A radical group in Italy called the Revolutionary Command claimed in 1974 to have injected toxic substances into Israeli grapefruits, and another group made the same claim in 1988 in support of Palestinian protests. Revolutionary groups in Uganda and Sri Lanka have publicized similar threats, all with the goal of disrupting the agricultural economy and harming the governments of the nations they oppose.

Food terrorism need not come only from international terrorists or religious cults. The British Animal Liberation Front allegedly poisoned products such as turkey and eggs to protest mistreatment of animals but announced the poisoning to avoid human casualties while still harming the food industry.[66] Certain environmental groups have on some occasions used violence against machines, buildings, and roads and might attempt to contaminate produce grown from genetically modified seeds.

Why might terrorists use food as a weapon against their enemies? For one, food contamination most often sickens rather than kills and disrupts rather than destroys. Terrorists may find contaminating food easier to justify morally than killing with bombs and bullets. For this reason, the Rajneesh cult rejected the use of a more dangerous pathogen in favor of a less dangerous one in its biological attack. If direct violence seems most appropriate for terrorist attacks on the armed forces, bacteria and contaminated food may seem more appropriate to some terrorists for attacking civilians. Less deadly attacks on food may, in particular, attract less extreme but still discontented groups.

In addition, contamination of food presents less risk to terrorists than direct attacks on people. Whereas people defend themselves, the objects of food terrorism lack awareness of the intent of others to harm them and the ability to respond to attacks. Crops, animals, and food products are passive, usually unprotected, and easy to contaminate. By the time the contamination affects humans, the terrorists will have disappeared. During times of heightened security, food terrorism may represent an effective alternative to using guns, bombs, and hijackings.

VULNERABILITY OF THE FOOD SUPPLY

Contaminating food with biological agents appears simple compared to the complexity of the September 11 attacks. Terrorists would first need an agent of infection and then access to food supply. Unfortunately, both the agent and the access are readily available and make the food supply vulnerable to a terrorist attack.

The CDC classifies agents into three types, two involving live organisms and one involving metals and chemicals.[67] The first type, Category A agents, includes bacteria and their toxins that represent the greatest threat to humans. The risk of death from the two food contaminants in this category, *Bacillus anthracis* (anthrax) and *Clostridium botulinum* (botulism), is particularly high. However, neither agent seems a likely source of terrorist attacks on food. Anthrax can do more harm to the public when breathed as a powder than when added to food, and the botulism toxin, one of the most deadly substances known to science, also threatens those who handle it.

Category B agents, although less deadly, are easier to obtain and disseminate than Category A agents. They include the most common and serious foodborne illnesses, such as *Salmonella*, *Shigella*, and *E. coli* O157:H7, which terrorists can obtain from biological supply houses. Other disease agents might be purchased on the black market. Terrorists with laboratory skills might not even need to purchase the diseases from others if they can find access to infected food and culture the agents. Highly skilled scientists working with terrorists might even use new drug-resistant or genetically engineered forms of the Category B agents.

The third category consists of heavy metals such as arsenic, lead, and mercury, and other chemicals such as pesticides, dioxins, furans, and polychlorinated biphenyls (PCBs). These agents are easier to obtain and store than the live agents and can cause serious harm in large doses. Recently, a Ukrainian presidential candidate Viktor Yushchenko became ill after eating food laced with dioxin (presumably by a political opponent).

Points of Contamination

With disease agents in hand, terrorists would have numerous choices about how to contaminate food. They might choose to attack at the start of the food chain by infecting animals or crops with the disease, expecting that it would eventually work its way into human food. With crops and cattle typically left unprotected, terrorists could gain easy access. They could then swipe healthy animals with disease agents or infect their food, and the close proximity of animals in modern animal farms would allow the disease to spread. They could also contaminate vegetables and crops by spraying them with high doses of dangerous chemicals.

For example, in 1996, liquid feed manufactured for dairy cattle in Wisconsin was contaminated with a lethal pesticide.[68] The contaminated product was shipped to 4,000 dairy farmers in four states. Although discovered and recalled before doing harm, the pesticide could have infected milk and milk products that would have been sold to consumers. In 1985, 1,400 people became sick from eating watermelon grown in soil treated with pesticide.[69] In similar ways, terrorist contamination of animals or soil could cause harm to the public.

The next point of vulnerability occurs in factories and warehouses that process and store food. Large amounts of meat butchered in a packing plant, vegetables and fruit stored in a warehouse, and food manufactured in factories would give a terrorist with access to the building the opportunity to infect large amounts of food. In 1998, more then 200 people became sick in several states from a rare form of *Salmonella* in packages of cold cereal that, for unknown reasons, were contaminated during production.[70] In 1981, more than 800 people died and 20,000 people were injured by the presence of a chemical agent in cooking oil produced and sold in Spain.[71] Still yet, a terrorist with entry into feed-manufacturing plants could infect animal feed with bacteria or perhaps meat protein with BSE, thereby spreading disease to animals and then to humans.

With modern distribution networks, tampering with food in a single factory or warehouse would affect people across the nation within a few days. In 1994, for example, ice cream premix was accidentally contaminated with *Salmonella* during transportation in a tanker truck that had earlier contained nonpasteurized liquid eggs. That an estimated 224,000 people across the nation later became sick from eating the ice cream illustrates the spread of disease during transport.[72] As noted by the Community Food Security Coalition, "In our present food system, the food we eat travels on average about 1,200 miles. This makes our food system tremendously vulnerable in the field, in storage, or in transit."[73]

Imports may present even greater opportunities for contamination than domestic shipments. Food produced in other nations may have fewer safeguards than food produced in the United States, allowing terrorists greater access to factories and warehouses. Given the huge amount of food imported into the United States, it is impossible to check it all for contamination.

A few import-related incidents illustrate the problem: "In 1989, approximately 25,000 people in 30 states in the U.S. were sickened by *Salmonella* in cantaloupes imported from Mexico. In 1996 and 1997, 2,500 people in 21 states in the U.S. and two Canadian provinces developed *Cyclospora* infections after eating tainted Guatemalan raspberries."[74] In another less serious but potentially deadly case, a phone call in 1989 warned that grapes shipped to the United States from Chile had been contaminated with the poison cyanide. The caller claimed the action served as a protest against the government and living conditions in Chile. After testing grape shipments and finding small amounts of the deadly chemical, the FDA stopped import of grapes and other fruit from the country. Without the phone call warning, the tampering might have killed Americans without the terrorists having even entered the country.

A last point of vulnerability occurs in restaurants and grocery stores that prepare and sell food. The deliberate contamination of a salad bar with *Salmonella* by the Rajneesh cult illustrates this possibility most clearly, but other instances, usually carried out by single individuals with criminal rather than terrorist intent, also demonstrate the risks. For example, in 2003 a supermarket employee intentionally poisoned 200 pounds of ground beef with an insecticide, leaving 111 people sick, including approximately 40 children. In China, nearly 40 people died and more than 200 were hospitalized in 2002 after the owner of a fast-food outlet poisoned a competitor's breakfast foods with rat poison.[75]

One other incident demonstrates terrorist intent to poison food. In January 2003, the U.S. Central Intelligence Agency described its investigation of a plot by one of al Qaeda's leading experts on chemical and biological warfare to poison food intended for British troops.[76] The investigation stemmed from the discovery of ricin, a dangerous toxin, in a London apartment. One suspected militant linked to the apartment worked for a catering company and others had been in contact with people who worked on a British military base. Although discovered early, the plan suggests the potential for harm through contamination of prepared food when even just a single employee works for a restaurant or catering company.

Regardless of the point of attack, any terrorist contamination of food would resemble a natural outbreak of foodborne illness. Without knowing that an outbreak was deliberately caused, officials would not recognize the need for immediate action to stop the terrorism and would create more opportunities for harm. For this reason, food terrorism can prove both more effective and difficult to stop than other types of terrorism.

Terrorist Attacks on Agriculture

Other types of terrorist attacks on food would not directly harm humans through food poisoning but might disrupt the supply of food available to Americans. Killing livestock and crops rather than people would slow the economy, raise food prices, and shake the confidence of consumers in the safety of food.

Experts worry about the use by terrorists of foot-and-mouth disease, a highly contagious and deadly viral disease of hoofed animals that does not affect humans, to damage the nation's animal agriculture. Careful monitoring of the disease has prevented a large natural outbreak in North America since the 1950s, but this success leaves livestock vulnerable to a new outbreak. If a terrorist infected even a few animals, the disease would spread quickly to the others in the herd and then to new herds. Farmers and agricultural officials would not know if the outbreak came from terrorist or natural causes and might not take immediate action to identify and stop the terrorist. Such a delay would create more opportunities to harm livestock.

A terrorist might find other relatively simple ways to attack the food supply. With fields left largely unguarded, a terrorist with a crop-dusting plane or even a car and spray-painting equipment could spread herbicide across crop fields. With access to storage facilities, a terrorist could mix crop diseases such as soybean rust with seed supplies. Spreading crop disease depends on the wind and good weather conditions and requires technical expertise, but the potential for this kind of terrorist attack remains.

Terrorist attacks like these examples have the potential to devastate agriculture.[77] The loss of income would harm not only farmers and ranchers whose animals or crops are infected but would affect other workers who depend on agricultural work. Rural towns would lose their major source of income, and those outside rural areas in the restaurant, transport, grocery, and agricultural supply businesses would suffer economically as well. For example, an outbreak of foot-and-mouth disease could cost producers billions in lost cattle and raise the cost of meat and dairy products. A small outbreak in Britain in 2001 cost the nation between £2.5 and £8 billion (about $4.5 to $15 billion).[78]

The economic harm of a terrorist attack on the economy would likely be worsened by a loss of consumer confidence in the safety of food. Even one incident of terrorists infecting livestock could lead consumers to avoid all meat products. The resulting decline in demand for certain foods might damage the industry more than the actual loss of animals or crops. The drop in demand would likely extend to exports: The World Trade Organization has rules that even a small outbreak of a contagious disease among livestock requires a ban on exports of that product. An attack on agriculture might lead people to distrust the ability of the government to prevent another, heightening concerns about food safety. If the public were to avoid even safe food, it would worsen the economic consequences of an attack.

In short, attacks on livestock and crops, even if they would not directly infect humans, could have devastating effects. One expert says that "response to an agricultural bioterrorism attack could require significantly more resources than the attack on the World Trade Center."[79]

PREVENTION

Protection of the food supply from deliberate terrorist attacks must rely to a large extent on efforts to ensure the safety of food from diseases caused by natural or accidental outbreaks. Yet government agencies have taken extra steps in recent years to combat terrorism more directly. President George W. Bush, responding to concerns expressed by outgoing Secretary of Health and Human Services Tommy Thompson that the food supply offers an easy target to terrorists, cited progress made so far but also admitted the need for more work to be done. Three organizations have major responsibility for preventing terrorist attacks on the food supply: the Food and Drug Administration, the Department of Agriculture, and the Department of Homeland Security. New regulations and laws also guide prevention efforts.

Ongoing Government Actions

Food and Drug Administration (FDA): This agency in the Department of Health and Human Services regulates food and medical products to ensure they are safe. After September 11, Congress allotted an additional $195 million in funds to the FDA in the 2002 and 2003 fiscal years, which allowed the agency to hire 655 new inspectors and expand its biological and chemical labs. The FDA has since doubled the percentage of food that is inspected to 2 percent.[80] Even with these additional resources, the vast majority of food is left uninspected. There is simply too much food for any more than a small portion to be checked.

To obtain help, the FDA has worked to form new alliances with intelligence agencies—relationships of little importance in the past. Since government employees cannot on their own protect the enormous amount of food transported across and within our borders, they must rely on information to concentrate resources at the points of greatest vulnerability. The Central Intelligence Agency, Department of Defense, and police agencies can provide information that would help the FDA prevent terrorist actions against food sources. If, despite these efforts, a terrorist attack should compromise the food supply, the FDA has developed emergency response plans—again in collaboration with other agencies—to deal with the crisis.

The FDA must also rely on the actions of businesses and consumers to protect food safety. Toward this end, it publishes guidelines on food security for those operating food-related businesses: Managers should investigate and report suspicious activity, teach workers to check for tampered products, perform background checks on employees, and protect their facilities from intruders. These recommendations are not only for establishments that produce and sell food but also for restaurants and caterers. The FDA similarly offers guides to transportation companies to prevent contamination of food en route from producers to sellers. Still yet, the agency urges consumers to follow proper food handling and cooking procedures.

U.S. Department of Agriculture (USDA): Since the September 11 attacks, this agency has added the threat of terrorism to its goal of protecting the safety of the food supply. It established an Office of Food Security and Emergency Preparedness to coordinate its activities in this area and now checks meat, grain, fruit, vegetable, and other agricultural produces for both natural disease agents and deliberate contamination. To improve inspections, Congress appropriated additional funds to the agency, but the immensity of the food supply means only a small portion of agricultural food products can be examined.

With additional funds, the USDA has increased its effort to prevent diseases in agricultural products from being brought across U.S. borders. It has also worked to create a surveillance system that can identify diseases before they can spread and to develop new ways to test for the presence of biological and chemical agents in food. In addition to these efforts, a blue-ribbon panel has offered dozens of recommendations to reduce the likelihood of a terrorist event against livestock. Among the many recommendations, the panel calls for a better tracking system of animal diseases—much like the incidence of human disease is tracked by the Centers for Disease Control and Prevention.

In addition, the USDA partners with private industry to protect the food supply. It offers guidelines to companies and inspectors for the transportation of meat, poultry, and egg products. The guidelines encourage businesses to assess vulnerabilities for attack, require all shipping documents to be checked carefully, put procedures for security in place, develop a recall plan if problems are identified, reject packages that appear to have been changed or have improper papers, install security devices in warehouses and factories, monitor all visitors, and assess employee behavior for appropriateness. Similar kinds of checks are needed in transporting food products from one place to another. These guidelines are effective only to the extent that businesses follow them, but they stress the importance of the issues to those who deal most closely with food.

Department of Homeland Security (DHS): Established after the attacks of September 11, 2001, this agency takes major responsibility for the prevention of bioterrorism. In fact, many agencies that had been part of other departments transferred to DHS in order to combine anti-bioterrorism activities. For example, members of the USDA border inspection force moved to DHS with employees of the Immigration and Naturalization Service, the Border Patrol, and the U.S. Customs Service to form the Customs and Border Protection Agency. Along with controlling movement of people across U.S. borders and stopping the entrance of terrorists into the country, this agency helps police the movement across borders of foods and bioterrorism agents.

To provide research and guidance in dealing with food-based terrorist attacks, the DHS has funded university centers of excellence. The University of Minnesota Homeland Security National Center for Food Protection and Defense will receive $15 million over three years for research on how to prevent and respond to food contamination events. The Texas A&M Homeland Security National Center for Foreign Animals and Zoonotic Disease Defense will receive $18 million over three years to address potential disease threats to animal agriculture. Zoonotic diseases refer to those that can be transmitted from animals to humans, including those transmitted via food products.

Partnerships with states as well as universities are crucial. The DHS has set up multistate partnerships to protect the food supply as part of its Agriculture Counterterrorism Project. The partnership helps states develop the best practices that other states can adopt. To foster coordination and communication across states in the event of a terrorist attack, the DHS maintains an operations center that gathers and distributes information on bioterrorism threats.

New Regulations and Laws

On June 12, 2002, President Bush signed into law the Public Health Security and Bioterrorism Preparedness and Response Act of 2002. Among its provisions, the act requires domestic and foreign food facilities to register with the FDA and to give advance notice of food they will import. It also charges the FDA with developing new methods to test for contaminated food and animal feed at ports of entry that do not unduly delay the distribution of food to domestic markets. The act charges other agencies with regulating biological agents and toxins to ensure they are registered, handled safely, and protected from misuse.

To supplement the new legislation, the White House released its own homeland security directive for food safety on January 30, 2004. The directive specifies duties and goals of the diverse agencies with responsibilities for maintaining U.S. food security. It directs the secretary of homeland security to set up monitoring and surveillance programs on animal diseases, plant diseases, and food quality for early detection of problems. The secretary should, however, consult with the attorney general, director of central intelligence, the secretary of agriculture, the secretary of Health and Human Services, and the administrator of the Environmental Protection Agency to enhance the information it receives on threats and possible methods of attack. Such efforts should increase the awareness throughout the government of potential problems and promote ways to prevent an attack.

The presidential directive also requires that plans be developed to respond to a terrorist attack on agriculture. If a terrorist assault on the food supply occurs, agencies need to isolate the problem and prevent further spread of the disease. With plans in place, they can coordinate their actions with other government agencies and private enterprises, and can maximize the effectiveness of the response.

Research and development represent important antiterrorism components. The presidential directive encourages agencies to develop and promote higher education programs to protect the food supply. Grants to universities should combine training in food sciences, agriculture, medicine, veterinary medicine, epidemiology, microbiology, chemistry, engineering, statistics, mathematics, and disease prevention. Researchers will need access to new laboratories and equipment such as special biocontainment laboratories to study contagious biological agents.

Despite these new laws and regulations, some experts believe that protecting the food supply from terrorist attacks requires much more. It requires an integrated and comprehensive system of surveillance for livestock, crops, food-processing plants, points of entry for imports, food transportation systems, and grocery stores and restaurants. It requires programs to better identify points of vulnerability and concentrate resources where the threat of attack is highest. And it requires a way to trace and recall infected products. Government agencies and businesses have taken steps toward these goals, but the enormity of the task—and the tiny fraction of food now being inspected—means that they remain inadequate.

Government officials in charge of homeland security note in response that a major terrorist attack on food has not occurred in two decades. They argue that their agencies have done well in using their limited resources effectively—the public is safer now from food terrorism than they were before the September 11 attacks. Given limited government resources and a current budget deficit, however, any more extensive efforts at prevention would have to compete with needs of the military, Social Security, and a variety of important programs for funds. It appears that the actions taken thus far will not be expanded in the near future.

FOOD ADDITIVES AND TOXINS

Polysorbate 60, BHA (butylated hydroxyanisole) and BHT (butylated hydroxytoluene), sodium nitrate, potassium bromate, olestra, acesulfame-K, propyl gallate, and stevia—although food chemists may know the nature and purpose of these substances, most consumers do not. Yet these and hundreds of other food additives—products not normally consumed as food but added in the food production process—remain part of our daily diet. Are they safe? The food industry, with support of the FDA, has assured the public that they are. Some health groups, however, believe that at least some of the additives commonly used today threaten the public's health. Many consumers are also suspicious of additives with names they cannot pronounce.

Debates over the safety of food additives in the United States actually date back more than a century.[81] For example, borax, a mineral that is poisonous in large amounts and used today to kill ants, had become widespread as a preservative in flour by 1900. Food manufacturers claimed that such preservatives caused no harm in small amounts and prevented food from spoiling. Yet the public naturally had doubts about even tiny doses of poison in their food. Aiming to settle the question, Dr. Harvey W. Wiley and government scientists in 1902 obtained volunteers to eat food that contained borax or several other possibly dangerous preservatives. Called the poison squad, these volunteers received free food prepared by a chef on-site at government offices in Washington, D.C. In return, however, they had to risk sickness from the additives being tested and collect their urine and feces for analysis. None of the volunteers died or experienced serious illness, but scientists concluded that borax and other poisonous preservatives could cause dangerous health problems by accumulating over time. Their findings were a first step in ending the use of borax and other poisonous additives in food.

Over the next 60 years, battles continued over the safety of other food additives. The Pure Food and Drug Act of 1906 allowed the federal government to regulate additives, and a year later Congress specified allowable food-coloring agents. These laws, however, did not end the controversy, because they didn't specify standards to evaluate the safety of products. Instead, courts often had to settle disagreements between companies and the government. In 1914, the Supreme Court ruled in the *United States v. the Lexington Mill and Elevator Company* that additives had to be shown to cause harm before the government could ban them.[82] The Federal Food, Drug, and Cosmetic Act, passed in 1938 after five years of debate, revised obsolete aspects of the 1906 act. It gave the FDA authority to regulate food additives and set allowable levels of toxic additives to prevent harm to the population. Still, the statute failed to provide specific guidance for what could be allowed and what could be banned.

During this time, food manufacturers declared that additives were essential to feeding the growing population. Without preservatives, they argued, food would spoil quickly, making consumers shop every day for fresh products and preventing the shipment of products grown faraway. Even food shipped and sold quickly might still change color and consistency in ways that would make it unappetizing. Small rural societies could make do without additives, but large, modern and industrial nations like the United States, where the population desired a variety of flavorful foods, needed something more. Manufacturers wanted to transport food over long distances without spoilage, and consumers wanted to buy food that remained wholesome when stored.

TESTING THE SAFETY OF ADDITIVES

The question became not whether food additives were necessary but how policies should balance possible harm from additives with the undeniable benefits. In 1958, some 20 years after the last legislation, Congress specified clear standards for the safety of food additives. The Food Additives Amendment made three important changes. First, it required manufacturers to demonstrate the safety of new additives before they added them to food products, rather than requiring the government to prove the harm of additives already included in food. Second, it demanded evidence that an additive have a reasonable certainty of safety when used as intended. (A stricter standard requiring proof of safety beyond any possible doubt or when misused would exclude most any food product.) Third, it made an exception in the standard for cancer-causing substances. It prohibited the use of additives shown to cause cancer in humans or animals, thus establishing a zero-tolerance standard.

The power given to the FDA to approve food additives led the agency to recognize the special responsibility it had.[83] The FDA already had procedures in place to approve drugs, but these were used only when drugs were prescribed, could be withheld from those particularly vulnerable to side effects, and were typically used for a limited period. Food additives were different. They were consumed by all persons who ate normal foods such as bread, meat, and chocolate and could not be withheld from at-risk groups such as pregnant women, young children, and sick elderly persons. The additives would further accumulate over decades of eating, particularly given that government officials could do little to control the amount of food and food additives people consumed. The FDA intended to evaluate food additives in a way that would gain the confidence of the public and assure them of the safety of their food.

After the 1958 legislation, the FDA began compiling a list of additives that, because of a long history of apparent use without harm, were listed as Generally Recognized as Safe (GRAS). GRAS additives such as salt, vinegar, baking powder, and spices did not require scientific proof of safety. Use of other additives already identified by the agency as safe could continue to be used; nitrates for preserving meat fell into this category. In 1969, the advancement of better testing procedures led the FDA to reevaluate its GRAS list. Despite discovering the need for more data on many GRAS additives, the list has expanded over the years to include more than 690 items.[84]

Since 1958, other food or color additives in processed food have required approval from the FDA.[85] Manufacturers wanting to use a new additive or one not on the currently acceptable list must petition the FDA for approval. The petition must contain scientific evidence that the additive has a reasonable certainty of being safe, and manufacturers must re-petition each time they decide to use the additive in other kinds of foods. The FDA evaluates the scientific validity of the evidence and its consistency with the intended use of the product. In providing approval, the FDA specifies the foods in which the additive can be used, the maximum allowable amount, and the information to be included on the label.

Most safety tests described in the petitions involve injecting large amounts of a substance into mice specially bred for testing purposes. Using small animals and large amounts of a food additive simulates over a short time-span the longer-term effects on humans of small amounts of a food additive. Although sometimes used for testing certain products, human subjects obviously cannot be exposed to tests involving additives that could cause cancer or serious illness. Besides minimizing human risks, animal tests err on the side of caution in the approval process: Huge amounts of additives are given to the test animals (exceeding what would be consumed realistically by humans), helping ensure the safety of food additives that pass the test.

In 1996, legislation modified the testing standard for some food additives. Complaints accumulated that the animal-testing standards for the cancer-causing potential of food additives were unrealistic. As measurement techniques improved, the zero-tolerance rule for cancer-causing food additives created problems. If food additives contained even the slightest amount of a carcinogenic chemical, an amount that could be measured in increasingly tiny units, it could not be used in processed food (although it could be allowed as pesticide residue on raw food, which fell under different legislation and a different regulating agency). With bipartisan support, the Food Quality Protection Act of 1996 changed the standard. It allowed the use of food additives that showed a negligible or insignificant foreseeable risk to human health resulting from its intended use, defined generally as less than one excess cancer case per million people exposed as its acceptable threshold. This change made for a clearer assessment standard, and most interest groups were comfortable with the new rule.

Also in the late 1990s, the FDA reorganized its food-additive review process. It had been criticized by food companies and questioned in 1995 congressional hearings for its backlog of petitions and slow approval process.[86] Critics of the agency worried that delays in approval would stifle innovation in food products. In response, the FDA established the Office of Food Additive Safety, with a separate Division of Petition Review that would speed the process. It also allowed for the use of unintentional food additives—such as what occurs when packaging materials migrate into food—without going through the petition process; companies could instead notify the FDA of their intention.

Given the approval and safety standards, the FDA and the food industry stress that consumers can have full confidence in the safety of food additives. What consumers need most is an understanding of the value of additives for food quality. Toward that end, the FDA summarizes the benefits of five main types of additives:

- Emulsifiers give products a consistent and appetizing texture and smoothness. Without them, salad dressings and peanut butter would separate, and salt and cocoa would clump. They include lecithin in chocolate, monoglycerides and diglycerides in ice cream, and lactic acid esters of monoglycerides and diglycerides in bakery products.

- Vitamins and minerals in milk, cereal, flour, pasta, and margarine fortify and enrich the nutritional value of the diet. For example, common additives include, ascorbic acid, or vitamin C; alpha-tocopherol, or vitamin E; beta-carotene (a source of vitamin A); calcium carbonate; zinc oxide; and iron.

- Antioxidants and other preservatives retard spoilage from mold, bacteria, and air. They prevent bread from becoming moldy and dry and prevent fats and baked goods from becoming rancid and sour. Examples include sodium nitrite in sausage and ham, calcium propionate in bread and other baked foods, and sulfur dioxide in wine and beer.

- Agents to control the acidity and alkalinity of products improve the taste, color, and texture of food. Yeast, sodium bicarbonate, citric acid, fumaric acid, phosphoric acid, lactic acid, and tartrates in cakes, cookies, crackers, butter, chocolates, and soft drinks serve this purpose.

- Natural and artificial flavors enhance the taste of food products, and color additives improve their appearance. Examples include butter flavoring in popcorn, vanilla flavoring in ice cream, artificial sweeteners in diet soda, and colors in soft drinks, butter, and soups. Artificial flavors may, according to literature of the Food Additives and Ingredients Association, improve on natural flavors.

Despite complex names, about 90 percent of additives are compounds found originally in nature.[87] Their popularity comes from the desires of consumers for food that tastes and looks good but is also convenient to buy, store, and use.

CONCERNS ABOUT APPROVED FOOD ADDITIVES

Despite a careful approval process, consumers remain suspicious of the use of additives. Even if uncertainty stems from unfamiliarity with chemical names and the benefits of additives, it has led to the growing popularity of natural and organic foods. Based on recent trends, consumer concerns will likely strengthen. Sometimes groups take advantage of these concerns with unverified and alarming claims about the harm of food additives. However, legitimate organizations focused on scientific evidence also express doubts about the safety of some additives.

The Center for Science in the Public Interest (CSPI), a health and nutrition advocacy group led by Michael Jacobson that is critical of the food industry and government regulators, agrees that chemicals are a necessary part of today's diet. It accepts most of the FDA's decisions to approve food additives and lists 42 widely used food additives on its web page as safe. It lists another 16 additives as nontoxic but, in large amounts, as contributing to bad nutrition; most people should cut back on products that contain additives such as corn syrup, hydrogenated vegetable oil, salt, and sugar. However, the CSPI offers differing views on some of the products approved by the FDA. It recommends that consumers avoid several additives that need better testing or appear unsafe from current testing. Consider these examples of such additives.[88]

Butylated hydroxyanisole (BHA) and butylated hydroxytoluene (BHT) are synthetic antioxidants that help maintain food color, taste, and odor. By reacting with oxygen, these antioxidants prevent meat and fats from oxidizing, which can turn food sour and unpleasant. Cereals, chewing gum, potato chips, and vegetable oil often include BHA or BHT. Although most animal studies show the additives are safe, some have indicated that they can cause cancer. Since residues of BHT can be stored in body fat, it suggests the potential for harm to humans. The CSPI suggests that consumers avoid products with these additives and urges food manufacturers to substitute safer additives or use other production techniques that make BHA and BHT unnecessary.

Aspartame (Nutrasweet), a low-calorie artificial sweetener that replaces sugar in diet soft drinks, diet foods, and Equal packets, received FDA approval on the basis of negative tests for cancer. However, its widespread use has resulted in reports of dizziness, hallucinations, and headaches. Scientific studies have not validated claims that aspartame causes these symptoms, nor have they provided evidence for other claims that aspartame causes diabetes, hypertension, arthritis, Alzheimer's disease, lupus, and brain tumors. Still, the CSPI argues that more thorough tests done by independent agencies are needed to validate the safety of this food additive. In the meantime, it recommends that consumers avoid products with aspartame.

Sodium nitrite and sodium nitrate are preservatives that maintain the coloring and flavoring of bacon, ham, frankfurters, lunch meat, smoked fish, and corned beef. Without these additives, most meat would look gray rather than red. These additives can lead to the formation of cancer-causing chemicals called nitrosamines. The risk is small in general but may be higher for children, pregnant women, and adults who already have cancer. The CSPI suggests that consumers avoid food with these additives and that the food industry develop safer alternatives.

Olestra is a synthetic fat developed by Procter and Gamble that the body does not absorb; instead it passes directly through the intestines. Products such as chips and ice cream with olestra have the feel of fatty products that people like but are similar to fat-free products because olestra does not reach the circulatory system. Replacing the intake of normal fats with olestra can reduce heart disease, obesity, some cancers, and other health problems. Scientists at Procter and Gamble point to a long history of thorough research on the product that includes more than 150 research publications in top peer-reviewed journals and to positive consumer reception.[89] In 1996, the FDA approved olestra as a food additive but also took the unusual step of requiring a warning about its use.[90] The agency noted that the unabsorbed fat could, much like some laxatives, prevent the absorption of vital nutrients, and the long-term consequences of digestive changes caused by the product are unknown. For these same reasons, Canadian Health authorities have not approved products with olestra in Canada. The CSPI and many other organizations recommend that consumers ignore the FDA approval and avoid any food with the additive.

Critics of the FDA argue that the food industry has exerted too much influence on Congress and the agency in getting new products such as aspartame and olestra approved and keeping BHA, BHT, sodium nitrite, and sodium nitrate in foods. The high profits from use of these additives motivate companies and industry groups to do what they can to influence scientific evaluations of the additives. In the case of olestra, for example, Procter and Gamble lobbied Congress to extend its patent while undergoing the long review process and hired consultants and experts to promote the safety of the product.[91]

As further evidence that the government safety standards are not thorough enough, the CSPI lists 29 food and color additives that, after being used for many years, were found to pose health risks and banned. If mistakes were made for these items, they may have been made for other items now approved.

CHEMICAL AND NATURAL TOXINS IN FOOD

Along with food additives meant to improve taste, texture, and freshness, other substances can become part of food as a by-product of modern farming, livestock production, and environmental pollution. Although not intended for human consumption, these chemicals still affect the safety of food. Three types of substances—pesticides, animal hormones, and chemical and metal pollutants—have generated the most concern. In addition, some chemical toxins occur naturally in food but also present a threat to food safety.

PESTICIDE RESIDUE IN FRUIT, VEGETABLES, AND GRAINS

Pesticides are chemicals designed to control insects (insecticides), fungi (fungicides), weeds (herbicides), and other diseases and pests that harm crops and animals. Insecticides often work by destroying the nerve system of insects, and other pesticides contain chemicals designed to kill plants, worms, and fungi. Such products can prove harmful for people as well. Above certain amounts, they can cause nerve damage, cancer, birth defects, and other diseases. The residue that ends up in food is small, but most people would prefer that their food contain no amount of poisonous substances. Why then is pesticide residue allowed on food?

Without pesticides, the amount, quality, and affordability of fruits, vegetables, and grains would decline substantially. Pesticides allow farmers to more efficiently grow crops and prevent the destruction of crops by pests before they are harvested. As summarized by the International Food Information Council, "Farmers must contend with approximately 80,000 plant diseases, 30,000 species of weeds, 1,000 species of nematodes [roundworms], and more than 10,000 species of insects. . . In the United States alone, about $20 billion worth of crops (one-tenth of production) are lost each year."[92] Without pesticides the problem would be even worse: Weeds would choke off soil nutrients and crowd out crops, mold and mildew brought on by heavy rains or high humidity would destroy crops in only a few days, and an explosion of insects would devastate a field in hours. Home gardeners know the damage pests can do to vegetables.

The benefit of pesticides comes, in short, from making an abundant and inexpensive supply of food available to the public. Without pesticides, much of the food we now get would never make it to market. Of the food that gets to market, much of it would be less appetizing. As one document on pesticide use states, "Imagine opening a fresh ear of gold corn, only to find it's already been half eaten by worms. Or biting into a bright red strawberry, discovering it's half rotten from a fungus."[93]

For these reasons, pesticide use will not disappear soon. Many farmers have begun using integrated pest-management techniques that minimize the use of chemicals. Planting pest-resistant plant varieties, spraying pesticides only when tests show they are necessary, and rotating crops to prevent pests from becoming established can help but do not eliminate the potential for pesticide residue. Washing fruits and vegetables likewise cannot remove all the pesticide from food. Even organic farming allows for use of natural pesticides and for residue from synthetic pesticides that have drifted from neighboring fields.

Although pesticide residue on food cannot be avoided, it can be regulated. In fact, pesticides may be the most regulated type of chemical product used in the United States. They fall under the jurisdiction of three federal agencies (the EPA, FDA, and USDA) and more than 14 separate regulations. The most important regulations come from the 1996 Food Quality Protection Act, which requires the EPA to reexamine currently allowed pesticides to ensure that they meet newly defined standards and will not harm infants and young children. According to the government's National Institute of Environmental Health Sciences (NIEHS), these regulations are both strict and effective.[94] They first require government scientists to estimate the maximum amount of a pesticide that, if ingested over a lifetime, would still not cause any harm. They then lower this level by a factor of 10 to 100 to ensure that, within a large margin of error, the pesticide is safe for children as well as adults. In a sense, this means that pesticides are 10 to 100 times safer than a level determined to have no toxic effect.

If a pesticide does not demonstrate this degree of safety, farmers cannot use it. Even those approved as safe can legally be used by farmers only in certain amounts and only following certain procedures. If misused in some way, spot tests of pesticide residue on food can identify excessive amounts, and government officials can withhold the products and others coming from the same source until farmers rectify the problem. Government officials also sample and test imported fruit, vegetables, and grains. In 1994, 99 percent of domestic samples and 96 percent of imported samples had residues below the allowable levels.[95] Tests for the presence of pesticides have become so sensitive and accurate in recent years that they can now detect the equivalent of one teaspoon of salt in one million gallons of water—a level well below any safety threshold.

Taking the evidence into account, experts generally believe that the health benefits of eating a variety of fruits and vegetables outweigh any risks from pesticide residue. A report from the NIEHS concludes, "While pesticides may be found in many products, the levels at which they are present fall far below the levels known to not cause any health effects."[96] Another scientist states that pesticide residue intake is so small relative to the amounts causing harm "that even the most restrictive assessments that take into account particularly sensitive groups (newborns, adolescents, the elderly, etc.) would lead to 100 percent safe results."[97]

Despite government claims of safety, many people and organizations remain unconvinced. A 1999 article published in *Consumer Reports* concludes that "it is surprisingly easy for children to eat fresh fruits and vegetables with unacceptable levels of some especially toxic pesticides."[98] The article reports that apples, grapes, green beans, peaches, pears, and winter squash have particularly high levels of toxins, likely because farmers use more pesticides on these crops. In nearly all instances, the observed pesticide levels fell below government safety standards, but this merely indicates the inadequacies of the standards.

Consumers, particularly pregnant women and parents of children, worried by these findings can take several steps to protect themselves from pesticide threats. Some experts say they should buy organic fruits and vegetables, which cost more but have only one-third the levels of pesticides of conventional products.[99] They should thoroughly wash rather than quickly rinse raw foods and even peel apples and pears to remove the part most likely to contain pesticides. Lastly, they should demand stricter standards in government evaluations of the safety of fruits and vegetables.

However, critics regard such claims as nonsense that needlessly scares parents. Officials of the Society of Toxicology, the nation's largest professional organization of toxicologists, say that *Consumer Reports'*s "conclusions concerning the dangers of pesticides in food are not credible and are unnecessarily alarmist."[100] They identify flaws in the methods used by the article and favor those adopted by government agencies, but media reports seldom understand or explain these details. As a result, reports can frighten consumers away from eating the variety of fruits and vegetables needed for good health.

Since the *Consumer Reports* article, the use of one of the offending pesticides, methyl parathion, has been restricted. New tests of the product mandated by the 1996 Food Quality Protection Act led the EPA to conclude that it represented an unacceptable risk. Reflecting the ongoing nature of the debate over pesticide residue on food, this action led congressional representatives of farm states to strongly criticize the EPA and prompted consumer groups to claim the reversal reveals the flaws in past methods.

Pesticide use thus presents a dilemma for those concerned about food safety. On one hand, pesticide residue on food results inevitably from modern farming methods that provide the fresh foods needed for good health. Government agencies have used a variety of scientific testing methods to determine that residues remain within safe limits. On the other hand, any pesticide on food worries many consumers. Organizations opposed to pesticide use endorse these worries, often criticizing government testing methods and relying on their own research to demonstrate the harm of pesticides.

ANIMAL HORMONES IN MEAT

Just as pesticides are used to protect and promote the growth of crops, certain hormones are used to protect and promote the growth of cattle and sheep. Hormones occur naturally in animals to help control development and reproduction, and extra doses of hormones can shorten the growth time of beef cattle and improve the milk production of dairy cattle. For example, several types of steroid hormones, including female sex hormones, are approved as growth promoters in cattle and sheep, and the bovine growth hormone, originally extracted from the cow pituitary gland and now created artificially using recombinant DNA technology, increases milk production.

However, the potential for hormone residue in meat and milk to cause breast cancer and other health problems in humans raises serious concerns. Because an increased risk of breast cancer is associated with lifetime exposure of women to the female hormone estrogen, it seems possible that the presence of similar hormones in meat could raise this risk. Milk from cows given the bovine growth hormone could do the same: It contains increased levels of a natural protein that may be associated with breast cancer and other health problems.[101] For these reasons, the European Union since 1989 has banned all meat from animals treated with steroid growth hormones and milk from cattle treated with the bovine growth hormone.

Scientific studies have not confirmed these fears. Although it may take many more years and better methods to know the long-term harm of hormones, the potential for problems seems small. The human body naturally produces amounts of steroid hormones many times larger than those eaten in meat and growth hormones many times larger than those consumed in milk. Thus, the Cornell University Program on Breast Cancer and Environmental Risk Factors in New York State, after noting the need for more research, concludes that "studies done so far do not provide evidence to state that hormone residues in meat or dairy products cause any human health effects."[102] Yet the European Union, in responding to accusations that it unfairly restricted sale of beef with hormones, formed a scientific committee to investigate the issue. The committee reaffirmed the claim that meat with hormones posed a risk to humans.

Scientific evidence or not, many consumers worry about hormone additives. Breast cancer survivors in particular want to avoid any food that might cause the return of their disease. Appealing more widely to those concerned about food additives, dairies often advertise that their milk is free of artificial hormones, and most stores sell organic milk. The popularity of such products has led to a counterresponse. In 2003, the Monsanto Company, which produces bovine growth hormones, sued to stop Oakhurst Dairy in Maine from advertising their products as free from artificial growth hormones. They claim that no differences exist between milk with artificial and natural hormones, and the FDA supports that claim. Under pressure from the suit, Oakhurst Dairy changed their milk labels.

CHEMICAL AND HEAVY METAL POLLUTANTS

Environmental pollution can cause food safety problems (along with other serious health problems). Chemical pollutants are not meant to get into food but inevitably affect plants and animals used for food. For example, perchlorate is an ingredient used in rocket fuel and manufacturing processes that makes its way into water and soil and then to lettuce and milk. Dioxins are poisonous chemicals that result from the commercial and local incineration of wood, coal, and oil that get widely distributed throughout the environment; they can be absorbed by plants, animals, and fish and enter the body through food consumption. Acrylamide, a chemical used for a variety of industrial purposes such as plastic manufacturing and wastewater treatment, has been detected in a wide range of food products and causes cancer in large doses among animals.

The FDA has recently begun to monitor the presence of these chemicals in foods. Although the chemicals have been around for many decades, the ability of scientific methods to detect their presence in food has improved. The agency does not make recommendations to avoid particular food because of these chemicals and argues more research is needed before making any policy changes that would require testing and control of the chemicals. In the meantime, the FDA recommends eating a varied diet to minimize overexposure to any of these chemicals.

Along with synthetic chemical pollutants, heavy metals such as cadmium, mercury, lead, and arsenic can contaminate food and cause health problems. Cadmium, a heavy metal often used in batteries, is released into the air in manufacturing and is released into the soil as part of fertilizers. It can be taken up by crops and vegetables and cause kidney damage in humans. Mercury compounds released into the environment during manufacturing processes accumulate in fish and in humans through fish consumption; the metal compounds can cause neurological damage but present the most risk to the fetuses of pregnant women. Lead, once a component of paint and gasoline, can seep into soil and plants and cause neurological damage. Arsenic, a strong poison, enters the air from the smelting and burning of fossil fuels and can be absorbed into plants through the soil and water and then into humans through food.

Given the source of these metals in food—environmental pollution— consumers can do little about these threats to food safety. Pregnant women should restrict the fish in their diet. Otherwise, the main recommendation for a healthy diet—to eat a wide variety of foods—applies here as well.

NATURAL TOXINS

Many foods contain natural toxins that present dangers similar to or worse than those of food additives. For example, as a result of natural chemicals in plants that help protect them from pests and plant-eating animals, natural pesticides are 10,000 times more common in the food people eat than manufactured pesticides.[103] Such figures surprise most people, who tend to worry more about artificial pesticides. Of special importance, the toxins are contained in organic as well as conventional food.

Natural toxins in small amounts are managed by the body's liver without harm, but in larger amounts, they can cause health damage. Here are some foods with toxins that affect food safety.

- Potatoes contain toxins called glycoalkaloids in small amounts that show up most obviously in a greenish tinge to the skin. These toxins irritate the mouth and stomach and have been reported to cause a few deaths overseas. Cooks should store potatoes in cool, dry places and remove green and bruised parts of potatoes before using them in recipes.
- Kidney beans contain toxins called lectins that can cause severe stomachaches, vomiting, and diarrhea. Raw kidney beans should be soaked for at least five hours and boiled to destroy the toxin, while canned beans can be used without further cooking.
- Peanuts, peanut butter, and corn can contain a toxin called aflatoxin that is produced by mold and can cause liver problems and cancer. Proper storing of these foods in dry conditions prevents the growth of the dangerous toxin, but consumers should avoid peanuts with mold and peanut butter from unknown manufacturers.

- Cabbage, cauliflower, Brussels sprouts, broccoli, kale, kohlrabies, turnips, radishes, mustard, and rutabagas contain glucosinolates that can, when digested, inhibit the uptake of iodine by the thyroid.
- Spinach, beets, celery, radishes, and rhubarb contain natural nitrates, substances also added to meats as a preservative and found to be carcinogenic in animals.
- Oysters, clams, scallops, and mussels can absorb toxins from algae in warm water that cause paralysis and breathing problems.

When consumed in moderation and with care in preparation, none of these foods presents a serious risk. Yet the presence of natural toxins demonstrates that issues of food safety go beyond problems of food additives.

FOOD ALLERGENS AND INTOLERANTS

In 1991, 12-year-old Umar Murtaza died in a Los Angeles hospital several hours after eating a piece of birthday cake that contained crushed pecans. He was allergic to nuts. . . In 1999, the day after hosting a cookout for his championship lacrosse team, 18-year-old Joe Murphy ate some pistachio nuts. The Boston-area resident knew he was allergic to peanuts but had no idea that he couldn't eat pistachios either. Murphy collapsed into anaphylactic shock, then fell into a coma. He died nine days later.[104]

As illustrated by these stories, small portions of the population—about 6 percent of children under three years old and 1.5 percent of adults—have clinically proven allergies to certain foods.[105] Although rare, these food allergies can be deadly: About 150 people die each year from allergic reactions to what they eat. The foods causing these deadly incidents are safe for most everyone else, but for individuals with these allergies, they become dangerous enemies.

A food allergy involves an abnormal immune response that is triggered by food. Like any allergy, a food allergy comes from the action of antibodies to destroy foreign substances, but in this case the antibodies act abnormally in responding to common foods, even in small amounts. These antibodies are formed during the first exposure to specific food, and the next exposure to the food leads the antibodies to release histamine chemicals that produce an allergic reaction (although sometimes an immune response builds more slowly). The reaction can lead to itching and swelling of the mouth, nose, and throat area; asthma and problems in breathing and swallowing; migraine headaches from swelling or spasms of blood vessels;

digestive problems such as stomach pain and diarrhea; and skin irritation in the form of hives.

The most dangerous consequence involves an allergic reaction called anaphylactic shock, a condition that produces a sudden drop in blood pressure, inability to breathe, and loss of body temperature. Each year, about 30,000 people with food allergies go into anaphylactic shock after eating the wrong food and about 150 die.[106] During emergencies, injecting epinephrine (or adrenaline), a quick-acting hormone, treats the shock by widening the passages to the lungs, constricting the vessels to increase blood pressure, and increasing the beating of the heart. Those with severe allergies need to carry epinephrine, particularly the form for injection, and get immediate medical care in the case of emergency.

Most food allergies are inherited. They occur more commonly in children, and many outgrow the problem as adults. If not obvious from an immediate reaction to a specific food, the source of the food allergy can be identified by physicians using a variety of tests. Once the source is identified, the treatment is simple in principle but often difficult in practice—avoid the offending food. Those with multiple allergies can follow special diets that rotate the type of foods consumed so that problematic substances do not build up in the body. Children with allergies depend on parents to carefully monitor and control their diets. However, even those vigilant about their allergy can unknowingly consume dangerous foods.

The FDA lists eight foods—all with high protein content—that most often cause allergic reactions: milk, eggs, fish, wheat, tree nuts (such as walnuts and pecans), peanuts, soybeans, and shellfish. Allergies to peanuts (actually a legume similar to beans and peas) and tree nuts appear most common and dangerous. Allergies for other foods often disappear after childhood, but those for nuts and peanuts persist, often affecting teenagers and young people. Most deaths involve contact with the food outside the home that, unknown to the victim, included small amounts of the nuts. For example, environmentalist and writer Robert Kennedy, Jr.'s, son Conor has such a strong peanut allergy that coming in contact with someone who has eaten a peanut butter sandwich can cause a severe reaction. By age six, he had been rushed to the emergency room 31 times and been hospitalized nine times.[107]

Even people without allergies can suffer from related health problems called food intolerance. Together, food allergies and food intolerances are called food sensitivities. Although sometimes used interchangeably with food allergy, food intolerance does not involve an allergic reaction of the immune system, produces milder symptoms, and is seldom deadly. The symptoms of food intolerance are many. One web page cites more than 70 medical conditions thought to be associated with food allergies and notes that "virtually any symptom can be associated with food allergy or intolerance."[108] Conditions include sinus irritation, sore throat, gastroenteritis, headaches, dry skin, arthritis, diabetes, fatigue, and overweight.

The diffuseness of the symptoms makes it hard to separate problems caused by food intolerance from those caused by something else. Yet several foods clearly trigger intolerance.[109]

- Lactose or milk sugar intolerance occurs in roughly 30 percent of the population that lacks enough of the enzyme lactase. Undigested lactose causes gas or diarrhea when it reaches the large intestines. Those who are lactose intolerant can usually digest small amounts of milk and eat cheese, ice cream, and yogurt or consume special lactose-free milk products.

- Sulfites additives used for preservatives in dried fruits, wines, and dried potato products like mashed potato flakes can cause serious breathing problems and death in some people. Until 1986, sulfites had been used commonly in salad bars to keep the fresh appearance of raw fruits and vegetables, but new regulations ended the practice that year. Although 1,132 serious reactions and more than a dozen deaths occurred between 1980 and 1999, most preceded the 1986 regulations, and no recorded deaths from sulfite intolerance have occurred since 1990.

- Monosodium glutamate (MSG), a saltlike flavor enhancer once commonly used in Chinese food, is reported to cause headaches, dizziness, and flushness. Despite much criticism of the additive, studies find that only a few people are sensitive to it, and the symptoms are extremely mild.

- Tartrazine (yellow dye no. 5) helps produce shades of cream, orange, and green in foods but also can cause itching or hives in some people.

- Gluten is a substance found in wheat and grain products, particularly bread. Some people lack an enzyme in the lining of the walls of the intestines that is needed to process gluten, a condition called celiac disease that causes nausea, loss of appetite, abdominal pain, and malaise.

Sulfites present the greatest threat to health, but even the less serious sources of food intolerance can cause discomfort.

Other symptoms often claimed to result from food intolerance, including hyperactivity, migraine headaches, arthritis, tension fatigue, and difficulty concentrating, present more controversy. As indicated by popular books on treating food allergies and sensitivities, many people believe that the health and psychological problems they and their children face stem from food allergies. Yet the scientific evidence of these effects remains meager, and most experts dismiss such claims.

As staples of the diet for most people, food allergens and intolerants cannot be regulated or restricted. Rather, individuals with sensitivities must do what they can to protect themselves by avoiding the food. They must read labels carefully and know about recipe contents to make sure they do not unknowingly eat products that are unsafe for them. At the same time, food manufacturers, government agencies, and restaurants can do more to ensure that those with allergies know what they are eating and limit food additives with the potential to cause allergies. Clear and complete labels can help save lives and reduce the pain and suffering of allergic reactions.

For many years, people with food sensitivity have complained that food labels are incomplete and unclear, which can put their lives and health at risk. The Food Allergen Labeling and Consumer Protection Act of 2004 addressed this problem. By January 2006, it requires new labels on all products that contain the major food allergens. The labels should describe food in plain English, using terms like eggs, milk, and wheat, along with the more technical terms of, respectively, albumen, casein, and semolina. It should also list all allergenic food ingredients rather than using broad categories such as flavoring, coloring, and spices. Consumers can then more easily determine if a product contains ingredients that can harm them.

The legislation aims to address another gap in food production safety. Food contamination can occur unintentionally by careless production process. Making products with and without food allergens in the same building and at the same time, or with the same equipment at different times can lead to contamination. Simple mistakes can do much the same. Ben and Jerry's, for example, had to recall ice cream in which tree nuts were accidentally added. The company worried that the nut ingredients, which the labels did not list, might cause serious allergic reactions in some customers. The legislation requires the secretary of Health and Human Services to investigate how cross-contamination can occur in production processes and how inspection or education can reduce the problems. It also requires gathering of better data on adverse events from food allergies, making it easier to chart progress in dealing with the problem. Critics believe that the food industry has not done enough on its own and hope this legislation will improve the situation.

Although food allergies and intolerance affect only a small part of the population, some experts argue that the problem has grown. Peanut allergies, for example, increased twofold among children from 1997 to 2002.[110] Perhaps with the fewer germs in the environment, the body's immune system devotes more resources to dealing with certain foods. If true, food sensitivity may become an increasingly serious threat to food safety.

TECHNOLOGICAL INNOVATIONS

Nukeburgers, cold pasteurization, frankenfood, damage-resistant crops—perceptions of threats to food safety depend much on the commonly accepted names of food technology. Two technological innovations to improve food safety—irradiation of food to kill pathogens and genetically modified crops to improve resistance to damage—have created controversy over the appropriate names. The slang terms *nukeburgers* and *frankenfood* make irradiated and genetically modified food sound bizarre, hazardous, and unappetizing, while cold pasteurization and damage-resistant crops sound familiar and comforting.

Names do not make food safe or unsafe—the chemical properties of irradiated and genetically modified food are critical. Yet debates over names reflect considerable controversy over the potential benefits and dangers of these technological innovations. Do these new developments represent a threat to food safety? As is often the case, it depends on one's viewpoint. In general, scientists and government experts remain steadfast in their support of the new technology, critics vocally oppose the techniques as a threat to health, and the public harbors suspicions.

The differing viewpoints reflect underlying debates over the value of technology. Those most concerned about food safety tend to distrust many other forms of technology and note a certain irony in the use of irradiated and genetically modified foods: The new products represent technological solutions to problems caused in the first place by technology. Over the last several decades, technologies have allowed cattle and chickens to be raised in huge farms, accelerated the growth of food animals with antibiotics and hormones, and made for efficient and quick slaughtering—all possible sources of the growing presence of dangerous pathogens in food. One solution, using radiation to kill the pathogens, involves more technology. Also over the last several decades, mass production of crops has required the use of large amounts of pesticides that, as residue on food, present a risk to consumers. One solution, using genetically modified crops that are resistant to damage from pests, again involves more technology. According to opponents, the solutions not only pose new risks to food safety but also direct attention away from the original technological causes of the problems.

Those more supportive of the new technologies see the developments as choices necessary to protect food safety in modern societies. The goals of feeding a growing world population while at the same time keeping costs down demand new technology that is both safe and effective. Supporters express optimism rather than distrust about new food technologies.

FOOD IRRADIATION

Food irradiation illustrates debates over the value of technology for food safety. When directed at raw food, high-dose radiation kills bacteria, parasites, and insects, just as high-dose radiation can kill humans (indeed, medical treatment narrowly targets radiation to kill cancerous cells). So, does the high-dose radiation change the food in ways that may be harmful?

Radiation refers to released energy that commonly takes the form of light and heat but also takes other forms such as microwaves and radio and television waves. Food irradiation refers to subjecting food to special forms of radiant energy such as gamma rays, electron beams, and X-rays. At the atomic level, these three forms of radiant energy (sometimes call ionizing radiation) have the property of dislodging electrons and producing a special type of atom called an ion. At the cellular level, the changes in electrons damage the genetic material of living organisms so that they die or are unable to grow and reproduce. In principle, food irradiation harms living organisms without damaging the food itself.

The idea for food radiation dates back more than 100 years.[111] In 1905, the first patents were issued to use ionizing radiation as a way to kill bacteria in food and prevent spoilage. Numerous experiments in the following decades examined the effects of the irradiation on a variety of foods, generally with positive results. After World War II and the development of the nuclear bomb, the U.S. Atomic Energy Commission and other government agencies, wanting to transform atomic energy into peaceful uses, began a more systematic program of research on food irradiation. Scientists determined the proper level of radiation to use, helped develop safe equipment, and examined the safety of irradiated food. With evidence and recommendations in hand, government agencies endorsed the process. The FDA approved irradiation to kill insects in wheat and flour in 1963, to prevent growth of sprouts in potatoes in 1964, and to sterilize packing material in 1971. In 1972, the National Aeronautics and Space Administration (NASA) began to use irradiation to sterilize food for astronauts in space.

During the 1980s, food irradiation spread to nations throughout the world. Of special importance, a committee of experts sponsored by the Food and Agricultural Organization of the United Nations, the International Atomic Energy Agency, and the World Health Organization recommended approval of irradiated foods and the adoption of worldwide standards for their use. Also in the 1980s, the FDA approved irradiation of pork, vegetables, spices, poultry, shelled eggs, and frozen uncooked meats, not only to kill microbes but also sometimes to extend shelf life.

Despite government approval and worldwide acceptance, the public in the United States has been slow to accept irradiated foods. By law, fresh irradiated foods must contain a label with an internationally accepted symbol of radiation and the phrase "treated by irradiation." Even with added reassuring phrases such as "to eliminate bacteria," the label scares buyers. Proposals from Congress to use the term *cold pasteurization* rather than irradiation aim, given the familiarity with pasteurized milk, to make the label less frightening. Processed foods that contain irradiated ingredients such as spices do not need to include an irradiation label. However, foods with the organic label cannot be irradiated or include irradiated ingredients.

The Case for Food Irradiation

Government agencies assert without any qualification that irradiated food is safe. The FDA, for instance, states the following on its web site:

> *Is irradiated food safe? Yes. The Food and Drug Administration has evaluated the safety of this technology over the last 40 years and has found irradiation to be safe under a variety of conditions and has approved its use for many foods. Scientific studies have shown that irradiation does not significantly reduce nutritional quality or significantly change food taste, texture or appearance. Irradiated foods do not become radioactive. Irradiation can produce changes in food, similar to changes caused by cooking, but in smaller amounts.*[112]

The CDC similarly states that, in well-controlled studies of both animals and people, "There is no evidence of adverse health effects."[113]

Some chemical changes admittedly occur in food that undergoes irradiation, but then chemical changes also occur in food during cooking. In fact, changes due to irradiation are quite small compared to those from baking, grilling, frying, or sautéing. Irradiation of food may destroy tiny amounts of some nutrients and vitamins or release some chemical by-products, but according to defenders, these changes pose no risk to health. Some consumers may believe that the process makes food radioactive, but this is not the case; radiation waves pass through the food rather than make it dangerous. Hundreds of tests reveal no short-term harm from eating irradiated food. After all, the astronauts experienced no problems eating irradiated food in space. Even tests giving large amounts of irradiated products to lab animals over many generations do not provide reliable evidence of cancer, birth defects, or other disease.

If the risks of irradiation are insignificant, the benefits are indisputable. The process destroys bacteria, parasites, molds, and insects that sicken millions and kill thousands when present in food. Of particular benefit, irradiation kills deadly *E. coli* O157:H7 and *Salmonella* that are commonly found in meat, poultry, and eggs. It does not eliminate the threat of these pathogens altogether or the need to thoroughly cook food and follow careful food handling procedures. It does, however, reduce foodborne disease. One figure suggests that sickness and deaths decline by 25 percent from irradiation of meat—a change that translates into thousands fewer hospitalizations and hundreds of saved lives.[114]

65

Irradiation also provides an alternative to chemical treatment of crops. Spices and herbs, for example, can contain microbes that in the past have been killed with chemicals, a process that leaves residue on the food; irradiation has replaced this process and leaves no harmful residue. Irradiation can similarly help control the infestation of insects and the growth of mold in stored grains, nuts, and peanuts without the use of pesticides. It can kill dangerous insects hidden in imported food and can extend the shelf life of fresh foods by preventing spoilage.

Government advocates of food irradiation view the technique as a supplement rather than replacement of other measures taken to ensure food safety. Even with irradiation, government inspectors need to do all they can to enforce cleanliness standards in plants and factories, and restaurants and home cooks need to do all they can to cook meat thoroughly and avoid spreading germs. Irradiation brings added safety to such efforts. Because microorganisms are a natural part of life and can never be eliminated altogether from food, use of irradiation as one more source of protection from foodborne illness should be welcome.

If, as advocates claim, irradiation of food is so beneficial, then why has the public not come to accept it? Misunderstandings of the process may contribute to suspicions about irradiated food (much as misunderstandings about pasteurized milk occurred earlier in the century). For example, one 1995–96 study found that the percentage of consumers likely to buy irradiated food increased from 57 percent to 82 percent after seeing a 10-minute video describing the value of the process.[115] A minority of people opposed to most technologies or unreasonably concerned about radiation will never purchase irradiated food. With education, however, the wider public may come to see the benefit of such products.

Those who distrust these optimistic claims made about food irradiation by agencies in the U.S. government can look to other nations for confirmation. More than 40 nations throughout the world—including many that prohibit routine use of antibiotics or hormones in food animals—have approved food irradiation.

The Case against Food Irradiation

Critics of food irradiation may sometimes exaggerate the failures of the federal government in making the case against food irradiation. Accusations that it ignored numerous studies of the harm of the practice, selected only a few favorable studies, and acted on behalf of large corporations that stand to profit from irradiation make little sense given the widespread approval of food irradiation by other nations, the World Health Organization, the Centers for Disease Control and Prevention, and the editors of the highly respected *New*

England Journal of Medicine. Presented in a less exaggerated form, however, arguments against food irradiation raise some telling questions.

One question concerns whether food irradiation might produce dangerous mutations in microorganisms. A mutation is an alteration in the genetic messages carried by a cell, and some forms of radiation are known to cause genetic mutation. Although a dangerous mutation in microorganisms from food irradiation does not occur often, the odds of it happening increase as more and more food undergoes irradiation. The Center for Food Safety cites studies that find irradiated food causes genetic or cellular damage in animals or people who eat them.[116] It is less clear how this damage occurs; perhaps genetic material damaged by food irradiation attaches itself to cells and proteins in the body and thus causes genetic or cellular damage in those who eat irradiated food. In any case, the potential for such damage worries critics.

Another question concerns whether food irradiation might produce dangerous chemical by-products. The Center for Food Safety cites evidence that irradiation of certain fats in eggs, beef, pork, chicken, and turkey produces chemicals called cyclobutanones. Comparisons of store-bought meat show the presences of cyclobutanones in irradiated products but not in conventional products. Worse, some studies suggest that these chemicals promote tumors in lab animals. The FDA says that it is examining this new evidence, but it has not responded publicly.[117]

Still one more question concerns whether food irradiation depletes nutrients and vitamins. Critics claim that irradiation results in the losses of A, C, E, and B complex vitamins in food and reduces the levels of beneficial antioxidant compounds in fruits and vegetables. Cooking may do the same, but the negative consequences of irradiation for fresh fruits and vegetables remain. In addition, using irradiation to extend the shelf life of food will reduce its nutritional value: The longer the period from harvest to table, the greater the natural loss of nutrients and vitamins.

Along with threats to health, food irradiation has other undesirable social and economic consequences according to critics. The use of irradiated food encourages lax enforcement of food-safety procedures in the production process—producers will expect that their errors will not matter if irradiation kills pathogens. Yet more rather than less emphasis on safety and sanitation remains the key to a health-promoting food supply. Economically, the widespread use of irradiation favors large corporate food companies at the expense of smaller farmers and companies. Only large companies can afford the extra expense of purchasing or using irradiation machines. If irradiation becomes common, it will advantage large companies, give them greater power and profits, and limit the supply of fresh, natural, and healthy food.

Along with offering evidence of long-term harm of food irradiation, critics dispute its supposed benefits. A 2003 study in *Consumer Reports* found that "Bacteria levels in the irradiated, uncooked ground beef and skinless chicken tenders were generally much lower than levels in the non-irradiated meat. But the irradiated meat still contained some bacteria. And, like any meat, irradiated meat can become contaminated if it is handled improperly."[118] Irradiated products thus do not deliver complete safety. In addition, tasters used in the study found the cooked irradiated meat to have slight, but noticeable unpleasantness in its taste and smell.

Opponents of food irradiation have found encouragement in the slow acceptance of irradiation by shoppers and the recent bankruptcy of one firm specializing in food irradiation. However, they worry that the government will take new measures to sway the public. For example, a switch in labels from "treated by radiation" to "cold pasteurization" could mislead the public, and the use of irradiated food in restaurants could expose unknowing customers to the product. Already, school districts have been given the option of ordering irradiated ground beef, and the USDA has set up programs to publicize the benefits of irradiated food among students and parents. Concerned consumers should therefore take care to avoid irradiated food and purchase organic products that guarantee no irradiation.

Advocates of food irradiation, of course, reject these claims. They argue that any long-term harm is, at best, debatable while the short-term benefits in terms of preventing foodborne illness are indisputable. Opponents nevertheless remain unconvinced. Suspicions about the treatment of food by new technology, distrust of food companies, and concerns about the potential for harm from irradiated food persist. As one critical report states, the FDA "should order a suspension of all ongoing food irradiation . . . Failure to do so could put the health of the American people at serious risk."[119]

GENETICALLY MODIFIED (GM) FOODS

It is not often that a single person can nearly shut down international trade in a food product as common and important as corn. In 2000, Larry Bohlen of the environmental group Friends of the Earth did just that. Suspecting that foods sold in the United States contained a genetically modified variety of corn, he bought corn chips, corn meal, corn flakes, and corn taco shells at a Safeway grocery store in Silver Spring, Maryland. Genetic lab tests confirmed that taco shells made by Kraft foods contained genetically modified corn, and on September 18, 2000, Bohlen and a coalition of groups opposed to genetically modified food announced the findings.[120]

Grocers soon pulled taco shells from their shelves, manufacturers recalled shipments of the products, and government officials tried to trace the source of the genetically modified corn. Giant food processors began to test shipments of corn it received for the presence of the genetic modifications and turned away rail cars filled with the product when tests were positive. Japan and European nations that had not approved the product threatened to embargo corn shipments. Farmers who grew the corn, and even those whose conventional corn was tainted by small amounts of the genetically modified brand, could not sell their harvest. About 50 million bushels of the corn throughout the Midwest had little use and sat on farms until Aventis, the biotechnology company that developed the corn, agreed to repurchase the worthless products. In the end, the developer of the corn suspended sales of its technology to seed companies.

Why the crisis? In short, the presence of this altered corn in the human food supply was unlawful. Some years earlier, the EPA had decided to give a split approval for this genetically modified crop. It declined to approve the genetically modified corn as safe for people and had insisted on rules to ensure that it did not enter the human food chain. It did allow the corn to be used as animal feed and transformed into ethanol for automobiles but required segregation of altered corn from conventional corn intended for human consumption. That the new corn ended up in human food did not shock critics, but it did demonstrate the failure to regulate genetically modified food.

The story of this genetically modified corn dates back to the early 1990s, when Aventis introduced a new corn product called StarLink that was resistant to insect damage. In studying bacteria that organic gardeners often used to protect their vegetables from insects, geneticists working for the company had isolated the gene for a protein that produced the natural insecticide. Using genetic-engineering techniques, the scientists spliced the protein gene (called Cry9C) from the bacteria and inserted it into the genes of corn. The genetically modified food crop, which would kill corn caterpillars but ideally not harm humans, might allow farmers to reduce the artificial pesticides they sprayed on their corn fields. The company petitioned the EPA, which has responsibility for pesticide safety, for approval of the product.

Although the EPA has approved other genetically modified foods, it had concerns about this one. Tests indicated that humans did not fully digest the Cry9C protein, and scientists worried that the undigested protein could cause allergic reactions. While not willing to risk human health, the EPA approved use of StarLink for animal feed and energy use. It required the company to have farmers grow, store, and sell the crop separately from other corn. The company in turn asked its distributors to explain this procedure and get signed statements from farmers that they would follow them.

In hindsight, the plan to segregate the corn appears naive. The company agreed to formal procedures required by the EPA but could not enforce the practices on the farms. Mistakes inevitably occurred: Distributors did not always explain the requirements, farmers did not always understand them, grain storage firms did not always know of the need for separation, and food processors did not always check the shipments they received for the altered corn. The EPA no longer allows the use of so-called split approvals. Any genetically modified food not approved for humans cannot be used for animals or other purposes.

Although all parties agree that the StarLink corn should not have been in human food, debate continues over whether the incident actually threatened food safety. When news about the Cry9C presence in taco shells came out, several diners concluded that the severe allergic reactions they had recently experienced came from eating the genetically modified food. Within 15 minutes of eating chicken enchiladas, Grace Booth of Oakland, California, experienced hotness, itchiness, and swelling. "I felt my chest getting tight, it was hard to breathe," she said.[121] An ambulance brought her to the hospital, where drugs moderated the allergenic shock, and she left the hospital soon after. In another case in Florida, Keith Finger experienced the same symptoms after a dinner of tortillas, rice, and beans. After hearing about the presence of traces of genetically modified corn in taco shells, the two notified the FDA about their allergic reactions.

Despite these and many other claims, scientists have not yet been able to demonstrate that reported allergic reactions actually resulted from the altered corn. The Centers for Disease Control and Prevention examined 51 persons who had suffered from allergic reactions soon after eating taco shells but found that the symptoms did not stem from StarLink corn.[122] Still, the debate continues over the safety of the product.

What Is Genetically Modified Food?

Given that no proven harm to humans has occurred from StarLink corn, the controversy over its entrance into the human food supply seems out of proportion. Why should farmers and businesses pay the enormous cost to remove a product that as yet appears harmless? The answer relates to the deeply held concerns about the safety of a new kind of food. Genetically modified (GM) or genetically engineered food comes from advances in biotechnology made in the last several decades that the public does not fully understand.

In the broadest sense, biotechnology can be defined as the application of biological knowledge and the use of live organisms to improve human life. This definition includes traditional forms of plant and animal breeding to create tastier food, hardier crops, and meatier cattle. However, the term has taken on a more common meaning today in regard to advances in the tools of genetic science. More narrowly, biotechnology involves methods to mod-

70

ify genetic materials of living cells to produce new substances and organisms. Genetic modification or engineering thus involves altering or transferring genes from one type of organism to another, and genetically modified or genetically engineered food involves the application of this process to plants and animals used for food. Sometimes the term *transgenic* is applied to a crop to indicate that it contains a gene transferred from another organism.

Biotechnology frightens many people. They worry about the creation and release of unknown and dangerous GM bacteria or the development of new and grotesque GM plants and animals. Critics used the term *frankenfood* to describe genetically modified food, implying that, like the creation of the Frankenstein monster, the product involves science gone to excess. And indeed, the creation of new organisms and food presents real and not fully understood risks. At the same time, however, biotechnology applied to food and other products has enormous potential for good.

The famous discovery of the double helix structure of DNA, the building blocks of genes, by James Watson and Francis Crick in 1953, revolutionized the understanding of cells and organisms. In the decades to follow, scientists not only deciphered the genetic code contained in DNA molecules but also learned how to change it. By the 1970s, they had developed technology to combine DNA from different organisms and by the 1980s, had begun testing genetically modified bacteria that could protect strawberries from frost damage. While the technology also led to DNA fingerprinting, cloning of animals (including pets), and genetic tests for diseases, it became particularly important for the development of new crops.

In 1994, the FDA approved the first genetically modified food, a tomato called Flavr Savr that did not spoil as quickly as conventional tomatoes. It could be allowed to ripen longer on the vine to fully develop its flavor and then be shipped and stored for longer periods without rotting. Although a new product, the food received approval without much evaluation. Two years earlier, the FDA had decided that GM foods did not require special regulations. The agency reasoned that GM crops did not differ all that much from crops such as hybrid corn that had been created in the past using cross-breeding techniques. Biotechnology allowed for more precision, speed, and control in creating new plant breeds than did traditional methods but otherwise did not change the essential nature of the food or present new problems of food safety. After all, both GM and conventional foods contained nearly all the same DNA and proteins. If tomatoes were generally considered as safe, then GM tomatoes would be as well.

The policy meant that GM foods would not have to undergo the same thorough testing as food additives. Rather, the FDA set up a voluntary process of consultation for companies wanting to market GM foods. The

FDA recommended that the GM food should look and taste the same as the conventional food, and have the same level of nutrients. It should also have no more toxins than conventional food, and any new protein contained in the food should be digestible. Otherwise, the FDA did not require tests of the long-term health effects on lab animals—agency officials reasoned that past history of safety for conventional foods applied as well to GM foods.

The policy also meant that GM foods would not require special labeling. As former FDA commissioner Jane E. Henney states, "We are not aware of any information that foods developed through genetic engineering differ as a class in quality, safety, or any other attribute from foods developed through conventional means. That's why there has been no requirement to add a special label saying that they are bioengineered."[123] There are some exceptions to the labeling policy. If a GM food causes allergies, the label would state that the product contains an allergen; or if genetic engineering produces a wholly new kind of food, the product would need to have a different name and special label. Otherwise, both traditional and bioengineered foods are subject to the same labeling requirements.

By the end of 1995, 35 applications to grow commercial GM crops had been approved. The market for the products looked promising, and companies hoped to profit from the billions of dollars they had invested in developing the new foods. However, the promise has been realized for only a few crops such as soybeans, corn, canola, and papayas. Otherwise, StarLink corn, Flavr Savr tomatoes, and GM potatoes have failed, and GM wheat, fruits, and vegetables have yet to reach the market or find success. As the director of the Pew Initiative on Food and Technology says, "Biotech crops have probably been the most rapidly-adopted agricultural technology in history. But the biotech revolution has stalled."[124]

How Common Are Genetically Modified Foods?

The United States leads the world in the production of GM crops. More than 7 million farmers worldwide have planted 167 million acres of GM products. Of that total, the United States grows 63 percent (with Argentina, Canada, Brazil, and China growing most of the remaining percentage).[125] GM crops are highly specialized, however. In 2004, 85 percent of soybeans and 45 percent of corn grown in the United States were genetically modified. About 54 percent of canola and 50 percent of papayas grown in the United States were genetically modified (although the acreage and amounts of these crops are small).

Despite the small number of GM crops, roughly 75 percent of processed foods on grocery shelves by some estimates contain genetically engineered ingredients.[126] Derivatives of GM soybeans may show up in bread, chocolate, cheese spread, vitamin E, tofu, soy sauce, chips, ice cream, fried foods, and enriched flour and pasta. Derivatives of GM corn may show up in corn syrup sweetener used in soft drinks, vitamin C, chips, salad dressings, cereals, margarine, and powdered sugar. Other foods are linked indirectly to GM products. Meat comes from cattle that are fed GM corn, and milk comes from cows that are given hormones derived from genetic engineering.

So far, GM foods have largely benefited farmers and companies rather than consumers. The resistance of StarLink corn to insect damage allowed farmers to use less pesticide and get higher yields than with conventional corn. The long shelf life of Flavr Savr tomatoes allowed companies to harvest the products later and groceries to store products longer. GM canola and soybean crops produce oils and fatty acids that are better suited to food processing. Roundup Ready, a GM soybean that is resistant to herbicides, allows farmers to use herbicides to kill weeds without harming the crops. None of these products improve the taste, safety, or wholesomeness of food but could benefit consumers by reducing the cost of products they buy.

To appeal more to consumers, the next generation of GM foods will likely have improved nutritional value. Genetic engineering may be used to add ingredients, flavors, and vitamins to foods that make them healthier and better tasting to consumers. Examples include strains of GM rice with greater levels of iron or vitamin A, GM tomatoes with higher levels of antioxidants, GM fruits and vegetables with higher levels of vitamin C and E, GM strawberries with increased levels of a potential cancer-fighting agent, and GM garlic cloves with increased levels of a cholesterol-lowering agent. Such advances could contribute to wider use of GM crops and greater sales to consumers.

In the meantime, consumers seldom know about the presence of GM ingredients in their food. If they knew more, it likely would reduce sales, as many people say they are opposed to the product. In a September 2004 poll, about 30 percent of respondents said GM foods are basically safe, while 27 percent said they are basically unsafe.[127] The survey found that most are unaware of the presence of GM products in the food supply and are willing to change their opinions given new information. That could produce changes in either direction: A scandal could harden attitudes against this food, while education and research could increase their favor.

Consumers in European nations oppose GM foods more strongly than they do in the United States. From 1998 to 2002, the European Union informally blocked the import of new varieties of GM foods until they could establish a new approval process. More recently they approved a few such foods, but European consumers remain wary of the products. Policies require clear labels and the ability to trace the origins of food shipped from the United States. American farmers view these rules as a way to limit competition, and U.S. officials have filed protests over the rules with the World Trade Organization. Yet attitudes about food technology in Europe remain negative enough to prevent a large market for GM foods from developing.

Health Risks of GM Foods

Critics of GM foods in the United States favor the European go-slow approach. They reject the FDA conclusion that GM foods do not differ substantially from natural foods and complain bitterly that this premature conclusion has stopped full tests of the safety of the products. They can point to only a few studies to support their concerns about the health risks of GM foods, but they express their views with strong conviction.

One proven threat to food safety from genetic engineering came from inserting genes from Brazil nuts into soybean genes. The idea behind this product was to make soybeans a more nutritious animal feed by increasing the level of a protein found in Brazil nuts. However, independent researchers discovered that the GM soybeans, should they get into the human food supply, might cause fatal reactions in humans who are allergic to Brazil nuts. The product was withdrawn from the market, but other GM foods may also produce unexpected allergies. Reported increases of reactions to soybeans, a food not traditionally a major source of allergies, may come from GM versions of the product.

More suggestive studies indicate other risks of GM foods, although they have provoked more controversy than consensus. A Scottish researcher, Dr. Arpad Pusztai, found that a GM potato developed to be resistant to pests was also poisonous to lab rats. Substances in the GM potatoes apparently damaged the organs and immune systems of the animals. The results of this study go beyond the particular GM potato that underwent testing but reflect risks inherent in all GM products. Although many scientists dismiss the study as based on flawed methods, the findings may indicate that GM products thought not to differ from conventional products can have unexpected and dangerous health consequences. The same problem found in the potatoes could affect many other GM crops.

Other claims, although more speculation than demonstrated fact, point to the indirect harm of GM foods on health. Crops genetically engineered to be resistant to herbicide allow farmers to use higher levels of artificial chemicals to kill surrounding weeds, but they can also leave greater residues of toxic chemicals on foods. GM-produced bovine growth hormone used in cows can cause chemical changes in the milk that may promote cancer in humans. And genetic engineering of animal feeds might contribute to the development of antibiotic-resistant bacteria in animals. Although unproven, these claims sound worrisome.

Introduction to Threats to Food Safety

Proof of major harm from GM foods has not emerged yet, but opponents believe such a result is inevitable. The only reason evidence of harm has not yet emerged, they say, is that the FDA and biotech companies have avoided the thorough testing required for other new food products. One critic of genetic engineering states the risks: "Without detailed, ongoing analyses, there is no way of knowing if hazardous consequences might arise . . . The genetically engineered crops now being grown represent a massive uncontrolled experiment whose outcome is inherently unpredictable. The results could be catastrophic."[128]

The real concern about genetic engineering, as reflected in this quote, is the unpredictability of the process. Scientists can never know exactly what type of new products will emerge from gene splicing. Many worry that the complexity of genetic materials and the efforts to combine genes from completely different types of organisms—such as bacteria and corn or tree nuts and soybeans—make the creation of new, dangerous, and little-understood substances not only possible but likely. For example, genes might get scrambled during the splicing process in ways that create new toxins, or inactive genes might get activated in ways that promote cancerous growth. Since no one can know for certain what consequences these products will have for health, opponents believe genetic engineering represents a serious threat to food safety, one that should lead the government to proceed more carefully.

Distortions and Lies

Given their convictions about the dangers of GM foods, critics strongly dispute FDA and business claims of safety. Some even say that claims of safety are part of a conspiracy to keep the public from getting the knowledge they should. Frances Moore Lappé, a famous author and advocate of vegetarianism, makes the case bluntly in stating that a handful of corporations "has used its enormous wealth, as well as intimidation and deception, to turn Americans into nutritional guinea pigs [and] forced without our knowledge . . . to consume staple foods that have been virtually untested as to their effects on our health."[129] In speaking of business goals of opening markets to GM food, author Jeffrey Smith states that "Just as the magnitude of the industry's plan was breathtaking, so too are the distortions and cover-ups."[130]

The distortions flow, according to those most opposed to GM foods, from efforts of companies to convince the public that they are helping to solve world problems when, in fact, they want only to increase their profits, size, and power. Companies claim that GM foods will end world hunger by allowing poor countries to grow more crops, but surplus food already exists—the problem is that poor countries do not get their share. Companies claim that GM foods will reduce pesticide use but could instead contribute

75

to the emergence of new pests. Companies claim that GM foods are safe but few studies have been conducted to demonstrate this safety.

The main villain in the eyes of critics, the company that has done the most in the United States to develop and promote GM foods, is the Monsanto Company, with headquarters in St. Louis. Monsanto makes Roundup Ready, a soybean product that is resistant to its herbicide Roundup, which farmers can use on weeds without harming the soybean crop. With that and other products it owns, many obtained through the purchase of smaller biotechnology firms, the company has become the world leader in the genetic engineering of food. It has pushed hard to promote GM foods, aiming to replace rather than merely supplement conventional crops. In so doing, its scientists have made some remarkable technological achievements, even receiving an award from former U.S. President Bill Clinton. At the same time, however, the company has received "an extraordinary barrage of skepticism, criticism, and outright condemnation."[131] Critics condemn the company for putting profits before safety and using its power to mislead the public about the potential harm of GM products.

The government, particularly the FDA, is seen by opponents as a willing accomplice in deceptions about GM foods. While pesticides and food additives go through a review process that allows for public comment and review of documents, no such process exists for GM foods. To the contrary, reviews occur through a voluntary consultation between the company and the FDA. The companies present data on the safety of GM foods and must be prepared to defend their results if sued. Otherwise, the FDA does not check the data, and the public does not participate in the consultation or have knowledge of the evidence—the FDA publishes only a summary of the manufacturer's evidence that the GM foods are as safe as conventional foods. Many demand that the FDA do more to evaluate independently the safety of GM foods and be given the power to prevent the planting of GM crops or the selling of GM foods.

Why is such a review not required by the government? The answer according to critics is the power and money of agricultural technology firms. Companies can afford to spend money on advertising and public relations to convince the public of the benefits of GM foods. They can also afford to spend money on legal action. Monsanto, a major advertiser on television and radio, can threaten action against stations planning to present negative stories on GM foods. Rather than present the risks of GM foods to the public, the media repeats the public relations statements of GM companies. The companies also have undue political influence, according to those opponents of GM foods. They contribute heavily to political campaigns and spend millions of dollars lobbying the government in favor of GM foods and against regulations.

Defenders of GM foods obviously reject the way opponents portray their activities. Monsanto, for example, presents its goals in a much more positive light: The company's web page lists as its mission the praiseworthy goals of developing products and solutions to meet the world's growing food needs, conserve natural resources, and improve the environment. The web page of the Biotechnology Industry Organization similarly disputes the myths that it believes GM opponents spread. Are GM foods safe to eat? Yes, defenders say. Not a single person has become sick from GM foods. Are GM foods tested? Again they say yes. Companies spend millions to test GM crops before they are brought to market. Are GM foods as nutritious as conventional foods? Yes, they are essentially the same. Respected research organizations such as the National Academy of Sciences and the British Medical Association have said as much.

If critics point to the Monsanto Company as a villain, supporters do the same with Jeremy Rifkin, an author and director of the Foundation on Economic Trends. Highly critical of the risks brought on by biotechnology, Rifkin has fought against GM products in Europe as well as in the United States. More successful in Europe, he helped persuade leaders to hold off further approval of GM crops until a better system of assessment could be established. In the United States, he filed a class-action suit against Monsanto in 1999 for, among other things, misleading farmers and selling an unsafe product. His persistent and highly publicized battle angers scientists who favor GM foods. One Monsanto scientist says of Rifkin, "He says genetic engineering is going to destroy the world; in fact, Jeremy Rifkin is going to destroy the world."[132]

The battle remains heated. Opponents disagree not only on the possible harm of GM foods but also on the tactics each side uses to present its case. Some say that the extreme positions have prevented reasoned and responsible debate. With one side claiming that GM foods are a completely safe solution to world food problems and the other side claiming that GM foods will result in a catastrophe, it can be hard to evaluate more specific benefits and risks. A more careful conclusion notes that GM foods have not yet caused serious health problems, but the potential for problems in the future remains.

RISKS OF TECHNOLOGY FOR FOOD SAFETY

Food irradiation and GM foods have so far done little to make food less safe—to the contrary, they have in some ways improved food safety. Since demonstrated harm to health of humans has not yet emerged, continued improvement and use of the technologies may make sense.

However, critics are less concerned about what has happened so far as they are about what could happen in the future. They ask the "what if" question: What if scientists discover something bad 20 years from now, something wholly unexpected and unstudied?[133] Compared to threats to food safety involving foodborne disease, threats to safety from technology right now are minimal. Still, they could become very serious in the future.

THE FUTURE OF FOOD SAFETY

Concerns about food safety will almost certainly expand in the decades to come. The risks of dying from foodborne infection, mad cow disease, terrorist contamination, cancer-causing additives, food allergies, and unknown food properties from genetic engineering and irradiation remain small relative to the major causes of death—heart disease, smoking-caused cancers, accidents, violence, and diseases common in old age. Still, the threats to food safety will take on added importance in the future. This claim follows from the idea that the better the health of members of a society, the more they concern themselves with smaller risks. Given healthier living, improved medical care, growing life expectancy, and declining deaths from heart diseases, deaths from diseases contained in food or perhaps associated with food additives become all the more tragic.

With the increased concern about the risks of food-based disease, spending on organic food has grown faster in the last decades than other parts of the food industry. According to recent reports, 43 percent of consumers say they buy organic foods, and organic sales have risen about 20 percent a year since 1997.[134] These products have become mainstream items, now widely available in traditional grocery stores as well as in natural grocery stores and local farmers' markets. Consumers wanting to stress food safety through purchase of organic products now have many options, and the trend in organic sales will no doubt continue.

The popularity of organic foods has led the government to clarify the meaning of the term. Since 2002, the National Standards Board of the USDA has required that foods using its organic label meet several agriculture requirements: They must be grown or raised without using sewer sludge fertilizer, most chemical fertilizers, synthetic pesticides, nonorganic animal feed, growth hormones, antibiotics in feed, genetically engineered organisms, and irradiation. Farms selling organic products worth more than $5,000 must gain certification from government-approved inspections to use the organic label. Foods with 70–94 percent organic ingredients can say they are "made with organic ingredients" but do not get to use the organic label. Natural foods typically do not include artificial additives but need not use organically grown ingredients and do not get to use the USDA label.

Even with a strict definition, organic foods cannot guarantee safety. Studies have found that organic foods have lower levels of pesticides than conventional foods but are not pesticide-free.[135] Organic foods also contain bacteria, although controversy exists over whether levels are lower than in conventional food. According to some critics, organic foods can be more dangerous than conventional food. They rely on fertilizers such as manure that, if not used properly, can spread dangerous bacteria to crops, and they fail to use fungicides that stop the growth of molds with dangerous toxins. Critics further dispute claims that organic food tastes better than conventional food (although organic food may have a flavor advantage since it tends to be eaten fresher than conventional food).

If the science can demonstrate only modest benefits of organic foods, this does not deter consumers, who nonetheless believe organic foods taste better and are healthier. They continue to buy organic food despite higher prices and claims of critics that the extra cost brings little benefit. As income rises in the future with economic growth, households will no doubt use more of their disposable income for food safety and willingly pay the higher prices of organic foods.

Media publicity may further generate interest among the public in organic foods. In 1989, the widely viewed television show *60 Minutes* presented a segment on the dangers of a chemical called Alar that when sprayed on apples helps them ripen on the tree. The show, which used information contained in a report from the Natural Resources Defense Council, claimed that high levels of Alar in apple juice could cause cancer. The claims gained enormous publicity. One famous parent, actress Meryl Streep, announced her intention to help keep children from eating apples or drinking juice and testified before Congress in opposition to Alar. Although scientific studies had been unable to clearly identify the harm of Alar, growers stopped using the chemical in response to the public outcry.

Now over 15 years old, this incident illustrates the power of media information for food safety concerns. Since then, consumer health groups have publicized studies and claims about the dangers of conventional food and the benefits of organic food, while the food industry and free-market advocates have criticized the studies and claims as unscientific and unproven. Government agencies investigate claims on both sides but cannot settle the debates. The attention paid to media reports and the effectiveness of consumer organizations in using the media to publicize its claims suggest the continued importance of this source of information about food-safety threats.

---

[1] Paul S. Mead, Laurence Slutsker, Vance Dietz, Linda F. McCaig, Joseph S. Bresee, Craig Shapiro, Patricia M. Griffin, and Robert V. Tauxe, "Food-Related Illness and Death in the United States," *Emerging Infections Diseases*, vol. 5, no. 5, September–October 1999, pp. 607–625. Available online. URL: http://www.cdc.gov/ncidod/eid/vol5no5/mead.htm. Downloaded in November 2004.

[2] Nancy Donley, Alex Thomas Donley," S.T.O.P.: Safe Tables Our Priority. Available online. URL: http://www.safetables.org/Victim_Support/stories/donley_alex.html. Downloaded in December 2004.

3 Linda Deasley, "Jimmy Deasley," S.T.O.P.: Safe Tables Our Priority. Available online. URL: http://www.safetables.org/Victim_Support/stories/deasley_jimmy. html. Downloaded in December 2004.

4 "Economics of Foodborne Disease," U.S. Department of Agriculture, Economic Research Service. Available online. URL: http://www.ers.usda.gov/briefing/ FoodborneDisease/features.htm. Downloaded in December 2004.

5 "The Most Dangerous Women in America," NOVA Science Programming On Air and Online. Available online. URL: http://www.pbs.org/wgbh/nova/typhoid/ about.html. Downloaded in December 2004.

6 Marion Nestle, *Safe Food: Bacteria, Biotechnology, and Bioterrorism.* Berkeley: University of California Press, 2003, pp. 66–67.

7 B. P. Bell, M. Goldoft, P. M. Griffin, M. A. Davis, D. C. Gordon, P. I. Tarr, C. A. Bartleson, J. H. Lewis, T. J. Barrett, J. G. Wells, et al., "A Multistate Outbreak of *Escherichia Coli* O157:H7—Associated Bloody Diarrhea and Hemolytic Uremic Syndrome from Hamburgers: The Washington Experience," *JAMA*, vol. 272, no. 17, November 2, 1994, pp. 1,349–1,353. Available online. URL: http://jama.ama-assn.org/cgi/content/abstract/272/17/1349. Downloaded in December 2004.

8 Pam Bellcuk, "Juice-Poisoning Case Brings Guilty Plea and a Huge Fine," *New York Times*, July 24, 1998, p. A12.

9 Elinor Levy and Mark Fischetti, *The New Killer Diseases: How the Alarming Evolution of Mutant Germs Threatens Us All.* New York: Crown Publishers, 2003, pp. 153–154.

10 Levy and Fischetti, *The New Killer Diseases*, p. 155.

11 "FoodNet—Foodborne Diseases Active Surveillance Network," Centers for Disease Control and Prevention. Available online. URL: http://www.cdc. gov/foodnet. Updated on June 23, 2003.

12 Nichols Fox, *It Was Probably Something You Ate: A Practical Guide to Avoiding and Surviving Foodborne Illness.* New York: Penguin Books, 1999, p. 66.

13 F. Y. Lin, J. G. Morris, Jr., D. Trump, D. Tilghman, P. K. Wood. N. Jackman, E. Israel, and J. P. Libonati, "Investigation of an Outbreak of *Salmonella* Enteritidis Gastroenteritis Associated with Consumption of Eggs in a Restaurant Chain in Maryland," *American Journal of Epidemiology*, vol. 128, no. 4, October 1988, p. 839.

14 Anthony E. Fiore, "Hepatitis A Transmitted by Food," *Food Safety*, vol. 38, no. 1, March 2004, pp. 705–715. Available online. URL: http://www.cdc.gov/ncidod/ diseases/hepatitis/a/fiore_ha_transmitted_by_food. pdf. Downloaded in December 2004.

15 Mead, et al., "Food-Related Illness and Death in the United States," pp. 607–625.

16 Nestle, *Safe Food*, p. 38.

17 Paul D. Frenzen, "Deaths Due to Unknown Foodborne Agents," *Emerging Infectious Diseases*, vol. 10, no. 9, September 2004, pp. 1,536–1,543. Available online. URL: http://www.cdc.gov/ncidod/EID/vol10no9/03-0403.htm#1. Downloaded in December 2004.

[18] Nestle, *Safe Food*, p. 36.

[19] "Preliminary FoodNet Data on the Incidence of Foodborne Illnesses—Selected Sites, United States, 2002," *MMWR Weekly*, vol. 52, no. 15, April 18, 2003, pp. 340–343. Available online. URL: http://www.cdc.gov/mmwr/preview/mmwrhtml/mm5215a4.htm. Downloaded in December 2004.

[20] Morton Satin, *Food Alert! The Ultimate Sourcebook for Food Safety*. New York: Facts On File, 1999, pp. 43–45.

[21] Satin, *Food Alert!* p. 43.

[22] "Antibiotic Use in Food Animals Contributes to Microbe Resistance," The National Academies News. Available online. URL: http://www4.nationalacademies.org/news.nsf/isbn/0309054346?OpenDocument. Posted on July 9, 1998.

[23] Sherwood L. Gorbach, "Antimicrobial Use in Animal Feed—Time to Stop," *New England Journal of Medicine*, vol. 345, no. 16, October 18, 2001, pp. 1,202–1,203.

[24] "Top Ten Fast Food Chains: How Clean Are They?" *Dateline NBC*. Available online. URL: http://www.msnbc.msn.com/id/7150482. Updated on March 11, 2005.

[25] "Fight Bac: Keep Food Safe from Bacteria," Partnership for Food Safety Education online. Available online. URL: http://www.fightbac.org/main.cfm. Downloaded in December 2004.

[26] "Microbiological Results of Raw Ground Beef Products Analyzed for *Escherichia coli* O157:H7," U.S. Department of Agriculture, Food Safety and Inspection Service. Available online. URL: http://www.fsis.usda.gov/Science/Ground_Beef_E.Coli_Testing_Results/index.asp. Downloaded in December 2004.

[27] "FDA Backgrounder: HACCP A State-of-the-Art Approach to Food Safety," Food and Drug Administration. Available online. URL: http://www.cfsan.fda.gov/~lrd/bghaccp. html. Posted in October 2003.

[28] "Interview: Patrick Boyle," *Frontline:* "Modern Meat." Available online. URL: http://www.pbs.org/wgbh/pages/frontline/shows/meat/interviews/boyle.html. Downloaded in December 2004.

[29] Eric Schlosser, "Bad Meat: The Scandal of Our Food Safety System," *The Nation*, vol. 275, no. 8, September 16, 2002, pp. 6–7.

[30] Philip Yam, *The Pathological Protein: Mad Cow, Chronic Wasting, and Other Deadly Prion Diseases*. New York: Copernicus Books, 2003, pp. 13–14.

[31] Richard Rhodes, *Deadly Feasts: The "Prion" Controversy and the Public's Health*. New York: Touchstone, 1998, p. 50.

[32] "Creutzfeldt-Jacob Disease," The Free Dictionary.com. Available online. URL: http://encyclopedia.thefreedictionary.com/Creutzfeldt-Jacob%20Disease. Downloaded in December 2004.

[33] Yam, *The Pathological Protein*, p. 107.

[34] Rhodes, *Deadly Feasts*, pp. 171–172.

[35] Yam, *The Pathological Protein*, p. 111.

[36] Andrew Rowell, *Don't Worry, It's Safe to Eat: The True Story of GM Food, BSE, and Foot and Mouth*. London: Earthscan Publications, 2003, p. 16.

37 "BSE 'Old Meat' Ban May End." BBC News Online. Available online. URL: http://news.bbc.co.uk/1/hi/uk/3050270.stm. Posted on July 7, 2003.

38 Douglas Powell, "Mad Cow Disease and the Stigmatization of British Beef," in James Flynn, Paul Slovic, and Howard Kunreuther, eds., *Risk, Media, and Stigma: Understanding Public Challenges to Modern Science and Technology.* London: Earthscan Publications, 2001, p. 222.

39 Patrick van Zwanenberg and Erik Millstone, "'Mad Cow Disease' 1980s–2000: How Reassurances Undermined Precaution," in Poul Harremoâes, David Gee, Malcolm MacGarvin, Andy Stirling, Jane Keys, Brian Wynne, and Sofia Guedes Vaz, eds., *The Precautionary Principle in the 20th Century: Late Lessons from Early Warnings.* London: Earthscan Publications, 2002, p. 173.

40 Yam, *The Pathological Protein*, p. 121.

41 Rhodes, *Deadly Feasts*, pp. 211–212.

42 "Probable Variant Creutzfeldt-Jakob Disease in a U.S. Resident—Florida, 2002," *MMWR Weekly*, vol. 51, no. 41, October 18, 2002, pp. 927–929. Available online. URL: http://www.cdc.gov/mmwr/preview/mmwrhtml/mm5141a3.htm. Downloaded in December 2004.

43 Powell, "Mad Cow Disease and the Stigmatization of British Beef," p. 222.

44 Andrew F. Hill, Melanie Desbruslais, Susan Joiner, Katie C. L. Sidle, Ian Gowland, John Collinge, Lawrence J. Doey, and Peter Lantos, "The Same Prion Strain Causes vCJD and BSE," *Nature*, vol. 389, no. 6650, October 2, 1997, pp. 448–450.

45 "Questions and Answers Regarding Bovine Spongiform Encephalopathy (BSE) and Creutzfeldt-Jakob Disease (CJD)," CDC National Center for Infectious Diseases: Bovine Spongiform Encephalopathy and Creutzfeldt-Jakob Disease. Available online. URL: http://www.cdc.gov/ncidod/diseases/cjd/bse_cjd_qa.htm. Updated on December 29, 2003.

46 Yam, *The Pathological Protein*, pp. 139–140.

47 "Probable Variant Creutzfeldt-Jakob Disease in a U.S. Resident," *MMWR Weekly*, pp. 927–929.

48 Sheila Rule, "Fatal Cow Illness Stirs British Fear," *New York Times*, May 20, 1990, p. A14.

49 "Oprah's Report on Mad Cow Disease," Show Transcript. Available online. URL: http://www.mcspotlight.org/media/television/oprah_transcript.html. Posted on April 15, 1996.

50 Sam Howe, "Talk of the Town: Burgers v. Oprah," *New York Times*, January 21, 1998, p. A10; "Jury Selection to Begin in Cattlemen's Suit against Oprah," CNN Interactive. Available online. URL: http://www.cnn.com/US/9801/20/oprah.beef. Posted on January 20, 1998.

51 Sam Howe, "Turf Was Cattlemen's, But Jury Was Winfrey's," *New York Times*, February 27, 1998, p. A10.

52 Matthew L. Wald and Eric Lichtblau, "U.S. Is Examining a Mad Cow Case, First in Country," *New York Times*, December 24, 2003, p. A1.

[53] Anne Veneman, "Statement," in *To Examine the Current Situation Regarding the Discovery of a Case of Bovine Spongiform Encephalopathy in a Dairy Cow in Washington State as It Relates to Food Safety, Livestock Marketing and International Trade. Hearing before the Committee on Agriculture, Nutrition, and Forestry, United States Senate, One Hundred Eighth Congress, Second Session.* Washington, D.C.: U.S. Government Printing Office, January 27, 2005, p. 19.

[54] Veneman, "Statement," p. 20.

[55] U.S. General Accounting Office, *Mad Cow Disease: Improvements in the Animal Feed Ban and Other Regulatory Areas Would Strengthen U.S. Prevention Efforts: Report to Congressional Requesters.* Washington, D.C.: U.S. General Accounting Office, 2002, p. 32. Available online. URL: http://www.gao.gov/new.items/d02183. pdf. Downloaded in November 2004.

[56] Lester M. Crawford, "Statement," in *To Examine the Current Situation Regarding the Discovery of a Case of Bovine Spongiform Encephalopathy in a Dairy Cow in Washington State as It Relates to Food Safety, Livestock Marketing and International Trade*, p. 23.

[57] Thad Cochran, "Statement," in *To Examine the Current Situation Regarding the Discovery of a Case of Bovine Spongiform Encephalopathy in a Dairy Cow in Washington State as It Relates to Food Safety, Livestock Marketing and International Trade*, p. 59.

[58] "BSE Test Results," USDA's BSE Testing. Available online. URL: http://www. aphis.usda.gov/lpa/issues/bse_testing/test_results.html. Downloaded in November 2004.

[59] Abigail Trafford, "Cow Madness Is Overblown," *Washington Post*, February 13, 2001, p. HE8. Available online. URL: http://www.washingtonpost.com/ac2/wp-dyn/A51502- 2001Feb9. Downloaded in April 2005.

[60] Linda Bren, "FDA Continues Work to Help Prevent Mad Cow Disease," *FDA Consumer*, vol. 35, no. 3, May–June 2002, pp. 31–32. Available online. URL: http://www.fda.gov/fdac/features/2002/302_bse.html. Downloaded in December 2004.

[61] "Mad Cow Disease," Center for Food Safety. Available online. URL: http://www. centerforfoodsafety.org/mad_cow_di3.cfm. Downloaded in December 2004.

[62] "New Rules Require Better Food Records," CNN.com. Available online. URL: http://blog.lib.umn.edu/archives/gruwell/publichealthliaison/012117.html. Posted on December 7, 2004.

[63] "Risk Assessment for Food Terrorism and Other Food Safety Concerns," U.S. Food and Drug Administration, Center for Food Safety and Applied Nutrition. Available online. URL: http://vm.cfsan.fda.gov/~dms/rabtact.html. Posted on October 13, 2003.

[64] "Risk Assessment for Food Terrorism and Other Food Safety Concerns," U.S. Food and Drug Administration; Jason Pate and Gavin Cameron, "Covert Biological Weapons Attacks against Agricultural Targets: Assessing the Impact against U.S. Agriculture," in Arnold M. Howitt and Robyn L. Pangi, eds., *Countering Terrorism: Dimensions of Preparedness.* Cambridge: MIT Press, 2003, p. 200.

[65] Pate and Cameron, "Covert Biological Weapons Attacks against Agricultural Targets," p. 200.

[66] Rocco Casagrande, "Biological Terrorism Targeted at Agriculture: The Threat to National Security," *The Nonproliferation Review*, vol. 7, no. 3, Fall/Winter 2000, p. 100.

[67] "Risk Assessment for Food Terrorism and Other Food Safety Concerns," U.S. Food and Drug Administration.

[68] Nicholas J. Neher, "The Need for a Coordinated Response to Food Terrorism: The Wisconsin Experience," *Annals of the New York Academy of Sciences*, vol. 894, 1999, pp. 181–183.

[69] "Epidemiologic Notes and Reports Aldicarb Food Poisoning from Contaminated Melons—California," *MMWR Weekly*, vol. 35, no. 16, April 25, 1986, pp. 254–258. Available online. URL: http://www.cdc.gov/mmwr/preview/mmwrhtml/00000721. htm. Downloaded in April 2005.

[70] "Food Poisoning Outbreaks Hit Hard Nationwide," CNN.com. Available online. URL: http://www.cnn.com/HEALTH/9807/10/summer.bad.food. Posted on July 10, 1998.

[71] "Risk Assessment for Food Terrorism and Other Food Safety Concerns," U.S. Food and Drug Administration.

[72] Thomas W. Hennessy, Craig W. Hedberg, Laurence Slutsker, Karen E. White, John M. Besser-Wiek, Michael E. Moen, John Feldman, William W. Coleman, Larry M. Edmonson, Kristine L. MacDonald, and Michael T. Osterholm, "A National Outbreak of *Salmonella Enteritidis* Infections from Ice Cream," *New England Journal of Medicine*, vol. 334, no. 20, May 16, 1996, pp. 1,281–1,286. Available online. URL: http://content.nejm.org/cgi/content/abstract/334/20/1281. Downloaded in December 2004.

[73] Peter Mann, "Why Homeland Security Must Include Food Security," Community Food Security Coalition. Available online. URL: http://www.foodsecurity. org/homeland_security.html. Downloaded in December 2004.

[74] "Risk Assessment for Food Terrorism and Other Food Safety Concerns," U.S. Food and Drug Administration.

[75] "Death Sentence over Chinese Poisonings," CNN.com/World. Available online. URL: http://archives.cnn.com/2002/WORLD/asiapcf/east/09/30/china.poison. Posted on September 30, 2002.

[76] James Risen and Don Van Natta, Jr."Plot to Poison Food of British Troops Is Suspected," *New York Times*, January. 24, 2003, p. A1.

[77] Peter Chalk, *Terrorism, Infrastructure Protection, and the U.S. Food and Agriculture Sector.* Santa Monica, Calif.: Rand Corporation, 2001, pp. 5–6.

[78] Pate and Cameron, "Covert Biological Weapons Attacks against Agricultural Targets," pp. 209–210.

[79] Danile G. Dupont, "Food Fears: The Threat of Agricultural Terrorism Spurs Calls for More Vigilance," ScientificAmerican.com. Available online. URL:

http://www.sciam.com/article.cfm?articleID=000D7192-62D3-1F6A-905980A84189EEDF. Posted on September 22, 2003.

[80] Mark B. McClellan, "Statement," in *Federal Biodefense Readiness, Hearing of the Committee on Health, Education, Labor, and Pensions, United States Senate, One Hundred Eighth Congress, First Session*. Washington, D.C.: U.S. Government Printing Office, July 24, 2003, p. 19.

[81] Carol Lewis, "The 'Poison Squad' and the Advent of Food and Drug Regulation," FDA *Consumer*, vol. 36, no. 6, 2002, pp. 12–15. Available online. URL: http://www.fda.gov/fdac/602_toc.html. Downloaded in December 2004.

[82] "FDA Backgrounder: Milestones in U.S. Food and Drug Law History," U.S. Food and Drug Administration. Available online. URL:http://www.fda.gov/opacom/backgrounders/miles.html. Updated on August 5, 2002.

[83] Donna U. Vogt, "Food Additive Regulations: A Chronology," CRS Report for Congress. Available online. URL:http://www.ncseonline.org/NLE/CRSreports/Pesticides/pest-5.cfm?&CFID=18010170&CFTOKEN=72878622. Updated on September 13, 1995.

[84] Beatrice Trum Hunter, "What is GRAS?" *Consumers' Research Magazine*, vol. 86, no. 6, June 2003, pp. 8–9.

[85] Some products such as container materials that migrate in small amounts into food can be used with notification to the FDA rather than prior approval.

[86] Vogt, "Food Additive Regulations: A Chronology."

[87] Sheila Globus, "Pros and Cons of Food Additives," *Current Health 2*, vol. 28, no. 2, October 2001, pp. 17–19.

[88] "CSPI's Guide to Food Additives," Food Safety Food Additives. Available online. URL: http://www.cspinet.org/reports/chemcuisine.htm. Downloaded in December 2004.

[89] Suzette J. Middleton, "Procter and Gamble Responds on Olestra," *Public Health Reports*, vol. 114, no. 1, January–February 1999, pp. 5–6.

[90] Marion Nestle, "The Selling of Olestra," *Public Health Reports*, vol. 113, no. 6, November–December 1998, pp. 508–520.

[91] Nestle, "The Selling of Olestra," pp. 508–520.

[92] "Background on Agriculture and Food Production," International Food Information Council: Agriculture and Food Production. Available online. URL: http://ific.org/food/agriculture/index.cfm. Posted in May 2004.

[93] "A Consumer's Guide to Pesticides and Food Safety," International Food Information Council: Educational Booklets and Brochures. Available online. URL: http://ific.org/publications/brochures/pesticidebroch.cfm. Posted in November 1995.

[94] "Pesticides," National Institute of Environmental Health Sciences. Available online. URL: http://www.niehs.nih.gov/external/faq/pest.htm. Downloaded in December 2004.

[95] "A Consumer's Guide to Pesticides and Food Safety," International Food Information Council.

[96] "Pesticides," National Institute of Environmental Health Sciences.

[97] P. Cabras, "Pesticides: Toxicology and Residues in Food," in J. P. F. D'Mello, ed., *Food Safety: Contaminants and Toxins.* Cambridge, Mass.: CABI Publishing, 2003, p. 123.

[98] "How Safe Is Our Produce?" *Consumer Reports,* vol. 64, no. 3, March 1999, pp. 28–31.

[99] "Organic. It's Lower in Pesticides. Honest." *Consumer Reports,* vol. 67, no. 8, August 2002, p. 6.

[100] Frances B. Smith, "Eat Your Fruits and Vegetables," Consumer Alert: Commonsense Consumer Column. Available online. URL: http://www.consumeralert.org/pubs/commonsense/Mar99Pest.htm. Posted in March 1999.

[101] "rBGH/Hormones," Center for Food Safety. Available online. URL: http://www.centerforfoodsafety.org/rbgh_hormo.cfm. Downloaded in December 2004.

[102] "Consumer Concerns about Hormones in Food," Cornell University Program on Breast Cancer and Environmental Risk Factors in New York State Fact Sheet. Available online. URL: http://envirocancer.cornell.edu/FactSheet/Diet/fs37.hormones.pdf. Posted in June 2000.

[103] Bruce N. Ames, Renae Magaw, and Lois Swirsky Gold, "Ranking Possible Carcinogenic Hazards," *Science,* vol. 236, no. 4799, April 17, 1987, pp. 271–280.

[104] David Schardt, "Food Allergies," Nutrition Action Healthletter. Available online. URL: http://www.cspinet.org/nah/04_01. Posted in April 2001.

[105] Ray Formanek, Jr., "Food Allergies: When Food Becomes the Enemy," *FDA Consumer,* vol. 35, no. 4, July–August 2001, pp. 10–16. Available online. URL: http://www.fda.gov/fdac/401_toc.html. Updated in April 2004. The percentages are, however, higher when including other types of food sensitivities.

[106] "Allergy Statistics." National Institute of Allergy and Infectious Disease Facts and Figures. Available online. URL: http://www.niaid.nih.gov/factsheets/allergystat.htm. Posted in December 2004.

[107] Schardt, "Food Allergies."

[108] "What Are Food Allergies and Why Do We Have Them?" Food-Allergy.org. Available online. URL: http://www.food-allergy.org/page1.html. Downloaded in December 2004.

[109] Schardt, "Food Allergies."

[110] "Food Allergy," American Academy of Allergy, Asthma, and Immunology, Patient/Public Education: Fast Facts. Available online. URL: http://www.aaaai.org/patients/resources/fastfacts/food_allergy.stm. Downloaded in December 2004.

[111] Robin Brett Parnes, William C. Idell, and Audrey L. Anastasia Kanik, "Food Irradiation: An Overlooked Opportunity for Food Safety and Preservation," *Nutrition Today,* vol. 38, no. 5, September/October 2003, pp. 174–185.

[112] "Food Irradiation: A Safe Measure," U.S. Food and Drug Administration. Available online. URL: http://www.fda.gov/opacom/catalog/irradbro.html. Posted in January 2000.

[113] "Frequently Asked Questions about Food Irradiation," Centers for Disease Control and Prevention. Available online. URL: http://www.cdc.gov/ncidod/dbmd/diseaseinfo/foodirradiation.htm. Updated on September 29, 1999.

[114] Robert V. Tauxe, "Food Safety and Irradiation: Protecting the Public from Foodborne Infections." *Emerging Infectious Diseases*, vol. 7, no. 3, Supplement, June 2001, pp. 516–521. Available online. URL: http://www.cdc.gov/ncidod/eid/vol7 no3_supp/tauxe.htm. Updated on April 21, 2003.

[115] "Food Irradiation," Center for Consumer Research, University of California, Davis. Available online. URL: http://ccr.ucdavis.edu/irr/index.shtml. Updated on May 7, 2000.

[116] "The Truth about Irradiated Meat," *Consumer Reports*, vol. 68, no. 8, August 2003, pp. 34–37.

[117] "Irradiation Revisited: As FDA Considers Expanded Use, New Health Concerns Arise," *Food Safety Review*, vol. 2, Winter 2002, p. 3.

[118] "The Truth about Irradiated Meat," pp. 34–37.

[119] Mark Worth and Peter Jenkins, "Hidden Harm: How the FDA Is Ignoring the Potential Dangers of Unique Chemicals in Irradiated Food," Public Citizen and Center for Food Safety. Available online. URL: http://www.mindfully.org/Food/Irradiation-FDA- IgnoringDec01.htm. Posted in December 2001.

[120] "StarLink Corn: How It Reached the Food Supply," Associated Press. Available online. URL: http://archive.showmenews.com/2000/dec/20001204busi011.asp. Posted on December 4, 2000.

[121] Jeffrey M. Smith, *Seeds of Deception: Exposing Industry and Government Lies about the Safety of the Genetically Engineered Foods You're Eating.* Fairfield, Iowa: Yes! Books, 2003, p. 165.

[122] "Transgenic Crops: An Introduction and Resource Guide. StarLink Corn," Department of Soil and Crop Sciences, Colorado State University. Available online. URL: http://www.colostate.edu/programs/lifesciences/TransgenicCrops/hotstarlink.html. Updated on March 11, 2004.

[123] Larry Thompson, "Are Bioengineered Foods Safe?" *FDA Consumer*, vol. 34, no. 1, January/February 2001, pp. 18–23. Available online. URL: http://www.fda.gov/fdac/features/2000/100_bio.html. Downloaded in December 2004.

[124] Michael Rodemeyer, "Science, Genetically Modified Foods, and the Rumsfeld Doctrine," Ogmius: Newsletter of the Center for Science and Technology Policy Research. Available online. URL: http://sciencepolicy.colorado.edu/ogmius/archives/issue_10/intro_to_exchange.html. Posted in January 2005.

[125] "Genetically Modified Crops in the United States," Pew Initiative on Food and Biotechnology Factsheet. Available online. URL: http://pewagbiotech.org/resources/factsheets/display.php3?FactsheetID=2. Posted in August 2004.

[126] "Genetically Modified Foods Eaten Regularly," AP Digital Associated Press. Available online. URL: http://www.stopgettingsick.com/template.cfm-7952. Posted on March 28, 2005.

127 "Americans' Opinions about Genetically Modified Foods Remain Divided, But Majority Want a Strong Regulatory System," Pew Initiative on Food and Biotechnology. Available online. URL: http://pewagbiotech.org/newsroom/releases/112404.php3. Posted on November 24, 2004.

128 Smith, *Seeds of Deception*, p. 75.

129 Smith, *Seeds of Deception*, p. iii.

130 Smith, *Seeds of Deception*, p. 3.

131 Bill Lambrecht, *Dinner at the New Gene Café*. New York: St. Martin's Press, 2001, p. 22.

132 Lambrecht, *Dinner at the New Gene Café*, p. 36.

133 Rodemeyer, "Science, Genetically Modified Foods, and the Rumsfeld Doctrine."

134 Joan Scheel, "New Product Trends: Driving Organic Growth," Prepared Foods. Available online. URL: http://www.preparedfoods.com/CDA/ArticleInformation/features/BNP__Features__Ite m/0,1231,131038,00.html. Posted on August 11, 2004.

135 Brian P. Baker, Charles M. Benbrook, Edward Groth III, and Karen Lutz Benbrook, "Pesticide Residues in Conventional, IPM-Grown and Organic Foods: Insights from Three U.S. Data Sets," *Food Additives and Contaminants*, vol. 19, no. 5, May 2002, pp. 427–442. Available online. URL: http://www.consumersunion.org/food/organicsumm.htm. Downloaded in December 2004.

CHAPTER 2

THE LAW AND THREATS TO FOOD SAFETY

Food-safety laws have accumulated over the last century in a way that has led politicians and experts to reach contradictory conclusions: The fragmented food-safety system both makes little sense and can't be changed. It makes little sense because laws have prevented a single agency from having primary responsibility for food safety. Senator Richard Durbin (D-Illinois) summarized the problem in his introductory statement to a 2001 hearing on the fractured food-safety system:

> Our government structure divides responsibility for food safety and security between at least a dozen Federal agencies operating under 35 different Federal statutes. It is a system of divided responsibility. It is a system of rivalry, in some aspects, when it should be one of cooperation. It is duplicative, it is costly and it is unduly complicated. It is impossible to explain.[1]

At the same time, Congress has not changed the system despite calls for a single or primary food-safety agency. Government officials and politicians seem unwilling to surrender any existing food-safety power to others or merge overlapping duties. Senator Durbin and others introduced bills after the September 11, 2001, terrorist attacks to create a single food-safety agency. As Senator Durbin argued,

> In an age where our Nation's food supply is facing tremendous pressure from emerging pathogens to an ever-growing volume of food imports, from changing food consumption patterns to an aging population susceptible to food-related illness and even potential food security risks, we must have a system in place to ensure the safety of our food.[2]

Yet the bills have not passed. A new tragedy involving the failure of the system to protect the population may change this, but food safety now relies on a patchwork of laws dating back over a century and a few court cases that generally have asserted the primacy of the laws.

As a result, inconsistencies abound in food laws and regulations. In one speech, President George W. Bush noted that "The way things work now, there is one agency that inspects cheese pizza. There is another that inspects pepperoni pizza. There is one agency that inspects food grown outside the United States, another for food grown here inside the United States."[3] Similarly, one agency inspects hotdogs and another inspects the bun that holds the hotdog; one agency inspects open-faced meat or poultry sandwiches and another inspects closed-faced sandwiches with the same ingredients; and one agency inspects eggs in shells and another inspects eggs in processed food.

With dozens of federal statutes in place, an overview of food-safety laws and regulations must be selective. Even a selective review faces complexities because legislation has never created a simple, logical organization of food-safety efforts. Rather, statutes have accumulated over time with one new law adding to and revising previous ones. In reviewing these complexities, this chapter highlights the most important laws and regulations in food safety and describes court cases that have contributed to the current form of the system.

LAWS AND REGULATIONS

FEDERAL

Food-safety laws and regulations first emerged in response to technology developed during the last decades of the 19th century. Before then, animals were slaughtered locally by butchers and sold to those in nearby communities. Not until large processing plants began to ship meat in refrigerated railroad cars did the government draw up national food-safety rules. With huge slaughtering houses located in cities like Chicago and with the transport of meat over long distances (even to other countries), buyers became separated from producers. Similarly, the use of new chemicals and additives in preparing food left consumers with little idea of the ingredients they were eating. These changes in the nature of food led to demands for a set of consistent, nationwide food standards.

Early Laws

Government food-safety regulations in the United States emerged slowly. In 1884, President Chester Arthur signed legislation that created the Bureau of Animal Industry and gave it responsibility for preventing the use of diseased animals for food. In 1890 and 1891, the government responded to calls from the meat industry for higher-quality standards in exported cattle and meat. Since foreign countries had adopted new safety rules for imported meat, new legislation ordered inspection of exported cattle and meat to ensure they met the rules.

Two legislative acts early in the 20th century extended federal government control of food safety in ways that continue to define today's policies. The 1906 Pure Food and Drug Act gave the Bureau of Chemistry in the U.S. Department of Agriculture (USDA) authority to determine if food specimens they examined had been mislabeled or adulterated. The law defined adulterated as taking the name of another product; mislabeling in a way to deceive buyers about the content, manufacturer, or size of the product; or adding poisons or ingredients that were injurious to health.

Different legislation would guide meat safety. The 1906 Federal Meat Inspection Act required inspection of cattle, sheep, swine, goats, and horses to be used for interstate and foreign commerce, thus extending inspection of exports to include meat transported across state lines (federal inspection of meat raised and sold within states would wait until 1967). It also required the inspection of meat-processing equipment and facilities. The USDA Bureau of Animal Industry carried out the inspections, seeking to make sure that diseased animals were not used for food and cleanliness standards were maintained.

The two pieces of legislation in 1906 defined separate spheres of authority that continue to this day.[4] The Bureau of Chemistry, which had been given authority under the Pure Food and Drug Act, became the Food, Drug, and Insecticide Administration in 1927 and then the Food and Drug Administration (FDA) in 1931. In 1940, the FDA was transferred to the agency that would become the Department of Heath, Education, and Welfare and then the Department of Health and Human Services. The Bureau of Animal Industry, which had been given authority under the Federal Meat Inspection Act, would eventually end up as the Food Safety and Inspection Service (FSIS) in 1981 and remain as part of the USDA.

Although specific in terms of goals, the 1906 legislation lacked details on how to decide if food and meat products met standards of purity and cleanliness. Judges thus had difficulty interpreting the law, and the government had difficulty enforcing it. The 1938 Federal Food, Drug, and Cosmetic Act attempted to update and overhaul some parts of the earlier legislation. It prohibited the addition of poisonous substances to foods except where unavoidable or required in production and, when necessary, specified allowable levels of such substances. It further allowed government agencies to inspect factories and enforce food standards, and it gave courts the power to stop production of foods in violation of the law.

The Meat Inspection Act of 1906 did not require inspection of poultry and eggs, which at the time were produced by local farmers on a small scale. The

Threats to Food Safety

1957 Poultry Products Inspection Act and the 1970 Egg Products Inspection Act extended the inspection authority of the government to these products. The old and new laws together created a full set of inspection requirements.[5] By law, plants, equipment, and operating procedures have to be safe and sanitary before slaughtering or processing of animals can begin. Federal employees have to check animals both before and after slaughter to look for signs of disease, contamination, and abnormal conditions. Processed meat for hotdogs, deli selections, prepared dinners, soups, and the like have to be inspected daily to check for cleanliness, correct ingredients, and proper factory procedures.

In the end, food-safety laws divided government responsibilities. The USDA has authority over meat, poultry, and certain egg products, both within and across states. The FDA has authority over most other products, including canned, frozen, or packaged foods containing meat, poultry, or eggs—but only when the products are shipped across state lines. As described by the agency, "FDA's jurisdiction covers approximately 80 percent of domestic and imported foods that are marketed in interstate commerce . . . [and] includes approval and surveillance for new animal drugs, animal feeds, and all food additives that can become part of food."[6] Otherwise, several other agencies have more specialized responsibilities: The Environmental Protection Agency (EPA) approves and regulates pesticides; the Bureau of Alcohol, Tobacco and Firearms in the Department of Treasury controls alcohol; the Centers for Disease Control and Prevention in the Department of Health and Human Services monitors foodborne disease; the Department of Commerce inspects fishing vessels; the Department of Justice prosecutes those suspected of violating food laws; and the Federal Trade Commission regulates unfair or deceptive food advertising.

Pathogen Reduction and HACCP Regulations (1995)

On July 25, 1995, the USDA's Food Safety and Inspection Service (FSIS) published detailed rules that drastically changed government food-safety enforcement—most likely for the better. The rules aimed to do no less than modernize meat and poultry inspection. Once based on approval by federal inspectors who relied on sight, touch, and smell to check meat, inspection would now change. It would rely more on companies to use scientific methods to identify and prevent pathogens (or disease organisms) from contaminating their meat and poultry. Guidance to companies would come from a system known as Hazard Analysis and Critical Control Points (HACCP), and the FSIS would replace direct meat and factory inspection with checks on records and test results.

The published regulations take up 185 pages of text in the *Federal Register* but highlight four important changes.[7] First, meat and poultry establishments needed to set up and follow written sanitary standard operating procedures.

92

The Law and Threats to Food Safety

The need for daily efforts to keep facilities and equipment clean, have employees maintain personal hygiene, and ensure use of proper food handling techniques would seem obvious. Yet studies had shown that sanitary operating procedures worked best when supervisors monitored performance, kept daily records to document completed work, and corrected any problems. The new regulations required all establishments to follow these steps and FSIS inspectors to use the records as one way to check for sanitary conditions.

Second, the regulations required daily microbial testing to prevent contamination of meat and poultry by fecal matter. The tests focus on the presence of *E. coli* O157:H7, bacteria found in feces that not only pose a significant hazard but also indicate the presence of other pathogens. Negative tests for *E. coli* indicate that slaughtering procedures did not allow the contents of animal intestines to spread to meat and poultry. Again, inspectors do not typically examine the meat or slaughtering process directly but instead check the outcomes of microbe testing.

Third, establishments must meet new pathogen reduction standards for the presence of *Salmonella* in raw meat and poultry. *Salmonella* bacteria are so common that they cannot be eliminated altogether, but the USDA aimed to reduce the levels. The regulations thus required that test results show the presence of the bacteria in no more than 7.5 percent of the samples. Higher levels would require that companies improve or risk losing USDA approval of their meat. However, an appeals court ruled in *Supreme Beef v. USDA* that this regulation exceeded the authority given to the agency by existing law. The agency now uses high levels of *Salmonella* to justify a more careful check of current procedures rather than to close down production.

Fourth, the regulations required establishments to develop and implement a system of controls known as Hazard Analysis and Critical Control Points (HACCP). The system consists of seven principles based on scientific methods of testing and measurement that will prevent or minimize contamination. Quoting an excerpt from FDA materials, establishments using HACCP must:

- *Analyze Hazards:* Potential hazards associated with a food and measures to control those hazards are identified. The hazard could be biological, such as a microbe; chemical, such as a toxin; or physical, such as ground glass or metal fragments.
- *Identify Critical Control Points:* These are points in a food's production—from its raw state through processing and shipping to consumption by the consumer—at which the potential hazard can be controlled or eliminated. Examples are cooking, cooling, packaging, and metal detection.
- *Establish Preventive Measures with Critical Limits for Each Control Point:* For a cooked food, for example, this might include setting the minimum cooking temperature and time required to ensure the elimination of any harmful microbes.

93

- *Establish Procedures to Monitor the Critical Control Points:* Such procedures might include determining how and by whom cooking time and temperature should be monitored.
- *Establish Corrective Actions to Be Taken When Monitoring Shows That a Critical Limit Has Not Been Met:* For example, reprocess or dispose of food if the minimum cooking temperature is not met.
- *Establish Procedures to Verify That the System Is Working Properly:* For example, test time-and-temperature recording devices to verify that a cooking unit is working properly.
- *Establish Effective Recordkeeping to Document the HACCP System:* This would include records of hazards and their control methods, the monitoring of safety requirements, and action taken to correct potential problems. Each of these principles must be backed by sound scientific knowledge; for example, publish microbiological studies on time-and-temperature factors for controlling foodborne pathogens.[8]

Companies unwilling or unable to follow these rules face punishment. The regulations state that "serious, repeated, or flagrant violations will result in immediate regulatory action, such as stopping production lines . . . and suspension or withdrawal of inspection."[9] Even if rules are followed, failing to maintain proper records or falsifying records represent serious violations. Since suspension of inspections virtually forces the plant to shut down, companies have strong motivation to adhere to the rules. Minor violations of rules result in more intense checks on plant procedures.

Food Quality Protection Act (1996)

Beginning in 1949, hearings chaired by Representative James T. Delaney of New York led eventually to three amendments that "fundamentally changed the character of the U.S. food and drug law: the Pesticide Amendment (1954), the Food Additives Amendment (1958), and the Color Additive Amendments (1960). With these laws on the books, it could be said for the first time that no substance can legally be introduced into the U.S. food supply unless there has been a prior determination that it is safe."[10] Of special importance, these amendments required manufacturers to prove the safety of their product before sale—rather than making the government prove the danger of a product after injuries had occurred.

The food- and color-additive laws included a condition that became known as the Delaney Clause and caused considerable controversy over the next 40 years. It stated that the FDA could not approve an additive as safe if studies found that it caused cancer in humans or lab animals. This zero-tolerance rule followed from the principle that no amount of a cancer-causing substance was safe. Yet many made the point that substances causing cancer in high doses posed no risk in tiny doses, a claim that would gain wider acceptance in decades to come. Controversy erupted, for example, with findings in the 1970s that large doses of saccharin, a popular artificial sweetener and sugar substitute, caused cancer in laboratory animals. Consistent with the Delaney Clause, the FDA proposed banning the sweetener (except as an over-the-counter drug), but public outcry led Congress to place a moratorium on the ban that still continues.[11]

The Delaney Clause also led to heated debate over pesticide residue on foods. In regulating the use of pesticides, the EPA allowed for residue on raw foods in amounts small enough not to appear to present a threat to human health. However, some pesticides had been shown to cause cancer in laboratory animals. When present on food, these pesticides met the definition of a food additive and violated the Delaney Clause. In 1989, the Natural Resources Defense Council brought suit against the EPA to enforce the zero-tolerance requirements of the law. The suit led to a settlement that required the EPA to phase out some cancer-causing pesticides but also led Congress to examine the issue.

Reaching consensus rare for most issues, Congress passed the 1996 Food Quality Protection Act with bipartisan and unanimous support. The act replaced the zero-tolerance standard for pesticides with a single standard of "reasonable certainty of no harm" that applies to pesticide residue on both raw foods and in processed food. In exchange for weakening the safety standard of some pesticides, the legislation offered a provision of special value to food-safety advocates: The standard of reasonable certainty of no harm, which defined the allowable levels of pesticide residue, would be set up to safeguard the health of infants and children. The standard would protect those most vulnerable to the harm of pesticides as well as healthy adults.[12]

With the need to define the standards more precisely, however, the consensus soon ended. The legislation gave the EPA responsibility for determining *tolerances*—a term used to mean the levels of pesticide residues that gave reasonable certainty of no harm—but the agency inevitably angered nearly all parties. All agreed that the EPA was proceeding too slowly in reassessing pesticide dangers and tolerances. Consumer groups wanted dangerous pesticides quickly banned or restricted, while farmers wanted clear advice on what pesticides to use. Both consumer and farm groups stood as plaintiffs in a 2001 suit against the EPA that would force the agency to meet the deadlines laid out in the legislation. To settle the suit, the EPA agreed in September 2001 (*Natural Resources Defense Council v. Whitman*) to adhere to a new schedule.

That agreement in turn angered some of the parties involved in the suit. Farm groups and members of Congress from farm states criticized the EPA for restricting use of some popular pesticides. They claimed that the agency bowed to outside pressure and media publicity rather than relying on scientific evidence in making some decisions. Consumer groups, including the organization that brought the 1999 suit, the Natural Resources Defense Council, accused the EPA of not living up to the agreement it signed to settle the suit. In 2003, the organization brought another suit against the EPA, as did the attorneys general from New York, Connecticut, Massachusetts, and New Jersey. These suits demanded that pesticide tolerances be set, as required by law, to protect the health of infants and children—a goal the EPA believes it is already meeting. The Food Quality Protection Act certainly changed the standard for the safety of pesticide residue on food but not the debate over how to define the standards.

Presidential Initiatives

New laws and regulations have not satisfied critics of the food-safety system. In a report on food safety, for example, the General Accounting Office called for a single agency to have responsibility for food safety. Such an agency would merge separate and overlapping duties and have more authority to enforce laws and regulations. In 2001 congressional hearings on the topic, experts testified on the benefits of such a change. As Congress has not passed legislation to reorganize the system, however, presidents Bill Clinton and George W. Bush both took steps to foster cooperation among the multiple food agencies.

In 1997, President Clinton announced with great fanfare an initiative called Food Safety from Farm to Table. The initiative proposed building a new national warning system for food disease outbreaks, improving the speedy response to outbreaks, developing new research methods to test for and treat foodborne illness, and improving the education of the public about food safety. To reach these goals, the initiative directed the USDA, FDA, EPA, CDC, and the Department of Commerce to form new interagency ties. For example, several agencies joined in the President's Council on Food Safety and cooperated on new surveillance and education programs. Still, the major divisions of responsibility for food safety remain in place.

In 2004, President Bush released a directive for food safety focused on security from terrorism. To help protect the safety of the food supply, this directive repeated previous calls for interagency cooperation. The Department of Homeland Security should work with the USDA, EPA, Justice Department, Central Intelligence Agency, and Department of Health and Human Services to obtain information on possible food tampering. In so doing, the agencies should avoid the competition and isolation that led to intelligence failures before the September 11 attacks. Again, however, the directive does not make major changes in the divided nature of the food-safety system.

STATE AND LOCAL

Food-safety activities of state and local government agencies complement and generally take the lead from the federal government. State and county departments of agriculture and health, for example, inspect dairy farms, meat- and poultry-slaughtering plants, groceries, other retail outlets, and restaurants within their jurisdiction. States also have responsibility for foods that are not shipped or sold across state lines and therefore not inspected by the FDA. The laws and standards enforced by state and local governments generally coincide with federal laws, but some of the major agricultural states such as California, which grows half the produce sold in the United States, have their own inspection systems and safety standards.[13]

The National Uniformity for Food Act, a recent bill approved by a committee in the House of Representatives aims to make state policies more consistent. It would require states to adopt food-safety warnings and product labels that match federal laws and regulations. Food industry groups argue that consistent wording will allow manufacturers to use the same labels throughout the country and help consumers to understand the labels better. Consumer groups, however, view the bill as a means to undermine strict food-safety laws in many states and strongly oppose the measure.

Perhaps most important, county health inspectors check food-safety procedures at restaurants. The laws, procedures, and requirements vary widely across counties and states but have become increasingly important as the popularity of eating out has grown. During typical visits, inspectors come unannounced to restaurants and observe the business during normal hours. They look for critical violations such as improper food temperature, presence of pests, poor sanitation, and inadequate hand washing. Although these routine inspections often get little attention, they remain a key part of food safety.

COURT CASES

TEXAS FOOD INDUSTRY ASSOCIATION, ET AL. V. MIKE ESPY U.S. DISTRICT COURT FOR THE WESTERN DISTRICT OF TEXAS, 870 F. SUPP. 143 (1994)

Background

Since at least 1974, when it won a suit brought against it by the American Public Health Association, the USDA had treated the presence of pathogens on meat as natural. Although not desirable and certainly distasteful from the point of view of consumers, having bacteria, viral agents, and parasites on raw meat was, the agency argued, unavoidable. Existing law states that the USDA has the authority to inspect and give approval to meat that is "wholesome, not adulterated." It further defines meat as adulterated when it has become contaminated due to unsanitary conditions or has been rendered to become injurious to health. The USDA approved meat even when it contained some types of foodborne diseases because it met these legal conditions. Given that the diseases existed on meat even in sanitary conditions, the meat was not adulterated; given that normal cooking procedures for the meat would kill the disease organisms, the meat did not cause health problems. The pathogens therefore were not adulterants or health risks that would be outlawed by federal law.

In 1994, however, the agency responded to the deaths of children from *E. coli* O157:H7 in undercooked hamburger by proposing new rules. The USDA would collect 5,000 samples of raw beef from meat establishments and retail outlets to test for this *E. coli* strain. Any samples testing positive for the pathogen would be considered adulterated, violate meat-safety requirements, and not receive approval for sale. In reversing its long-standing policy, the USDA in essence treated this one microbe as an adulterant. The Texas Food Industry Association and several other organizations representing meatpackers, retailers, grocers, and distributors brought suit to prevent the USDA from making this change.

Legal Issues

The food industry plaintiffs recognized that the sampling and testing program presented challenges for getting their meat approved. Under the new policy, products that appeared on the surface as fresh, wholesome, and clean might not gain approval if microscopic tests found *E. coli* O157:H7. The plaintiffs opposed the change, alleging that 1) the USDA did not allow for proper notice and comment time for the new rule, 2) the rule was arbitrary and capricious, and 3) microbe tests exceeded the authority of the agency under federal law. The USDA disputed the legal validity of each of these claims.

First, new regulations that present a substantial burden on the affected parties require a notice-and-comment period, which the USDA did not provide in their *E. coli* testing policy. In its defense, the USDA argued that the testing represents an inspection procedure rather than a new regulation. It involved more in the way of a change in the interpretation of a rule rather than a change in the rule itself. In addition, the new policy did not place a burden on meat and poultry establishments, as the sampling and testing could be carried out quickly and easily. Therefore, the policy change did not require a notice-and-comment period.

Second, the plaintiffs argued that the testing imposed excessive new costs on businesses that already did all they could to ensure safe meat. Such an imposition was both arbitrary and capricious. It was arbitrary in the choice to test only one product (ground beef) for one pathogen *(E. coli)* when other pathogens occur on other meat products. It was capricious in that the USDA did not provide a rational explanation for the new policy. In response, the USDA argued that the policy had a rational basis: The testing and threat of regulation would spur the industry to use better prevention measures, and the recent deaths from new forms of *E. coli* in hamburgers warranted the attention to this particular pathogen and meat.

Third, the plaintiffs adopted earlier arguments of the USDA, claiming that *E. coli* did not meet the two legal characteristics of an adulterant. It was not added to meat and, when cooked properly, did not harm health. The USDA therefore overstepped its authority in treating *E. coli* as an adulterant that could prevent approval of meat for sale. The USDA countered with evidence that many Americans preferred their ground beef cooked rare, medium rare, or medium, which would not kill all the pathogens. As a result, the pathogen could injure the health of consumers and fell under the legal inspection authority of the USDA.

Decision

The Texas District Court denied the plaintiff's appeal to stop the USDA testing and approval procedures, rejecting each of the arguments in turn. It first ruled that the agency could conduct testing without a notice-and-comment period. Since the testing itself does not affect the establishments or compel them to take any action, it does not require notice and comment. It next rejected claims that the decision to test for *E. coli* and treat its presence as an adulterant was arbitrary and capricious. Testing for *E. coli* makes sense as a way to understand and address the threats to health caused in recent years by this pathogen. Lastly, the court ruled that *E. coli* fits the definition of an adulterant given its potential to cause serious health problems and that the USDA had proper authority to make this determination.

Impact

This decision paved the way for the USDA to implement its Pathogen Reduction and HACCP regulations. With microscopic testing allowed for at least this one pathogen, the USDA could revamp its inspection procedures. Old methods based on seeing, touching, and smelling meat could be replaced by more scientific methods. The USDA further hoped that testing meat samples would, given the potential of positive results to shut down a meatpacking plant, lead establishments to do testing of their own. Consumer groups, including one consisting of relatives of victims of the 1993 Jack in the Box deaths from hamburger infected with *E. coli*, praised both the USDA's policies and the court decisions. Although another court decision would limit the ability to declare other bacteria as adulterants, this decision would do much to improve meat safety.

ALLIANCE FOR BIO-INTEGRITY, ET AL. V. DONNA SHALALA, ET AL. 116 F. SUPP. 2D (2000)

Background

In 1992, the FDA concluded that genetically modified, or GM, foods did not differ substantially enough from normal food to justify special treatment. If, for example, tomatoes or soybeans were generally recognized as safe, then GM tomatoes or soybeans would likewise be generally recognized as safe. The policy meant that GM foods would not undergo the thorough safety review required of new food additives. Instead, the FDA requested that producers of GM foods consult with them before marketing their products. The FDA could step in to regulate a GM product that appeared unsafe but did so only on a case-by-case basis rather than routinely. The FDA further reasoned that since GM foods differed little from nonmodified foods, they did not require special labels.

Opponents of GM foods had protested the FDA policy for many years but had made little headway in changing the position of the agency. In 1998, a coalition of diverse groups called the Alliance for Bio-integrity, all united by their opposition to the policy, filed suit against Secretary of Health and Human Services Donna Shalala, who had oversight responsibility for the FDA. The suit alleged that, in setting the GM food policy, the FDA did not follow proper procedures. The agency further reached decisions that were arbitrary and capricious and violated the religious rights of the public. The coalition aimed to force the FDA to regulate 36 individual GM foods on the market—in other words, to thoroughly evaluate their safety and require special labels for their sale.

The plaintiffs expressed a variety of concerns about GM foods. Many worried that GM foods contained unexpected toxins or allergens that would harm consumers. Given the lack of labeling, those troubled about this risk could not act on their concerns when shopping. Along with the worry over health risks came another concern. Some plaintiffs believed that GM foods violated their religious beliefs. Products might mix genetic material from nonkosher food with kosher food, perhaps leading Jewish consumers to unknowingly violate their dietary laws. GM foods might also violate the beliefs of those opposed on religious grounds to the creation of what they view as unnatural foods. Yet believers could not act on their beliefs without labels for GM foods.

The Law and Threats to Food Safety

Legal Issues

The plaintiffs offered multiple claims objecting to the FDA policy on GM foods, but three legal issues stand out. First, the plaintiffs accused the FDA of not following proper procedures in making a policy decision of such importance. Although agencies must give early notice of new regulations and allow for a comment period, the FDA did neither in declaring that GM foods did not differ materially from nonmodified food. In addition, major federal actions require an environmental impact analysis, but the FDA failed to do this for GM foods. As a result of these procedural violations, the plaintiffs wanted the policy set aside.

The defendants responded that this particular policy required neither the notice-and-comment period nor the environmental impact analysis. The FDA policy merely stated that GM foods would be presumed to be safe unless evidence to the contrary appeared. The treatment of GM foods by the FDA represented more of an announcement than a major action or policy change—not something that required special procedures.

Second, the plaintiffs attacked the reasoning behind FDA claims of GM food safety. According to food-safety laws, any substance that might affect the characteristics of food shall be deemed an additive and require a scientific review of safety. Genetic engineering affects the characteristics of food and therefore cannot be deemed safe without thorough evaluation. According to the plaintiffs, the decision to do otherwise was arbitrary and capricious. Just as arbitrary and capricious was the decision of the FDA to not require labels for GM foods. Consumers have legitimate fears about the safety of GM foods. If the government does not take action to test the products, they should at least let consumers make informed judgments.

The defendants responded that genetic engineering does not add any new substance to food. Rather, it involves adding genetic materials that are already part of all foods. Not only are these genetic materials safe, but they are necessary for survival. The FDA would thoroughly examine the rare instance of a completely new substance triggered by genetic engineering; otherwise, trading DNA proteins is not the same as adding artificial preservatives or colorings to food. If the genetic engineering does not involve adding new substances to food, then another conclusion follows: Special labels for GM foods are unnecessary. Although some consumers may want more information on GM foods, the FDA argued that it does not have legal authority to require labels in the absence of demonstrated harm.

Third, the most creative and original claim made by the plaintiffs against the FDA policy on GM foods involves religious freedom. They argued that lack of knowledge about the presence of GM ingredients in food products violates their rights to the free exercise of religion. If eating GM foods violates religious convictions, then failing to provide labels prevents the exercise of their religion. Just as courts have ruled that the government has to meet religious diet restrictions of prisoners, the government must act in the interests of religious groups by labeling GM foods.

The FDA argued in response that the policy was not specifically directed at any one religion but applied to everyone. Since the policy did not require eating GM foods, it could not violate the right to free exercise of religion. To the contrary, only if the FDA began labeling food and setting its policies to aid in the practice of particular religions would it violate this right.

Decision

Before the suit went to trial, the coalition bringing the suit and the FDA filed motions for a summary judgment on the plaintiff's multiple claims. In a summary judgment, the court makes a decision without a trial. Typically, the parties agree on the facts but differ on the interpretation of the law, and the court reaches a decision based on the evidence and statements presented in the legal documents. Agreeing to the motions for a summary judgment, the U.S. District Court for the District of Columbia then decided in favor of the FDA on all counts. It held that the GM food policy did not violate the Constitution, federal laws, or administrative regulations. The decision that GM foods do not differ materially from nonmodified foods was not arbitrary and capricious. The FDA did not violate the right of the free exercise of religion in concluding that GM foods need not be labeled.

Impact

This decision represented a major defeat for the opponents of GM foods. Trying to overturn the FDA policy represented the best opportunity to have GM foods tested by the government and labeled in stores. Farmers had already been growing large amounts of GM crops, and stores already sold a wide variety of products with GM crops. According to the Grocery Manufacturers of America, roughly 75 percent of U.S. processed foods contain some GM ingredients.[14] With a voluntary change in policy by the FDA unlikely, the court decision allowed these trends to continue. However, plaintiffs took solace because the court decision ruled on a narrow application of the law. The court did not address the question of the safety of GM food or the value of the FDA policy not to regulate the food. Rather, it concluded that the policy fell within the legal rights of the agency. The Alliance for Biointegrity interprets the case in the best possible light by stating:

> *On balance, our lawsuit accomplished a lot by exposing the FDA's fraud and revealing the unsoundness of its policy and the irresponsibility of its behavior.*

Even though we failed to overturn the FDA's policy, the court's ruling refutes the standard claims of the biotech industry about the rigor of FDA oversight and the proven safety of its own products.[15]

The use of the suit to publicize the FDA's policy may be a moral victory but only a small one. GM foods remain both common and unlabeled and, despite the debate over their safety, the FDA policy remains in place.

SUPREME BEEF PROCESSORS V. USDA
U.S. COURT OF APPEALS FOR THE FIFTH CIRCUIT 275
F.3D 432 (2001)

Background

When the Food Safety and Inspection Service (FSIS) of the USDA published plans to implement the HACCP system of food control in 1995, it planned to test meat products for *Salmonella* much as it did for *E. coli* O157:H7. Resistance to the new testing emerged quickly, however. The Supreme Beef Processors plant in Texas failed the FSIS tests—47 percent of the meat samples contained *Salmonella*. Supreme Beef took measures to improve its performance, but a new round of tests still revealed *Salmonella* in 21 percent of samples. The company promised to bring the levels down to the required 7.5 percent but failed to provide details about how it would do so. The FSIS decided to suspend inspections, which in essence would stop plant production.

Asserting that the FSIS had overstepped its authority, Supreme Beef filed suit and asked for a restraining order to prevent the removal of inspectors. The Texas District Court granted the motion for a restraining order and then sided with Supreme Beef in ruling that the agency had indeed exceeded its authority in enforcing *Salmonella* standards. The USDA then appealed the decision.

Legal Issues

The Supreme Court had earlier set a standard for how government agencies should comply with legal statutes. In general, if the interpretation of the law by government agencies does not conflict with the plain language of the law's text, then judges should defer to the agency in their decision. In this case, the USDA relied on the legal definition of an adulterant (or harmful additive) to justify regulations on *Salmonella* testing. The relevant clause states that meat is adulterated "if it has been prepared, packed or held under unsanitary conditions whereby it may have been contaminated with filth, or whereby it may have been rendered injurious to health." Since *Salmonella* often makes people sick, the USDA claimed that it met the *injurious to health* definition of an adulterant, and meat with high levels of the pathogen could not be stamped as inspected and approved.

The plaintiff, Supreme Beef, rejected this reasoning. The company argued that *Salmonella* was all but impossible to eliminate from food. It shows up in eggs and other foods besides meat, exists even in the most sanitary conditions, and does not harm people who properly cook food. Indeed, the company believed that *Salmonella* came from contaminated carcasses brought into the plant rather than from unsanitary plant operations. If so, positive tests would not be the fault of the company, and the FSIS should not treat the bacteria as an adulterant. Rather than test for its presence on meat, *Salmonella* should be regulated by checking the cleanliness of the meat-handling procedures.

The USDA responded with a variation on its legal argument. It claimed that even if *Salmonella* is not itself an adulterant, its presence is associated with other adulterants that come from fecal matter. Regulating *Salmonella* through microscopic tests in essence regulates a variety of other unhealthy contaminants that would be considered adulterants.

Decision

In considering whether to affirm or overturn the district court decision, the appeals court emphasized the importance of unsanitary conditions for adulterated meat. If the company maintained sanitary conditions and did nothing to cause the spread of *Salmonella*, but the bacteria existed in the raw materials sent to the plant, then the food is not adulterated according to the law. The company would therefore not be responsible for the presence of *Salmonella*. In these circumstances, the USDA would not have the authority to withhold approval of the meat, even if testing disclosed the presence of *Salmonella* in the final product.

Following this reasoning, the court identified flaws in the arguments of the USDA. It noted the agency did not answer the plaintiff's claim that the beef it purchased for use in its plant comes from "trimmings" that tend to have higher levels of *Salmonella*. By relying on outcome tests, the USDA in essence was regulating the purchase of beef rather than the plant conditions. Yet the law does not give USDA inspectors authority over incoming meat. If concerned about how bacteria spread during processing, inspectors should do something more than test the final products. They should, for example, measure differences in *Salmonella* levels before and after processing. The court thus concluded that the tests do not do what the agency claims they do—measure factory contamination of meat.

It next rejected the claim of the USDA that *Salmonella*, if not an adulterant itself, should be treated as one because its presence is associated with other adulterants. This claim contradicted many published statements from the USDA—the agency in fact wanted to use *Salmonella* testing to protect food from that particular pathogen rather than from other pathogens. If concerned with other adulterants, the agency should, according to the court, test for them directly.

The appeals court thus affirmed the district court decision in favor of Supreme Beef and remanded (sent back) the case to the district court for final judgment. The court made no judgment about the value of *Salmonella* testing for food safety, the goals of the USDA to protect consumers, or larger societal and economic concerns. Rather, it compared the actions of the agency to those allowable under the law and concluded that the USDA's decision about Supreme Beef conflicted with the plain language meaning of the law.

Impact

The decision allows the USDA to continue testing for *Salmonella* but prevents the agency from using the results to shut down a plant. In limiting the power of the USDA, the ruling represented a setback to the food-safety goals and regulations contained in the Pathogen Reduction and HACCP rules. The agency has publicly minimized the importance of the decision, arguing that it can maintain food safety in other ways. It can, for example, use high levels of the pathogen to more carefully evaluate the plant and perhaps identify specific violations that justify shutting down the plant. It can also continue its policy of requiring that meat products remain free of *E. coli* O157:H7. As a result, the agency has not appealed the decision.

Consumer groups viewed the decision differently. They are outraged by the ruling and view it as a major obstacle in efforts to protect the public from foodborne disease. Carol Tucker Foreman of the Consumer Federation of America states: "It's hard to overrate it's [the Supreme Beef decision] importance. It could be interpreted as saying there is no amount of disease-causing bacteria in raw meat or poultry that would cause it to violate the law."[16] A statement from a coalition of consumer groups similarly concludes that the decision "severely undercuts the integrity of USDA's new meat and poultry inspection system, increases the risk of food poisoning and jeopardizes public confidence in the safety of the nation's food supply."[17] The coalition calls for legislation to counter the ruling by requiring continuous *Salmonella* testing and giving authority to the USDA to shut down plants that do not meet testing standards. Although such legislation was introduced in 2002, it has made little progress in Congress.

Threats to Food Safety

NATURAL RESOURCES DEFENSE COUNCIL, ET AL. V. CHRISTINE TODD WHITMAN
C-99-3701 CAL (2001)

Background

In 1989, the Natural Resources Defense Council (NRDC) sued the EPA over residues of carcinogenic pesticides on food, arguing that the Delaney Clause prohibited additives that in any amount caused cancer. The EPA had held that the amount of pesticides on raw food was so small that it presented no harm to humans. The suit sought instead to enforce the zero-tolerance standard and ban carcinogenic pesticides. In 1995, the Clinton administration agreed to settle the suit. The EPA would evaluate whether residue amounts in 36 pesticides already known to be carcinogenic violated the Delaney Clause and determine if 49 others were carcinogenic. The agreement itself did not ban any pesticides, but applying the Delaney Clause to pesticides would likely have this result.

Congress entered the dispute with the 1996 Food Quality Protection Act. This legislation designated new rules for the EPA to use in determining allowable pesticide tolerance levels. Rather than applying a zero-tolerance standard of the Delaney Clause, the new law allowed the EPA to approve use of a pesticide if residue on food presented only negligible harm. However, the harm should be evaluated not for adults but primarily for infants and children who are most vulnerable to chemicals. In addition, the legislation required the EPA to reassess tolerances for 9,728 pesticide uses by August 3, 2006. Along with examining cancer-causing effects, the EPA would also need to investigate whether any pesticides had an estrogenic (or estrogen-like) effect on the human endocrine system. Scientists had found that some chemicals can act like estrogen and thereby disrupt the hormonal balance in the body and perhaps increase the risk of breast cancer. New studies of this possible harm would need to be started.

The legislation did not, however, end the disputes over pesticide residue on food. On August 3, 1999, the NRDC, the Breast Cancer Fund, CalPIRG Charitable Trust, Pesticide Watch Education Fund, Pesticide Action Network North American Regional Center, San Francisco Bay Area Physicians for Social Responsibility, and United Farm Workers of America of the AFL-CIO sued the EPA. The suit alleged that the EPA had failed to meet the deadlines for reassessing pesticide residue tolerances. It further alleged that the agency had failed to set new tolerances for the riskiest pesticides first and had not implemented the endocrine screening program required by the legislation.

For several reasons, the EPA hoped to settle the suit. It worried that loss of the suit might turn pesticide control and estrogenic screening over to the court, but more important, the EPA expressed the desire to improve its performance. It therefore entered into a consent decree, an agreement to correct actions without admitting guilt. The decree set a series of deadlines for reassessing pesticide tolerances, required early decisions about pesticides of special concern to health groups, and mandated annual reports on their progress. The EPA also entered into a settlement agreement—an agreement to come to terms in a suit without a court decision—that would lead to tests for the estrogenic effects of pesticides. On January 19, 2001, the EPA and NRDC filed a joint motion to accept the consent decree and, given the settlement agreement, dismiss the count about studying estrogenic effects.

Legal Issues

The district judge needed to approve the consent decree on the basis of whether it was "fair, reasonable, and equitable and does not violate the law or public policy." As a legally binding agreement, any consent decree must not contain language that conflicts with existing statutes. When a government agency is involved in a consent decree, the judge must consider another requirement. The consent decree in this case could not hamper the EPA's long-term ability to exercise its judgment and expertise or tie the agency's hands in future matters.

Several groups representing farmers and pesticide users opposed the decree. The American Farm Bureau Federation, the American Crop Protection Association, and the American Chemistry Council had initially joined in the suit against the EPA. They complained that the lack of timely pesticide tolerance reassessment left them uncertain about their use of pesticides. When the NRDC and EPA agreed on the consent decree, however, these plaintiffs opposed it. They claimed that the EPA did not consider relevant information in reaching an agreement, violated its own administrative procedures, and acted in an arbitrary and capricious manner.

Decision

The district judge approved the consent decree and dismissed the count of the suit focused on estrogenic screening. He determined that the consent decree was fair and reasonable, did not unduly tie the hands of the agency, and did not violate existing law. The decision noted that the decree had safety valves to allow for flexibility in meeting its goals, gave public notice of the plans and time for public comment, and had a limited period of four years. The decree further appeared consistent with congressional intentions and seemed based on acceptable legal principles and reasoned compromise.

The judge also rejected the claims of farm and pesticide groups opposed to the consent decree. In response to the allegation that the mediation discussion between the NRDC and the EPA improperly excluded other groups, the judge ruled that ample public comment time had been made available to the other groups. This made it unnecessary for the groups to participate directly in the negotiations and meant they were not unfairly excluded. In response to the claim that the decree deadlines came too quickly to allow for scientific evaluation of the safety issues and would lead to arbitrary and capricious decisions that overstate the risks of pesticides, the judge ruled that it made no sense to object to decisions as unscientific before they had been made. With deadlines far enough ahead for all parties to present scientific data on the issues, a fair evaluation of the risks of pesticides could be made.

Impact

The decision initially appeared to satisfy those concerned about the threat of pesticides in food. An NRDC representative said they were pleased "that EPA now is committed to carrying out many of its key legal duties mandated unanimously by Congress in 1996 to protect children, farm workers, and the general public from dangerous pesticides."[18] The EPA has published annual reports that, as required by the consent decree, described assessments of the risks and tolerances of the pesticides tested. Despite initial hopes, however, critics later came to argue that the EPA continued to violate the provisions of the Food Quality Protection Act. They were in particular concerned about methods used to define pesticide tolerances that protect children. In a September 2003 suit brought against the EPA, the NRDC claimed that the agency had relied on confidential computer models developed by the industry to determine pesticide risk. The agency should instead have used the tenfold safety factor for infants and children required by the law.[19] The EPA denies the accusation, and battles over the safety of pesticides on food thus make the consent decree less valuable than originally hoped.

[1] Richard Durbin, "Opening Statement," in *Food Safety and Security: Can Our Fractured Food Safety System Rise to the Challenge? Hearing before the Oversight of Government Management, Restructuring, and the District of Columbia Subcommittee of the Committee on Governmental Affairs, United States Senate, One Hundred Seventh Congress First Session.* Washington, D.C.: U.S. Government Printing Office, October 10, 2001, p. 19.

[2] Durbin, "Opening Statement," p. 2.

[3] Quoted in Rosa L. DeLauro, "Testimony," in *Food Safety and Security*, p. 9.

[4] "Agency History," U.S. Department of Agriculture, Food Safety and Inspection Service. Available online. URL: http://www.fsis.usda.gov/About_FSIS/Agency_History/index.asp. Downloaded in December 2004.

[5] Jean M. Rawson, "Meat and Poultry Inspection Issues," CRS Report for Congress. Available online. URL: http://www.ncseonline.org/NLE/CRSreports/Agriculture/ag-30.cfm. Downloaded in December 2004.

[6] Lester M. Crawford, "Statement," Committee on Governmental Affairs, U.S. Senate. Available online. URL: http://www.senate.gov/~gov_affairs/043002crawford.pdf. Posted on April 20, 2002.

[7] Food Safety and Inspection Service, "Pathogen Reduction; Hazard Analysis and Critical Control Point (HACCP) System; Final Rule," *Federal Register*, vol. 61, no. 144, July 25, 1996, p. 38806.

[8] "HACCP: A State of the Art Approach to Food Safety," FDA Backgrounder. Available online. URL: http://www.cfsan.fda.gov/~lrd/bghaccp.html. Posted in October 2001.

[9] "Pathogen Reduction," U.S. Department of Agriculture, Food Safety and Inspection Service, p. 38822.

[10] "The Story of the Laws Behind the Labels, Part II: 1938—The Federal Food, Drug, and Cosmetic Act," U.S. Food and Drug Administration, FDA Consumer. Available online. URL: http://vm.cfsan.fda.gov/~rd/histor1a.html. Downloaded in December 2004.

[11] John Henkel, "Sugar Substitutes: Americans Opt for Sweetness and Life," FDA Consumer. Available online. URL: http://www.fda.gov/fdac/features/1999/699_sugar.html. Revised in December 2004.

[12] Linda Jo Schierow, "Pesticide Legislation: Food Quality Protection Act of 1996," CRS Report for Congress. Available online. URL: http://www.ncseonline.org/NLE/CRSreports/Pesticides/pest-8.cfm?&CFID=18344197&CFTOKEN=10723000. Posted on September 11, 1996.

[13] "Background on Food Safety and New Technologies," International Food Information Council, Food Safety and New Technologies. Available online. URL: http://www.ific.org/food/safety/index.cfm. Posted in May 2004.

[14] "Genetically Modified Foods Eaten Regularly," AP Digital Associated Press. Available online. URL: http://www.stopgettingsick.com/template.cfm-7952. Posted on March 28, 2005.

[15] "How a U.S. District Court Revealed the Unsoundness of the FDA's Policy on Genetically Engineered Foods: A Report on the Results of *Alliance for Bio-Integrity v. Shalala, et al.*," Alliance for Biointegrity. Available online. URL: http://www.biointegrity.org/report-on-lawsuit.htm. Posted on October 1, 2003.

[16] Carol Tucker Foreman, "Interview," *Frontline*, PBS Online. Available online. URL: http://www.pbs.org/wgbh/pages/frontline/shows/meat/interviews/foreman.html. Downloaded in December 2004.

[17] American Public Health Association, et al., "Regarding Bush Administration and Congressional Response to the Supreme Beef Ruling," Consumer Federation of America. Available online. URL: http://www.consumerfed.org/sfccomment_draft.pdf. Posted on December 19, 2001.

[18] "Court Approves NRDC-Led Coalition's Settlement with EPA; Agency Must Meet Legal Obligation to Regulate Pesticides," National Resources Defense Council. Available online. URL: http://www.nrdc.org/media/pressreleases/010927.asp. Posted on September 20, 2001.

[19] "NRDC Sues EPA (Again) for Failing to Carry Out Pesticide Control Law," National Resources Defense Council. Available online. URL: http://www.nrdc.org/media/pressreleases/030915a.asp. Posted on September 15, 2003.

CHAPTER 3

CHRONOLOGY

This chapter presents a time line of significant events related to a variety of threats to food safety—foodborne disease, mad cow disease, terrorism, food additives, chemical and natural toxins, food allergies, irradiation, and genetically modified (GM) food.

1860s

- French microbiologist Louis Pasteur develops pasteurization as a method to destroy unwanted and often dangerous microorganisms in wine and milk.

1884

- President Chester Arthur signs legislation to create the Bureau of Animal Industry, giving it responsibility for preventing the use of diseased animals in food.

1885

- German bacteriologist Theodor Escherich identifies *Escherichia coli (E. coli)* bacteria, which is normally present in human intestines. Certain strains of the bacteria can, however, cause diarrhea and gastroenteritis.

1888

- German bacteriologist August Gaertner isolates *Salmonella enteritidis* bacteria from both the meat of a cow slaughtered while sick with diarrhea and the body of a man who died from food poisoning after eating that meat.

1890–91

- In response to the adoption of higher-quality standards for imported meat by European countries, new U.S. legislation orders inspection of cattle and meat to ensure that exports meet these standards.

111

1902

■ Government scientists have volunteers eat food that contains borax or several other possibly poisonous preservatives as a way to test for the safety of some commonly used food additives. The tests are a first step in ending the use of dangerous additives in food.

1905

■ The first patents are issued to use ionizing radiation as a way to kill bacteria in food and prevent spoilage.

1906

■ American writer and socialist Upton Sinclair publishes *The Jungle*, a novel based on his observations of activities in a slaughterhouse and meatpacking plant. Although fiction, the book's description of the filthy conditions in the Chicago stockyards appalls readers and leads to new food-safety laws.

■ Congress passes the Pure Food and Drug Act, which gives the Bureau of Chemistry in the U.S. Department of Agriculture (USDA) authority to check for food specimens that have been mislabeled or adulterated.

■ Congress passes the Meat Inspection Act, which requires inspection of cattle, sheep, swine, goats, and horses that are shipped across state or national boundaries. It also requires inspection of meat-processing equipment and facilities.

1907

■ Immigrant cook Mary Mallon, soon to be known as Typhoid Mary, is put under house arrest and quarantined for spreading typhus bacteria to food she prepared. Called the most dangerous woman in America, she helps publicize the dangers of foodborne disease.

1914

■ The Supreme Court rules in the *United States v. The Lexington Mill and Elevator Company* that additives must be shown to cause harm before the government can ban them, which makes it difficult to enforce the Pure Food and Drug Act.

1920

■ German neurologist Dr. Hans Creutzfeldt publishes an article that describes the case of a woman whose leg spasm prevented her from walking steadily. Around the same time, the head of a German psychiatric state

112

hospital, Dr. Alfons Jakob, identifies several patients with similar symptoms. These descriptions would lead to the disease being called Creutzfeldt-Jakob disease.

1931

- The Food and Drug Administration (FDA) replaces the Food, Drug, and Insecticide Administration (which had earlier replaced the Bureau of Chemistry). It receives the power to enforce the Pure Food and Drug Act.

1938

- Congress passes the Federal Food, Drug, and Cosmetic Act. The act revises obsolete aspects of the 1906 Pure Food and Drug Act and gives authority to the FDA to regulate food additives, set acceptable levels of possibly toxic additives, and protect the safety of food sold across state lines.

1953

- With their famous discovery of the double helix structure of DNA, the building blocks of genes, American biologist James Watson and British biologist Francis Crick revolutionize the understanding of cells and organisms. Among many other things, their discovery eventually leads to genetic engineering of food.

1957

- The Poultry Products Inspection Act extends the authority of the USDA to inspect poultry products.

1958

- The Food Additives Amendment passed by Congress includes the Delaney Clause, which prohibits the use of food additives shown to cause cancer in humans or animals. The law establishes a zero-tolerance standard for cancer-causing food additives.

1963

- The FDA approves irradiation to kill insects in wheat and flour.

1964

- Irradiation is first used in the United States to extend the shelf life of white potatoes.

1969

- Using the latest testing procedures, the FDA begins to reevaluate its list of Generally Recognized as Safe (GRAS) food products and additives, eventually expanding the list to include more than 690 items.

1970

- The Egg Products Inspection Act extends the new inspection authority of the USDA.

1972

- The National Aeronautics and Space Administration (NASA) begins to use irradiation to sterilize food for astronauts in space.

1974

- In the *American Public Health Association v. Butz,* a U.S. appeals court rules that the USDA is not required by law to place labels on raw meat packages that warn of the risks of bacterial infection and the need for thorough cooking. The association had claimed that existing inspection procedures did not guarantee the safety of meat.

1976

- Dr. D. Carleton Gajdusek receives the Nobel Prize in medicine for his discovery of a disease called kuru that is found among a New Guinea tribe and has similarities to Creutzfeldt-Jakob disease. His research found that the disease was spread by the eating of the brains of deceased relatives during funeral rituals.

1977

- The FDA proposes banning the use of the artificial sweetener saccharin in food and beverages after a study of lab animals suggests that it may cause cancer. However, given negative reaction and dispute over the validity of the study, Congress mandates a moratorium on the ban.

1978

- Members of the Arab Revolutionary Council inject a poisonous liquid into oranges being exported from Israel to Europe. The terrorist action injures only 12 people who ate the oranges but leads to a 40 percent drop in sales of Israeli fruit. This action represents an early instance of food bioterrorism.

Chronology

1982

- University of California, Berkeley, professor Stephen Lindow requests permission to test genetically engineered bacteria that would control frost damage in potatoes and strawberries.

1983

- The FDA approves a new artificial sweetener, aspartame (Nutrasweet), for use in soft drinks. Critics complain that the approval was given without full scientific study and recommend that consumers avoid products with the additive.
- The FDA approves irradiation of spices and seasonings.

1984

- A farmer in southern England reports to his veterinarian that one of his dairy cows has started to aggressively menace other cows and stagger when walking. The disease shown by the cow would come to be known as mad cow disease.
- The followers of Bhagwan Shree Rajneesh, a leader of a religious commune in Oregon, cause the illness of 751 people by poisoning a salad bar with *Salmonella*. No one dies from the poisoning, but the action illustrates the ability of terrorists to infect the food supply.

1985

- The National Research Council, a highly respected scientific organization, recommends that the food inspection system be improved and criticizes the existing sight, touch, and smell methods as inadequate and unscientific.
- About 1,400 people become sick from eating watermelons grown in soil that had been treated with pesticide.
- The FDA approves irradiation to prevent trichinosis in pork.

1986

- Congress passes a law that gives new inspection responsibilities to meat-processing companies and allows government inspectors to have more choice in deciding how often they should inspect plants. However, critics claim that the law makes meat less rather than more safe.
- A disease spreading among cattle in Britain is identified and given the name "mad cow disease" by farmers and veterinarians in Britain.

1987

- A published article uses the term *bovine spongiform encephalopathy* (BSE) to refer to mad cow disease. "Bovine" refers to cows, "spongiform" to the sponge-like change in tissue, and "encephalopathy" to a disease of the brain.
- Investigation suggests that BSE is spread by the consumption of cattle feed that contains meat and bone meal from infected cows.

1988

- Based on evidence that the practice is the source of spreading mad cow disease, the use of cattle- and sheep-derived protein for cattle feed is banned by the British government. Although the ban will prevent the spread of the disease to new cattle, it does not deal with cattle that already have the disease.

1989

- The United States prohibits imports of live cattle from nations where BSE already exists.
- A phone call to the U.S. embassy in Santiago, Chile, warns that grapes shipped to the United States from Chile have been contaminated with cyanide as a protest against the government and living conditions in Chile. After testing grape shipments and finding small amounts of the deadly poison, the FDA stops the import of grapes and other fruit from the country.
- The European Union bans the meat of animals treated with steroid growth hormones and milk from cattle treated with the bovine growth hormone. Since hormones are commonly used for animals in the United States, this blocks the export of many of its meat and milk products.
- The widely viewed television show *60 Minutes* presents a segment on the dangers of a chemical called Alar that is commonly sprayed on apples to help them ripen on the tree. Although scientific studies have not been able to verify the claims, the publicity from the show leads growers to stop using the chemical.
- The Natural Resources Defense Council (NRDC) sues the Environmental Protection Agency (EPA) to enforce the zero-tolerance requirements of the Delaney Clause for cancer-causing pesticides on food. The suit leads to a settlement that requires the EPA to phase out some common pesticides.

1990

- The death of a Siamese cat from symptoms that resemble mad cow disease suggests that the disease can cross species and might affect humans. Publicity about the death creates much concern among the British public.

- British agriculture minister John Grummer, hoping to dramatize the safety of British beef, eats a hamburger with his four-year-old daughter Cordelia in front of a television camera.
- Congress passes the Organic Foods Production Act of 1990, which attempts to establish national standards for organic foods and encourage interstate commerce in organic foods. Rules for labeling organic foods would not, however, become final until more than a decade later.

1992

- The FDA concludes after internal review and debate that GM foods do not differ substantially enough from normal foods to justify special treatment or testing.

1993

- Undercooked hamburger meat that contains a dangerous new strain of *E. coli* bacteria is sold by Jack in the Box restaurants. It results in 501 reported incidents of food poisoning, 151 hospitalizations, and three deaths.
- Food industry groups found the International Food Safety Council to counter the concerns over the safety of food products and the dangers they present to the public.
- Sixteen-year-old Vicky Rimmer falls into a coma caused by a human form of mad cow disease, the first such case identified in the United Kingdom and the world.

1994

- The Food Safety Inspection Service (FSIS) announces a new policy to test for *E. coli* O157:H7 in ground meat. Beef found to contain the bacteria will be considered adulterated and unfit for sale.
- The USDA requires that labels on all packages of meat and poultry include instructions for safe handling and cooking to minimize the chance of bacterial illness.
- In *Texas Food Industry Association, et al. v. Mike Espy, et al.*, a Texas district court upholds the plans of the government for mandatory testing of ground meat for *E. coli*.
- Ice cream premix is accidentally contaminated with *Salmonella* during transportation in a tanker truck that had earlier contained nonpasteurized liquid eggs. An estimated 224,000 people across the nation become sick from eating the ice cream.
- The FDA approves the first GM food, a tomato called Flavr Savr that does not spoil as quickly as conventional tomatoes.

Threats to Food Safety

1995

- Stephen Churchill, a 19-year-old from Great Britain, becomes the first known human to die of variant Creutzfeldt-Jakob disease from eating BSE-infected beef.
- The USDA's Food Safety and Inspection Service (FSIS) publishes detailed rules that will drastically change government food-safety enforcement. The rules require that a Hazard Analysis and Critical Control Point (HACCP) system replace direct meat and factory inspection and that the FSIS rely on inspection of records and test results rather than direct inspection of food.
- The Clinton administration settles a suit brought against the EPA by the Natural Resources Defense Council (NRDC). The EPA agrees to evaluate whether residue amounts in 36 pesticides already known to be carcinogenic violate federal law and determine if 49 others are carcinogenic.
- By the end of the year, 35 applications to grow commercial GM crops have been approved by the FDA.

1996

- The makers of Odwalla fruit juice recall 13 types of juice after an outbreak of *E. coli* is linked to their unpasteurized juice. One 16-month-old girl dies, several children develop life-threatening kidney ailments, and 70 persons become sick.
- President Bill Clinton approves new regulations for the Hazard Analysis and Critical Control Point (HACCP) system, the new comprehensive program for food safety that officials expect will modernize their inspection system.
- The secretary of state for health in the United Kingdom, Stephen Dorrell, announces that a variant form of Creutzfeldt-Jakob disease has been found in humans and most likely is caused by the consumption of beef from cattle with BSE.
- Approximately 4.5 million cattle are destroyed in Britain to ensure the safety of beef and dairy products from BSE.
- TV talk show host Oprah Winfrey devotes one of her shows to mad cow disease and its potential to infect Americans. The show generates much controversy, leads to a lawsuit against Oprah, and raises awareness of the risks of the disease in the United States.
- The Food Quality Protection Act of 1996 allows the use of food additives that show a negligible or insignificant foreseeable risk to human health resulting from its intended use, defined generally as less than one excess cancer case per million people exposed. It replaces the zero-tolerance standard for carcinogens mandated by the 1958 Delaney Clause.

118

Chronology

- The FDA approves olestra, a synthetic fat substitute that the body's circulatory system does not absorb, as a food additive, but it also takes the unusual step of requiring a warning about its use. Some food experts argue that, despite approval, olestra is unsafe.

1997

- Contaminated frozen strawberries transmit the hepatitis A virus to 262 persons in five states.
- Dr. Stanley B. Prusiner receives the Nobel Prize in medicine for his discovery of prions, a disease agent that destroys nerve cells in the brain and causes varied forms of Creutzfeldt-Jakob disease.
- The FDA bans the use of animal protein in feed for cattle and other grazing animals in order to help prevent the spread of mad cow disease.
- An outbreak of *E. coli* O157:H7, which sickens 20 people, leads to a recall of 25 million pounds of suspected contaminated beef from Hudson Foods Company, the largest such recall in U.S. history.
- President Clinton announces an initiative called Food Safety from Farm to Table, which proposes to build a new national warning system for food disease outbreaks, develop new research methods to test for and treat foodborne illness, and improve the education of the public about food safety.
- A campaign called "Fight BAC!" creates partnerships among government, industry, and consumer groups for the purpose of educating consumers and food industry workers about the problem of foodborne illness.
- The FDA approves the use of irradiation to kill *E. coli* in red meat.

1998

- An outbreak of food poisoning caused by *Shigella* bacteria is traced to imported parsley that was harvested in unsanitary conditions. The outbreak illustrates the risks of foodborne disease in uncooked vegetables.
- Reflecting the risks of eating raw shellfish, 368 persons become ill from *Vibrio parahaemolyticus* bacteria after eating raw oysters harvested from Galveston Bay on the Texas Gulf Coast.
- In considering a lawsuit brought by Texas cattlemen, a jury rules that talk show host Oprah Winfrey and guest Howard Lyman, a former rancher turned vegetarian, had no liability for the drop in beef prices that followed Winfrey's show on mad cow disease.
- Nearly 200 people become sick in several states from a rare form of *Salmonella* in packages of cold cereal that, for unknown reasons, had become contaminated during manufacturing.

■ A report of the General Accounting Office says that federal efforts to ensure the safety of imported foods are inconsistent and unreliable. It recommends that legislation give the FDA more authority to address the problem.

1999

■ The American Public Health Association urges the FDA to ban the use of antibiotics in animals for nonmedical purposes. Used to help fatten food animals quickly and efficiently, low-dose antibiotics may also contribute to the presence of resistant bacteria in human food.

■ The Natural Resources Defense Council (NRDC) sues the EPA to force the agency to meet deadlines for testing and setting guidelines for the safety of pesticides found on food. To settle the suit, the EPA agrees to adhere to a new schedule.

2000

■ ConAgra Beef Company of Greeley, Colorado, voluntarily recalls 19 million pounds of beef that are contaminated with *E. coli* O157:H7, leading some to question the effectiveness of government meat-safety regulations.

■ As part of an effort to prevent the spread of mad cow disease to American cattle, the U.S. government bans the import of animal protein products, the source of the disease's transmission.

■ More than 60 people contract *E. coli* illness from a salad bar at a Milwaukee Sizzler Steakhouse after restaurant employees use the same knives to cut watermelon that they had used earlier to slice tainted beef. Fifteen of the victims are children; three develop severe kidney failure, and one three-year-old girl dies.

■ An environmental group, Friends of the Earth, uses genetic lab tests to confirm that taco shells made by Kraft Foods and sold in local grocery stores contain GM corn. The corn was approved for animal but not human consumption.

■ A U.S. district court rules in favor of the FDA in a suit (*Alliance for Bio-Integrity, et al. v. Donna Shalala, et al.*) that challenged the agency's rules on GM foods. The decision allows current policy, which does not require special testing and approval for the foods, to continue.

■ The sale of irradiated meat becomes legal.

2001

■ *June 5:* The FDA announces that it will reorganize the office that handles premarket approval of food additives. The Office of Food Additive

Chronology

Safety will have a division of petition review to help speed the process of review for new food additives.

- *September 11:* Terrorists use airplanes to attack buildings in New York City and Washington, D.C., and kill 3,021 persons, raising new concerns about the safety of the U.S. food supply from biological terrorism.
- *October 10:* A Senate hearing addresses problems of the food-safety system in light of the recent terrorist attacks. New calls for a single, central authority for food safety emerge but ultimately fail to produce legislation.
- *November 26:* A study by Harvard University concludes that the chances of BSE entering the United States and posing a risk to consumers and the agricultural industry are "extremely low."
- *December 6:* In *Supreme Beef v. USDA*, the Fifth Circuit Court of Appeals rules that the USDA has overstepped its authority in threatening to shut down a beef plant after tests revealed high levels of *Salmonella* in its meat.

2002

- *April 18:* The first U.S. case of variant Creutzfeldt-Jakob disease is announced by the Florida Department of Health and the Centers for Disease Control and Prevention. However, the victim grew up in Britain, where she likely consumed the meat that gave her the disease.
- *June 12:* President George W. Bush signs the Public Health Security and Bioterrorism Preparedness and Response Act of 2002, which gives the FDA new authority to protect the nation's food supply from terrorist acts.
- *October 21:* The USDA implements its new National Organic Standards program, which defines special production and handling rules for organic foods. To be labeled "organic," a product must come from a farm certified as organic by a government-approved inspector.

2003

- *January:* The U.S. Central Intelligence Agency releases a report describing an al Qaeda plot to poison food intended for British troops. The report further warns of the risk of a terrorist attack on the American food supply.
- *April 4:* The FDA lowers the level of mercury thought to be safe in the human body. Health threats from mercury in fish appear all the more serious.
- *May 22:* McDonald's chief executive, Charlie Bell, stresses the importance of food safety, which has become a particular concern to the company given declining sales in Europe over fears of mad cow disease.

121

- *August:* An article published in *Consumer Reports* summarizes the results of an analysis of irradiated meat bought in local stores. The analysis finds that the meat contains bacteria and, according to expert tasters, has an unpleasant flavor.
- *September 15:* The attorneys general of New York, Connecticut, Massachusetts, and New Jersey sue the EPA to set pesticide tolerances that protect the health of infants and children—a goal the EPA believes it is already meeting.
- *December 23:* The USDA announces that a cow in Washington State imported from Canada has BSE—the first confirmed case in the United States. Agriculture Secretary Ann M. Veneman assures the public that the agency will take actions to keep American beef safe.
- *December 30:* Agriculture Secretary Veneman announces new actions to further protect the safety of meat from slaughtered cattle. The actions include a ban on downer cows (i.e., those that cannot walk properly) from the food system and tighter restrictions on the use of brain and spinal cord parts for food.

2004

- *January 30:* The White House releases a homeland security directive for food safety that specifies the duties and goals of the diverse agencies with responsibilities for maintaining U.S. food security.
- *March 15:* Agriculture Secretary Veneman announces that the USDA will test more than 200,000 cattle a year for BSE.
- *June 30:* President Bush signs the Child Nutrition and WIC Reauthorization Act. Among other things, the act requires schools to increase food safety inspections and places restrictions on use of irradiated ground beef in schools.
- *July 28:* Tiny amounts of poison are found in two jars of baby food sold in southern California. The jars had notes that the food had been contaminated. No one was harmed, but police begin the search for the culprit behind the tampering.
- *August 3:* President Bush signs the Food Allergen Labeling and Consumer Protection Act of 2004, which requires new labels by 2006 on all products that contain major food allergens. The legislation also aims to prevent the cross-contamination of allergens in food production and to gather better data on the incidence of allergic reactions to food.
- *August 25:* The EPA releases a report stating that one of every three lakes in the United States and nearly one-quarter of the nation's rivers contain enough pollution to contaminate fish. It warns people to limit or avoid eating fish caught in many bodies of water throughout the country.

Chronology

- **September 17:** California governor Arnold Schwarzenegger vetoes the right-to-know bill, AB 1988, which would require that use of irradiated food in school lunches be made public.
- **September 20:** The FDA proposes new rules to make egg producers responsible for lowering the presence of *Salmonella* in their products.
- **September 30:** The House Committee on Energy and Commerce approves the National Uniformity for Food Act, which would require states to adopt food-safety warnings and product labels that match federal laws and regulations. Viewed by opponents as a way to end stronger state laws, the legislation has not passed the House or Senate.
- **December 3:** On resigning as the secretary of Health and Human Services, Tommy Thompson talks candidly about his worries over a possible terrorist attack on the food supply. "For the life of me," he states, "I cannot understand why the terrorists have not attacked our food supply because it is so easy to do."
- **December 6:** The FDA announces new rules for food companies that will allow better tracking of the sources of food contamination in the case of a bioterrorism attack. Records on where foods came from and were shipped to would make a quick response to such an attack possible.

2005

- **January 3:** Canada announces that it has confirmed a new case of mad cow disease in an Alberta herd of dairy cattle. The announcement generates concern in the United States over a plan to reallow the import of young cattle from Canada, which had been closed off since 2003.
- **January 20:** Reports of a study suggest that the prion protein responsible for mad cow disease can be spread from infected animals to others through the liver and kidney, not just the brain and nervous system, as previously thought. The study suggests even greater danger of diseased meat.
- **March 11:** The television show *Dateline NBC* airs information on critical health violations in 100 fast-food restaurants in each of 10 chains. The show reports that Subway, Dairy Queen, KFC, Burger King, Arby's, Hardee's, and McDonald's had critical violations ranging from 98–126 violations per 100 inspections.
- **April 13:** The European Union announces that it is drafting stricter rules to prevent the import from the United States and other countries of animal feed with GM corn. The action reflects the high degree of concern in Europe about the safety of GM crops.
- **June 24:** Secretary Johanns confirms a second case of BSE in an American cow. As a downer, the cow was blocked from use for human food. Johanns

123

argues that the disposal of the animal even before testing results had determined it had mad cow disease demonstrated the effectiveness of the system, but critics remain unconvinced of the safety of food from mad cow disease.

- *July 14:* A federal appeals court overturns a ban on the import of cows from Canada, a ban put in place in 2003, when cases of mad cow disease were found in Canadian cattle. Secretary of Agriculture Johanns states his belief that the imports will not threaten the health of American cattle, but some American cattlemen oppose the change.
- *August 29:* The FDA offers tips to Hurricane Katrina victims, who must deal with lack of fresh water, power supply, and grocery stores, on how to ensure food safety during the aftermath of the natural disaster.
- *October 4:* The FDA announces new measures to prevent the spread of BSE to American cattle. High-risk feed that may contain infected tissue, which has been banned for cattle, sheep, and other ruminants since 1997, will also be banned from feed for other animals such as pigs and pets. The policy should prevent contaminated feed from unintentionally making its way to animals likely to contract BSE.
- *October 6:* The *Washington Post* reports that the FDA is expected to approve the sale of milk and meat from cloned animals or their offspring. Despite concerns from consumer groups about the safety of such food, scientific studies find little difference between the meat and milk of cloned and normal animals. The FDA, which has been examining the issue for several years, did not make a formal announcement but appears to have decided to support the use of cloned animals for commercial purposes.
- *November 22:* The two major government food-safety agencies, the FDA and the USDA Food Safety Inspection Service, agree to meet as a way to improve consistency in national food-safety rules. The meeting is a response to critics who claim that threats to food safety require an overhaul of the fragmented food regulation system.

2006

- *January 3:* A report from the USDA inspector general criticizes the agency for lax oversight of field trials of genetically modified crops. The USDA had granted permits to grow these crops but did not always check to see if farmers followed agency rules. The agency says it has already taken steps to address the problems raised by the report. Some say, however, that the problems show the inability of the government to protect the public from the risks of GM crops.
- *March 8:* The *New York Times* reports that the number of chickens with *Salmonella* bacteria has risen 80 percent since 2000. Critics blame the increase on lack of regulation by the USDA.

Chronology

- *March 14:* A third U.S. cow is confirmed to have mad cow disease. The Alabama cow, one of 650,000 tested over the last 18 months, did not enter the food chain and does not present any risk to humans or other animals. Still, the USDA will test other cows that in the past shared the same feed as the infected cow. This announcement brings less worry to the public than past discoveries of infected cows, but some consumer groups call for added precautions to stop any further the spread of the disease.
- *June 27:* A report released by the Democratic staff of the House Committee on Government Reform accuses the FDA of lax efforts to stop food safety violations. The report cites statistics that the FDA sent out 54 percent fewer food-safety warning letters than five years earlier. Critics claim the agency favors the commercial interests of the food industry over the food-safety concerns of citizens. The FDA responds that it focuses on warning the most serious violators of food safety regulations and has improved compliance in recent years.

CHAPTER 4

BIOGRAPHICAL LISTING

This chapter contains brief biographic sketches of persons who have participated in important events and controversies involving food-safety threats in the United States. They include scientists and researchers who have made food-safety discoveries, politicians and government officials who have set policies, and advocates and citizens who have worked for changes in food safety.

Bruce N. Ames, professor of biochemistry and molecular biology at the University of California, Berkeley. Along with developing the Ames test to identify chemicals that can cause cancer, he also discovered that many ordinary and commonly consumed foods are mild carcinogens. His studies demonstrated that natural pesticides in plants, which help protect them from pests and plant-eating animals, are 10,000 times more common in the food people eat than manufactured pesticides.

Chester Arthur, 21st president of the United States, from 1881 to 1885. He signed legislation that created the Bureau of Chemistry, the forerunner of the Food Safety and Inspection Service. The bureau was charged with preventing diseased animals from being used as food.

Larry Bohlen, director of health and environment programs of the environmental group Friends of the Earth. In 2000, he presented evidence that foods sold in local supermarkets in the United States contained a genetically modified (GM) variety of corn that had been approved for animal but not human food. The announcement leads grocers to pull taco shells from shelves, manufacturers to recall shipments of corn products, and government officials to trace the source of the GM corn. In the end, the developer of the corn suspended sales of its technology to seed companies.

Patrick Boyle, president and CEO of the American Meat Institute, the industry's national trade association. He has defended the safety of American meat from accusations that it is hazardous and poorly regulated. He argues that the cooperation of the meat industry with the Food and Drug

Administration (FDA) has done much to lower the risks to health from microbial contamination of meat, noting that the industry has become one of the most heavily regulated in the country.

George W. Bush, current and 43rd president of the United States. In response to the terrorist attack on September 11, 2001, he signed into law the Public Health Security and Bioterrorism Preparedness and Response Act of 2002. Among its provisions, it aimed to protect the safety of food from terrorist attacks. To supplement the new legislation, the White House released its own homeland security directive for food safety in 2004. The directive specifies duties and goals of the many agencies that help protect American food security.

Earl Butz, secretary of agriculture from 1971 to 1976. He was the defendant in a suit brought against the U.S. Agriculture Department (USDA) by the American Public Health Association (APHA). Given that meat inspection did not require microscopic exams, the suit demanded that raw meat packages have labels warning of the risks of bacterial infection and the need for thorough cooking of meat. In *APHA v. Butz*, an appeals court ruled in 1974 that the USDA could choose education over warnings and leave its inspections, approvals, and package labels unchanged.

Stephen Churchill, English teen who became the first known person to die from variant Creutzfeldt-Jakob disease caused by consumption of meat from a cow with BSE. After developing symptoms that reminded his parents of diseased cows shown in the news, he died in 1995 at age 19.

William Clinton, 42nd president of the United States, from 1993 to 2001. In his administration, which began about the same time as the deadly *E. coli* outbreak from undercooked Jack in the Box hamburgers, he approved two major food-safety initiatives: One involved use of HACCP procedures to improve the safety of food production procedures, and another involved a program called Food Safety from Farm to Table.

Thad Cochrane, senator and the chairman of the Committee on Agriculture, Nutrition, and Forestry. Taking the lead in Senate hearings on the potential for mad cow disease to spread to cattle and humans in the United States, he reassured the public of the safety of American beef.

Lester Crawford, former deputy commissioner and commissioner of the FDA. While deputy commissioner, he testified before the U.S. Senate on the policies in place to protect the American public from mad cow disease. As acting commissioner, he continued to give priority to this goal.

Hans Creutzfeldt, German neurologist who studied brain disorders common in elderly people during the first part of the 20th century. He described the symptoms of the disease that would take his name—Creutzfeldt-Jakob disease—after observing a young woman who was hospitalized in 1912 because her legs would jerk with spasms and cause her to walk unsteadily. The woman fell into a deep coma before dying in 1913, and Creutzfeldt described the case in a 1920 article.

Francis Crick, English Nobel Prize–winning molecular biologist. Working with James Watson at Cambridge University in England, he attempted to determine the chemical structure of all living matter. Their 1953 discovery that DNA, the basic material of genes, takes the form of a double helix revolutionized the study of biology and genetics. It made possible the recombinant DNA techniques used today in the biotechnology industry to create GM foods.

James T. Delaney, former Democratic New York representative from Queens during the 1950s who chaired a House Select Committee to investigate the use of chemicals in food products. He sponsored an amendment to the 1958 Food Additives Amendment that became known as the Delaney Clause. It prohibited the use of processed food additives that could cause cancer. The clause created controversy when it led to bans on the artificial sweetener saccharin and certain farm pesticides. Congress replaced the zero-tolerance standard of the Delaney Clause in 1996 with a standard of reasonable certainty of no harm.

Rosa L. DeLaura, Democratic representative from Connecticut. As a two-year-old, she nearly died from *Salmonella* poisoning, which later contributed to her interest in food-safety issues in Congress. Also concerned over deaths from *E. coli*–contaminated food, she has aided in efforts to require better food-safety enforcement by federal agencies.

Nancy Donley, president of Safe Tables Our Priority (S.T.O.P). Her son, Alex Donley, died from an infection he acquired from eating an undercooked hamburger that contained bacteria-laden cattle feces. With other victims of the *E. coli* outbreak, she founded S.T.O.P., an organization devoted to protecting the public from illness and death caused by foodborne disease. Besides serving as president of this organization, Donley has become a member of the National Advisory Committee on Meat and Poultry Inspection and has received several honors for leadership on meat safety reforms.

Stephen Dorrell, former British secretary of state for health. In 1996, he announced to Parliament and the world that a variant form of Creutzfeldt-Jakob disease had been discovered among humans and that it most likely stemmed from eating beef from cattle with BSE. The announcement confirmed worries of the public that they were at risk from British beef, and it contradicted claims made for many years that no such risk existed.

Richard J. Durbin, Democratic senator from Illinois since 1996 and Assistant Minority Leader since 2004. While carefully noting that American food is the safest in the world, he remains a critic of the U.S. food-safety system. He calls it duplicative, costly, fractured, and unduly complicated, and he believes it can be improved. Toward that end, he has worked on legislation to form a single food-safety agency, but the legislation has so far failed to pass Congress.

Lawrence J. Dyckman, director, Natural Resources and Environment in the U.S. Government Accountability Office (GAO). In developing legislation, the U.S. Congress depends on the GAO for evaluation of programs and policies. Dyckman has authored reports on numerous food-safety issues: protection against mad cow disease, school lunches, meat and poultry inspection, and the benefits of a single food-safety agency. He also testifies often before Congress on food-safety issues.

Bertha Elschker, first person to be labeled as having what would come to be known as Creutzfeldt-Jakob disease. She was hospitalized in 1912 because her legs would jerk with spasms, and she walked unsteadily. Over the next year, the symptoms worsened. She would fall over while standing, refuse to eat or bathe, scream that she was possessed of the devil, and appear dazed and confused. Falling into a deep coma, she died in 1913. Dr. Hans Creutzfeldt described the case in a 1920 article.

Carol Tucker Foreman, director of the Food Policy Institute at the Consumer Federation of America, a consumer advocacy organization. Foreman argues that the meat supply in America is not safe enough and that the government needs more authority to shut down unclean meatpacking plants. She has also criticized the USDA and Bush administration for not taking additional steps to protect cattle and the public from mad cow disease.

D. Carleton Gajdusek, Nobel Prize–winning physician. He studied an unusual disease called kuru, a word referring to trembling, that was common in the Fore Tribe region of New Guinea. After visiting the region, living with the tribe, and performing autopsies on kuru victims, Gajdusek concluded that the disease was spread by eating the brains of deceased relatives. After ending this cannibalistic tradition, the disease largely disappeared within a generation. Gajdusek won the Nobel Prize in medicine in 1976 for this discovery.

Daniel Glickman, former congressional representative from Kansas and secretary of agriculture from 1995 to 2001. While secretary of agriculture in the Clinton administration, he implemented the HACCP system for meat safety and several other food-safety initiatives. Since leaving this position, he has argued for a single food-safety organization and more government power to enforce food-safety regulations. He believes that the safety of the food supply has continued to improve, but the increasing centralization of food production raises the potential for error.

John Grummer, former British agriculture minister. In 1990, he hoped to dramatize the safety of British beef by eating a hamburger with his

129

four-year-old daughter Cordelia in front of a television camera. At the time, concerns had emerged that mad cow disease might spread to humans. Officials denied this possibility and downplayed the risk of eating beef, but events would later prove them—and Grummer—wrong.

Jane E. Henney, commissioner of the Food and Drug Administration from 1998 to 2001. As commissioner, Henney defended the safety of GM foods and also strengthened the premarket review of these foods to convince the public of their safety. Although critics claim that the review simply involves notification of intent to market a GM food rather than careful evaluation and testing, Henney continued to support the FDA policy and GM foods more generally.

Michael Jacobson, executive director of the Center for Science and the Public Interest (CSPI), a nutrition and food-safety organization. He has been a leading critic of the FDA for approving what he views as dangerous food additives, lax meat-inspection standards, and unproven technologies such as food irradiation and GM foods. Critics claim that he exaggerates the risks of popular foods.

Alfons Jakob, German psychiatrist who headed a state hospital. Observing several patients in the 1920s who initially complained of weakness in their legs, later had difficulty walking, and still later exhibited loss of mental capacity, he identified a new disease that would take the name Creutzfeldt-Jakob disease, or CJD. Like Dr. Hans Creutzfeldt, Jakob noticed that the brains of victims of the disease were spongy in nature and had nerve cells with holes.

Mike Johanns, former governor of Nebraska who was appointed secretary of the Department of Agriculture in 2005. In his position as secretary, he has listed three top priorities for funding, all related to food safety. The first is to protect against an outbreak of BSE and increase funding for testing cattle and developing a national animal identification system. The second is a food and agriculture defense system to protect against intentional terrorist threats or unintentional contamination. The third is to improve the nation's food inspection system and reduce the incidence of foodborne disease.

Frances Moore Lappé, author, well-known vegetarian, and founder of the Small Planet Institute. Her book *Diet for a Small Planet* argues that meat consumption contributes directly to world hunger by devoting excessive grain production to animal feed. She has worked on behalf of ending world hunger and more recently has addressed issues of GM foods, which many believe can help solve the problem by allowing farmers in poor countries to plant hardier and more nutritious crops. However, Lappé views GM foods as a threat to health, food safety, and the environment.

Biographical Listing

Howard Lyman, executive director of the Humane Society's Eating with Conscience program. As a guest on the *Oprah TV* show on mad cow disease, the former rancher turned vegetarian told Oprah that parts of dead cattle were still being fed to live cattle in the United States, a practice that could spread BSE much as it did in Britain. Along with Oprah Winfrey, he was sued by Texas cattlemen for making what they said were false and defamatory remarks about beef; he was acquitted by a jury.

Mary Mallon, Irish immigrant known as Typhoid Mary. A carrier of typhus bacteria who, unusually, did not get sick from typhoid fever, she still passed the disease from her hands to the food she prepared and caused others to get sick. Perhaps suffering from mental illness, she refused to stop cooking when told about being contagious. In 1907, she was arrested, quarantined, and called the most dangerous woman in America. Released in 1910 after promising not to cook for the public again, she continued to do so anyway, spreading typhoid fever through food wherever she went.

Mark B. McClellan, commissioner of the Food and Drug Administration from 2002 to 2004. During his tenure, he responded to two major problems involving food safety. First, he addressed concerns about the safety of beef caused by the discovery of a cow infected with BSE. The FDA made efforts to ban from human foods and dietary supplements any tissues from cattle with a high risk of BSE infection. Second, he increased inspections of domestic food facilities and imported foods to prevent contamination by terrorists.

Elsa Murano, undersecretary for food safety at the USDA from 2001 to 2004 and currently vice chancellor of agriculture for the Texas A&M University System, dean of the College of Agriculture at Texas A&M University–College Station, and director of the Texas Agricultural Experiment Station. An advocate of the use of science-based efforts to reduce foodborne illness, Dr. Murano used her background as a microbiologist to help cut the incidence of foodborne illness by 36 percent and reduce the number of food recalls. She also emphasized the importance of educating consumers about food safety.

Marion Nestle, professor and director of public health initiatives in the Department of Nutrition, Food Studies, and Public Health at New York University. She has criticized the food industry for failing to meet the health needs of the public with the products it sells and for focusing primarily on its economic interests. Her writings on topics ranging from GM crops to biotechnology, foodborne illness, and bioterrorism emphasize the inadequate attention given by corporations and the government to food safety.

Stanley B. Prusiner, Nobel Prize–winning physician. While doing research on CJD in his medical residency, he failed to find any evidence of

131

the presence of a virus. However, he later discovered an unusual, deformed protein in the brain cells of CJD victims that he called a prion. The prion seemed to disrupt the normal operation of other proteins in the brain, ultimately destroying nerve cells and producing holes in infected brains. For this discovery, Prusiner received the 1997 Nobel Prize in medicine.

Arpad Pusztai, scientist and researcher in Scotland. His research found that a GM potato developed to be resistant to pests was also poisonous to lab rats. Arguing that the results of this study reflect risks inherent in all GM products, he has become a leading critic of genetic engineering. However, many scientists dismiss his findings as based on flawed methods, and his claims have led to much controversy.

Bhagwan Shree Rajneesh, leader of a religious commune in Oregon. Members of his group caused the illness of 751 people by poisoning a salad bar with *Salmonella* in the hope, however illogical, of influencing a local election in their favor. Fortunately, no one died from the poisoning, but the ability to make people sick by infecting restaurant dishes illustrates the potential danger of food terrorism.

Tom Ridge, former governor of Pennsylvania, the first director of the Office of Homeland Security, from 2001 to 2003, and the first secretary of the Department of Homeland Security, from 2003 to 2004. In his homeland security positions, he responded to the September 11, 2001, terrorist attacks by working on a coordinated strategy to protect the country from future attacks. Among many other things, he attempted to implement polices to protect agriculture and the food supply from terrorism.

Jeremy Rifkin, author and director of the Foundation on Economic Trends. Highly critical of the risks brought on by biotechnology, he has fought against GM products in Europe as well as in the United States. In Europe, he helped persuade leaders to hold off further approval of GM crops. In the United States, he filed a class-action suit against Monsanto, a company developing biotech products.

Vicky Rimmer, the first known victim of variant Creutzfeldt-Jakob disease, the human form of mad cow disease. After experiencing unusual health problems, the 16-year-old Welsh girl fell into a coma in 1993 and died in 1997.

Theodore Roosevelt, 26th president of the United States, from 1901 to 1909. Repulsed by the slaughterhouse practices described in Upton Sinclair's novel *The Jungle,* he became actively involved in government efforts to improve food safety and was instrumental in overcoming resistance in Congress to passing new food-safety laws. He signed two major pieces of legislation in 1906, the Pure Food and Drug Act and the Meat Inspection Act.

Biographical Listing

Morton Satin, molecular biologist, author, and former chief of Agricultural Industries and Post-Harvest Management Service of the Food and Agricultural Organization of the United Nations. In that position, he helped promote the use of food irradiation, particularly in the developing world, as a means of limiting the risks of foodborne disease.

Eric Schlosser, award-winning journalist and correspondent for the *Atlantic Monthly*. A critic of food companies and their products, he has described in many magazine articles and in the book *Fast Food Nation: The Dark Side of the All-American Meal* that factory farms and meatpacking plants need to supply the huge demand for fast food. He argues that ineffective federal oversight leads to contamination of this food and makes eating in the United States "a high-risk behavior."

Upton Sinclair, author of the 1906 exposé, *The Jungle*. Based on his observations of activities in a slaughterhouse and meatpacking plant, the novel described the filthy conditions used to produce meat for sale. At least in part a response to his book, Congress passed the Pure Food and Drug Act and the Meat Inspection Act in 1906.

Robert Tauxe, the chief of the Foodborne and Diarrheal Diseases Branch of the Centers for Disease Control and Prevention. In his position, he helps track and control the incidence of foodborne disease. He notes that after rising from the 1950s to the 1980s, foodborne illness appears to have declined since the 1990s. He advocates the use of technology, including irradiation, to protect food from contamination by bacteria and viruses.

Tommy Thompson, secretary of Health and Human Services from 2001 to 2004. On resigning as secretary, he talked candidly about his worries over a possible terrorist attack on the food supply, noting that it would be easy for enemies of the United States to do. The comments created controversy because they might have led terrorists to consider such an attack, but experts agree that a serious risk for food terrorism remains.

Abigail Trafford, health columnist and former health editor of the *Washington Post*. In one column, she called fears about getting mad cow disease from eating beef irrational, arguing that other foodborne illnesses are much more common and more likely to do harm. She believes that Americans should worry about these other more serious and immediate food-safety problems.

Ann Veneman, Department of Agriculture Secretary from 2001 to 2005. She announced in December 2003 the discovery of the first case of mad cow disease in the United States and then quickly acted to identify the source of the disease and prevent it from spreading. New policies and procedures implemented the next year banned downer animals from the food system and tightened restrictions on the use of brain and spinal cord parts for food.

James Watson, American Nobel Prize–winning molecular biologist. Working with Francis Crick at Cambridge University in England, he attempted to determine the chemical structure of all living matter. Their 1953 discovery that DNA, the basic material of genes, takes the form of a double helix revolutionized the study of biology and genetics. It made possible the recombinant DNA techniques used today in the biotechnology industry and to create GM food.

Christine Todd Whitman, former governor of New Jersey and administrator of the Environmental Protection Agency (EPA) from 2001 to 2003. In her position, she settled a suit over the lack of progress of the EPA in evaluating acceptable levels of pesticide residue on food. The EPA also entered into a settlement agreement—an agreement to come to terms in a suit without a court decision—that would lead to new tests for the harmful effects of pesticides.

Harvey W. Wiley, physician, scientist, and, in the view of many, founding father of the FDA. To demonstrate the risk of some food additives, he obtained volunteers in 1902 to eat food that contained borax or several other poisonous substances used as preservatives. He and his scientists concluded that these preservatives could cause dangerous health problems by accumulating over time. Their findings were a first step in ending the use of dangerous additives in food.

Oprah Winfrey, popular television talk show host who devoted one of her shows to mad cow disease. Soon after the 1996 announcement from the British government that eating beef with BSE likely caused several deaths from vCJD, she invited several guests on the show, including Howard Lyman, who claimed that BSE represented a major public health threat. In learning that cattle eat food made from other cattle, Oprah said, "That just stopped me cold from eating another burger." The day after the program was broadcast, cattle prices dropped more than 10 percent, causing the industry to lose an estimated $36 million in two weeks. Responding to the loss, a group of Texas cattlemen used a 1995 Texas statute to sue Oprah and Lyman for estimated losses of $12 million. However, a Texas trial cleared them of all charges.

CHAPTER 5

GLOSSARY

Since many of the terms needed to understand food-safety issues have specialized meanings, this chapter lists and defines the terms for general readers.

acrylamide A cancer-causing chemical used for a variety of industrial purposes, such as plastic manufacturing and wastewater treatment, that has been detected in a wide range of food products.

adulterate To make impure by adding an inferior or harmful substance that deceives buyers about the content, manufacture, safety, or size of the product.

aflatoxin A natural toxin sometimes found in peanuts, peanut butter, and corn that is produced by mold and can cause liver problems and cancer.

agroterrorism The use of biological weapons by terrorists to destroy animals, crops, and food in order to harm societies or governments.

Alar A chemical no longer in use that when sprayed on apples helps them ripen on the tree but, according to some disputed evidence, can cause cancer in children.

allergen A substance that causes an allergic or immune system response.

anaphylactic shock A life-threatening condition that produces a sudden drop in blood pressure, inability to breathe, and loss of body temperature in response to a severe allergic reaction.

antibiotic A drug that kills bacteria and is used to treat many infectious diseases.

antibody A protein that is produced by the body to destroy or neutralize pathogens but which sometimes reacts to harmless food among those with food allergies.

antioxidant Food preservative that prevents or slows oxidation and can retard spoilage from mold, bacteria, and air (e.g., bread from becoming moldy and dry, and fats and baked goods from becoming rancid and sour).

arsenic A strong poison that enters the air from metal extraction during manufacturing and the burning of fossil fuels and from there can get into plants through soil and water and then into humans through food.

135

aspartame (Nutrasweet) A low-calorie artificial sweetener that replaces sugar in diet soft drinks, diet foods, and Equal packets; despite some controversy, the FDA has approved it as safe.

bacterium Small, single-celled organism that reproduces quickly and often causes illness.

biological agent A bacterium, virus, or toxin used in bioterrorism or biological warfare.

biotechnology The application of biological knowledge to improve human life; it includes traditional forms of plant and animal breeding as well as genetic engineering of food.

bioterrorism The use of living agents, such as human-made or natural biological agents, to attack people, animals, and plants.

borax A mineral that is poisonous in large amounts and used today to kill ants but was once used as a preservative in flour and other foods to prevent them from spoiling.

bovine growth hormone Given to cows to increase milk production, it was originally extracted from the cow pituitary gland but is now created artificially using genetic engineering.

bovine spongiform encephalopathy (BSE) The scientific name for mad cow disease, with "bovine" referring to cows, "spongiform" to the spongelike change in tissue, and "encephalopathy" to a disease of the brain.

butylated hydroxyanisole (BHA) A synthetic antioxidant added to food that reacts with oxygen and helps maintain the color, taste, and odor of the food.

butylated hydroxytoluene (BHT) A synthetic antioxidant added to food that reacts with oxygen and helps maintain the color, taste, and odor of the food.

cadmium A heavy metal often used in batteries that is released into the air during manufacturing and into the soil as part of fertilizers; it may be absorbed by crops and vegetables and cause kidney damage in humans.

Campylobacter jejuni A bacterial species spread by food, typically poultry contaminated with fecal matter, that causes diarrhea among more than a million persons each year.

carcass The dead body of an animal, especially one slaughtered for food.

carcinogenic Capable of causing cancer.

cholera A bacterial disease caused by ingestion of infected water or food that causes diarrhea, abdominal cramps, nausea, vomiting, and dehydration.

chronic wasting disease A form of transmissible spongiform encephalopathy that infects wild and captive deer and elk in several parts of the country but does not yet appear to be a threat to humans.

Clostridium botulinum A bacterial species that remains dormant until it finds low oxygen and acid conditions—the environment of canned prod-

Glossary

ucts—in which it can produce a nerve toxin that causes botulism, a disease characterized by paralysis, breathing failure, and death.

cold pasteurization An alternate name for food irradiation used by advocates to make the process sound familiar and comforting.

contaminate To make impure or unclear by introducing substances that are harmful or unfit for use.

counterterrorism A strategy intended to prevent terrorism.

Creutzfeldt-Jakob disease (CJD) A rare neurological disease that causes mental deterioration, involuntary movements, blindness, extremity weakness, and death in the later stages of life. See also variant Creutzfeldt-Jakob disease (vCJD).

cross-contamination The transfer of disease or toxic elements from one source to another, such as the transfer of allergens in one food to other foods during manufacturing.

Cry9C A gene from bacteria that was inserted into a corn gene to create a new insect-resistant genetically modified crop.

Cryptosporidium A microscopic parasite that lives in the intestines of animals and humans, is spread through contaminated drinking water and food, and causes diarrhea for one to two weeks.

cyanide A highly toxic and fast-acting poison when ingested in large doses.

cyclobutanone A chemical that is produced by food irradiation and may promote cancerous tumors.

Cyclospora cayetanensis A single-cell parasite that has been found to infect water and fresh produce, particularly in developing countries, and causes diarrhea, cramps, bloating, weight loss, and persistent fatigue.

dioxin A poisonous chemical that results from commercial incineration and burning of wood, coal, and oil. It can be widely distributed throughout the environment and can harm humans who eat plants, animals, and fish with the substance.

Deoxyribonucleic acid (DNA) A molecule found primarily in the nucleus of cells that carries the instructions for making all the structures and materials the body needs to function.

double helix Twin, parallel spirals that form the structure of DNA.

downer Term referring to a cow that, for a variety of reasons, cannot stand or walk, is more likely than others to have BSE, and has been banned from the food system in the United States.

E. coli **O157:H7** A strain of the normally harmless bacteria that is resistant to antibiotics, poisons the blood supply and organs, and can cause death, particularly among young children.

emulsifier Additive that allows oil and water to form a stable mixture and produce a consistent and appetizing texture and smoothness in foods such as salad dressings, peanut butter, salt, and cocoa.

epinephrine A quick-acting hormone that treats anaphylactic shock by widening the passages to the lungs, constricting the vessels to increase blood pressure, and increasing the beating of the heart.

Escherichia coli (E. coli) A species of bacteria found in the intestines of warm-blooded animals and necessary for the proper digestion of food.

factory farm A large-scale farming enterprise that raises livestock, poultry, and fish in small areas and uses hormones, antibiotics, and processed feed.

fecal Having to do with feces or solid waste from the digestive tract of humans or animals.

feline spongiform encephalopathy A form of prion disease that affects cats; the first case suggested that BSE had crossed species from cattle to cats (and therefore could cross species to infect humans).

Flavr Savr A genetically modified tomato that does not spoil as quickly as conventional tomatoes, can be allowed to ripen longer on the vine and fully develop its flavor, and can be shipped and stored for longer periods without rotting.

food additive A substance not normally consumed as a food by itself or as a food ingredient but which is added to food by the manufacturer to improve the appearance, texture, flavor, quality, production, or nutritional value of foods.

food allergy An abnormal immune response that is triggered by food and results in swelling, itchiness, sneezing, and sometimes difficulty in breathing and swallowing.

foodborne disease Illness caused by ingesting food with harmful bacteria, viruses, parasites, or toxins.

food intolerance A typically discomforting but sometimes life-threatening response to certain foods and additives that does not involve an allergic reaction of the immune system but can produce similar symptoms.

food irradiation Subjecting food to special forms of radiant energy such as gamma rays, electron beams, and X-rays (sometimes call ionizing radiation) that kill or damage microorganisms in food.

food poisoning An acute, often severe gastrointestinal disorder characterized by vomiting and diarrhea and caused by foodborne diseases.

food sensitivity A term referring to either a food allergy or food intolerance.

food terrorism A form of bioterrorism that involves contaminating food to infect consumers with disease.

frankenfood A slang term for genetically modified food that is used by opponents to make the food sound bizarre, hazardous, and unappetizing.

fungicide Chemical designed to control fungi that harm crops.

genetically modified (GM) Characteristic of a plant or animal organism that has altered or transferred genes from another type of organism.

genetic engineering Altering or transferring genes from one type of organism to another.

Glossary

glucosinolates A natural toxin found in small amounts in cabbage, cauliflower, Brussels sprouts, broccoli, kale, kohlrabies, turnips, radishes, mustard, and rutabagas that can inhibit the uptake of iodine by the thyroid when digested.

gluten A substance found in wheat and grain products, particularly bread, that some people cannot digest and which can cause nausea, loss of appetite, abdominal pain, and malaise.

glycoalkaloids A natural toxin that can show up as a greenish tinge on the skin of potatoes, irritate the mouth and stomach, and, more rarely, cause death.

hepatitis A A viral disease that can infect people through food; takes several weeks to develop; begins with symptoms of diarrhea, nausea, and fever; and later inflames the liver and produces jaundice.

herbicide Chemical designed to control weeds.

histamine Chemical released by the body during an allergic reaction.

hormone A naturally occurring chemical in the body that helps control growth, development, and reproduction; extra doses given to cattle can shorten the growth time and improve milk production.

human growth hormone A natural hormone that regulates growth of the body and in a synthetic form can be used to stimulate growth; its use appears to be related to Creutzfeldt-Jakob disease.

immune system Parts of the body responsible for fighting diseases by identifying foreign substances (bacteria, viruses, or parasites) and developing a defense against them.

infection A disease state resulting from the invasion of the body by harmful microorganisms.

insecticide Chemical designed to kill insects.

integrated pest management Methods to minimize the use of chemical pesticides, including planting pest-resistant crops, spraying pesticides only when tests show they are necessary, and rotating crops to prevent pests from becoming established.

ionizing radiation Special forms of radiant energy such as gamma rays, electron beams, and X-rays used in food irradiation.

kuru A term for an unusual disease once common in the Fore Tribe region of New Guinea that was spread by eating the brains of deceased relatives; it was shown to be a form of Creutzfeldt-Jakob Disease.

lactose A sugar found in milk that many have trouble digesting and which is a common source of food intolerance.

lead A heavy metal that was once a component of paint and gasoline and can cause neurological damage when ingested through food or other means.

lectins A natural toxin contained in kidney beans that can cause severe stomachaches, vomiting, and diarrhea.

Listeria monocytogenes   A bacterial species found in a wide variety of foods that does not harm most people but is highly dangerous to small parts of the population.

mad cow disease   The informal name of BSE, a brain disease of cattle first identified in England, in which victims have trouble walking and behave unusually; it is related to variant Creutzfeldt-Jakob disease (vCJD) in humans.

meatpacking   Process of slaughtering, processing, and packaging meat products for sale.

mercury   A heavy metal that when released into the environment by manufacturing accumulates in fish and in humans through fish consumption; in sufficient amounts, it can cause neurological damage, particularly to the fetuses of pregnant women.

microbe   An organism too small to be seen without a microscope.

microbiology   The study of microorganisms—those too small to be seen by the naked eye—such as bacteria, viruses, and molds.

monosodium glutamate (MSG)   A saltlike flavoring agent that has been reported to cause headaches, dizziness, and flushness in some people.

mutation   An alteration in the genetic material of a cell caused by, among other things, irradiation and some chemicals.

natural food   Food that does not include artificial additives but which does not necessarily use organically grown ingredients.

Norwalk virus   A foodborne virus belonging to a family of similar diseases called noroviruses that causes vomiting, nausea, abdominal pains, and diarrhea for a period of one or two days.

nukeburger   A slang term for irradiated burgers or meat that is used by opponents to make the food sound bizarre, hazardous, and unappetizing.

olestra   A synthetic fat that the body does not absorb and which passes directly through the intestines to stools. It may improve health by replacing the intake of normal fats; however, some view the product as unsafe.

organic food   Food that is grown or raised without using sewer sludge fertilizer, most chemical fertilizers, synthetic pesticides, nonorganic animal feed, growth hormones, antibiotic-laced feed, genetically engineered organisms, or irradiation.

pasteurization   The process developed by Louis Pasteur of heating milk or other liquids to destroy microorganisms that can cause disease or spoilage.

pathogen   A disease-causing organism such as a bacterium, virus, or parasite.

perchlorate   An ingredient used in rocket fuel and manufacturing processes that makes its way into water and soil and then can contaminate vegetables and milk.

pesticide   Chemical designed to control insects (insecticide), fungi (fungicide), weeds (herbicide), and other diseases and pests.

Glossary

prion A deformed protein often transmitted through infected food and thought to cause several forms of neurological disease related to Creutzfeldt-Jakob disease and mad cow disease.

protein Along with carbohydrates and fat, a major source of calories in the diet; it most often comes from meat, helps to build muscle and body mass, and sometimes is added to feed to speed the growth of food animals.

al Qaeda An international Islamic terrorist network that claimed responsibility for the September 11 attacks and, before then, had bombed U.S. embassies in Kenya and Tanzania and the USS *Cole;* despite efforts since September 11 to destroy the group, it remains a worldwide threat.

quarantine The separation or isolation of persons, animals, or plants to prevent the spread of communicable diseases or pests.

radiation Released energy that commonly takes the form of light and heat but can also take the form of microwaves and radio and television waves.

radioactive Giving off dangerous forms of radiant energy.

Roundup Ready A genetically modified soybean that is resistant to herbicides and allows farmers to use herbicides to kill weeds without harming the crops.

ruminants Grazing animals such as cows, sheep, goats, and deer.

Salmonella A family of bacteria often found in the intestines of animals that is a major source of food poisoning when transferred to meat, poultry, and eggs.

scrapie A prion disease among sheep that leads them to scratch themselves intensely and eventually begin to stagger, shake, go blind, and die; it does not infect humans but is similar to mad cow disease.

Shigella A family of bacteria usually associated with poor sanitation and hygiene that causes diarrhea in humans.

sight, touch, and smell methods Procedures to examine the safety of meat and food without the use of microscopes and other advanced equipment.

sodium nitrate A preservative that maintains the color and flavor of bacon, ham, frankfurters, lunch meat, smoked fish, and corned beef.

sodium nitrite A preservative that maintains the color and flavor of bacon, ham, frankfurters, lunch meat, smoked fish, and corned beef.

species A distinctive group of related organisms that have similar form and characteristics.

StarLink A brand name for genetically modified corn approved for consumption by animals; it created much controversy when it turned up in food sold for humans.

steroid A family of organic compounds that includes sex hormones and can affect the growth of muscle mass; some are approved as growth promoters in cattle and sheep.

stockyard Enclosed area where livestock such as cattle, pigs, and sheep are kept, often before being slaughtered for food.

sulfite An additive used to preserve dried fruits, wines, and dried potato products that can cause severe allergy-like reactions in some.

surveillance Close observation or monitoring of behavior or health, as in the surveillance of cattle for BSE.

tartrazine (yellow dye no. 5) An additive that helps produce shades of cream, orange, and green in foods but also can cause itching or hives in some people.

technology The application of science to commercial, industrial, or practical goals.

terrorism The unlawful or threatened use of force or violence with the intention of intimidating or coercing societies or governments, often for political reasons.

tolerance The level of exposure to potentially harmful amounts of a substance that does not produce an adverse effect.

toxicology The study of the toxic or harmful effects of chemicals and substances on the body.

toxin A poisonous substance that can cause illness, injury, or death.

Toxoplasma gondii A parasite that proliferates in cats but also can be spread to humans by undercooked pork, lamb, beef, and wild game, where it can cause flu-like symptoms and sometimes more severe sickness.

transgenic Term applied to a crop that contains a gene transferred from another organism.

transmissible spongiform encephalopathy (TSE) Strains of prion-caused brain disease in which tissue becomes sponge-like in texture; it includes scrapie, BSE, and vCJD.

typhoid fever A life-threatening bacterial infection caused by *Salmonella typhi* that is often transmitted by contaminated water, food, or milk.

variant Creutzfeldt-Jakob disease (vCJD) A new form of CJD likely caused by the prion proteins contained in beef from cows with BSE.

Vibrio parahaemolyticus A bacterial species that resides in coastal waters and infects shellfish inhabiting those waters; it typically infects humans who eat raw oysters and clams in the summer months.

virus A piece of DNA wrapped in a thin coat of protein that replicates in the cells of living hosts, often causes disease, and is not affected by antibiotics.

Yersinia enterocolitica A bacterial species that is spread to humans most often from undercooked pork and other food coming in contact with the unwashed hands of cooks handling pork products.

zero tolerance Strict enforcement of rules that, for example, defines the presence of potentially harmful pesticides in any amount as unacceptable.

PART II

GUIDE TO FURTHER RESEARCH

CHAPTER 6

HOW TO RESEARCH THREATS TO FOOD SAFETY

Because threats to food safety come from so many sources, the topic covers a wide variety of issues. Bacteria, mad cow disease, terrorist contamination, chemical additives, pesticide residue, natural plant toxins, food allergens, and new technologies such as food irradiation and genetic engineering all define a large field of study. They present enough in the way of literature—and controversy—to overwhelm those new to the topic. As a help to research on threats to food safety, this chapter offers some general suggestions, followed by more specific advice about where to find material and what Internet and print resources to consult.

To get started, review the general orientation provided by the first chapters of this volume. Skim this material and then use it as a guide for subsequent reading. Next examine the annotated bibliography in chapter 7 and the list of organizations concerned with food safety in chapter 8. These chapters can help identify key references and organize the vast amount of available information. Even with this help, however, those doing research on food safety will face several challenges.

First, writings on the topic span a variety of fields of study. Food safety relates to general issues of microbiology, meat processing, animal disease, homeland security, food chemistry, public health, public policy, nutrition, law, and food technology. It depends on knowledge of the long-term harm of food additives and technology, effectiveness of government enforcement, certain legislation and court decisions, the epidemiology of diseases, and many other specialized topics.

Second, the literature on the topic reflects economic interests and strong political views that often make it hard to separate facts from beliefs. These views come into play, for example, in debates over the proper degree of government intervention in farming and food production. All agree that a certain amount of government control is essential for food safety, but much

145

Threats to Food Safety

disagreement exists otherwise. On one side, consumer advocates criticize businesses for focusing more on profits than food safety and demand greater government power to enforce food safety laws. Liberals and Democrats who generally favor greater government regulation of the marketplace tend to take this view, as do leaders from urban states and areas that have large populations of consumers and few producers. On the other side, businesses and trade associations claim that current policies work well, complain that accusations made against them about food safety are exaggerated or plain wrong, and believe that changes will do more harm than good. Similar views come from conservatives and Republicans, who generally promote business interests and the free market, and from leaders of states and areas with large farm economies.

Third, studies of threats to food safety often cover technically difficult material. In some cases, the difficulties come from the terminology of microbiology, disease, and food chemistry. In other cases, they come from trying to determine the long-term harm of certain foods and additives. Sometimes the harm is immediate and apparent, such as when food contains life-threatening *E. coli* O157:H7 bacteria or less dangerous *Salmonella* bacteria. More often, however, the harm is less immediate. No one has contracted vCJD from meat eaten in the United States; the threat from food terrorism is real but as yet unrealized; and the harm from food additives, food irradiation, and GM foods may not appear for decades. Future risks from these threats can only be estimated and even then the validity of the estimates is hard to evaluate.

How can researchers overcome these challenges? Some helpful tips include:

- **Define the Topic and Questions Carefully:** Rather than researching the general topic of foodborne disease, instead research more precisely defined topics such as the new threats from *E. coli* O157:H7, the effectiveness of the government meat inspection system, or the risks of disease from eating sushi and rare meat. Similarly, researching the risks of mad cow disease spreading to the United States, the vulnerability of imported food to contamination by terrorists, or the scientific evidence on the risks of pesticide residue on food would be better than researching broad topics such as mad cow disease, bioterrorism, or food additives. With so many choices available, making the research manageable requires care and precision in selecting topics. Doing so can help avoid feeling overwhelmed by all the material on food safety and allow for an in-depth treatment of the selected topic.
- **Consider the Underlying Perspectives:** Relying on a variety of sources will help make sense of the differing economic interests and political beliefs that shape views on food safety. Toward that end, the annotated lit-

146

erature review in the next chapter includes a wide selection of readings that represent all perspectives. In addition, however, it helps to note the background and potential biases of the authors. Such information can help separate opinions from facts and emotion from reason.

• **Search for Balance:** Since complex questions about threats to food safety seldom have simple answers, do not accept claims at face value. Rather, search for balanced presentations based on evidence—even if highly technical—and careful weighing of the alternatives. Researchers should seek, for example, a balanced understanding of both the risks to the population from food dangers and the costs of prevention and enforcement. They need not fully understand the scientific issues debated in studies of food safety but can recognize the need to treat all sides of the debates fairly.

The rest of this chapter reviews various types of research resources. It considers online resources, print resources, and resources related to law and legislation.

ONLINE RESOURCES

GENERAL SITES

Given its ease in providing information, the Internet offers a good place to begin research on food safety. The web contains a wide variety of research, reference, and opinion pieces on the topic that can be easily accessed with an Internet connection. Useful facts and perspectives on nearly any aspect of threats to food safety can be found by patiently working through even a small portion of available web pages. Finding one suitable page suggests links to others, which in turn lead in new directions. Innovative ideas and fresh information emerge in this process.

However, the extraordinary wealth of information that the Internet makes available to researchers can be overwhelming. For instance, a Google search of the term "food safety" results in nearly 8 million hits—an impressive but dauntingly large number. The advice to define narrow topics for research applies particularly to using the Internet. Otherwise, combing through all the web sites listed by searches can result in wasted effort. In addition, the information obtained does not always meet standards of reliability and balance. Users must take care in using materials obtained from web sites and inquire into the background of the site sponsors. With these qualifications in mind, Internet research can proceed in several ways.

Popular and general search engines such as Google (http://www.google.com), Yahoo! (http://www.yahoo.com), Altavista (http://www.altavista.com), Excite (http://www.excite.com), MSN (http://www.msn.com), Lycos (http://www.lycos.com), Ask Jeeves (http://www.ask.com), and many others can identify web sites that contain food-safety terms. Using these search engines requires thoughtful selection of search terms and patient effort to find sometimes unexpected and intriguing information.

The web also includes directories or indexes relevant to food safety. In Yahoo!, a helpful directory of web sites, information, and organizations can be found by going to the Yahoo! home page. Click "Directory," then type in general search terms such as "food safety" and more specific terms such as "foodborne disease" or "mad cow disease."

Google also has a directory with a broad list of topics. On the Google home page, click "More" and then "Directory." At this point, type search terms in "Directory" or click "Science," "Technology," "Food Science," and "Food Safety."

Other directories besides those of Yahoo! and Google are available. Of particular interest, About.com (http://www.about.com) provides background information on a variety of food-safety topics. Simply search for appropriate terms from the home page.

The medical and scientific nature of food-safety topics warrants use of web encyclopedias. For example, the Medline Plus Medical Encyclopedia (http://www.nlm.nih.gov/medlineplus/encyclopedia.html) contains information on types of food-based diseases, bacteria, viruses, and many medical terms. Users can browse entries alphabetically or search for specific keywords.

ORGANIZATION SITES

Knowledge of key organizations—government, business, consumer, and research—is crucial for researching threats to food safety. Chapter 8 lists a wide variety of such organizations, but consulting the home pages of a few particularly important ones can help get the research started.

Two key government agencies deal extensively with food-safety issues: the Center for Food Safety and Applied Nutrition (http://vm.cfsan.fda.gov/list.html) and the Food and Drug Administration (http://www.fda.gov). The American Meat Institute (http://www.meatami.com) and the Center for Science and the Public Interest (http://www.cspinet.org) can be expected to take opposite views on most food-safety issues. Two research organizations also tend to take differing views: The International Food Information Council (http://www.ific.org) tends to favor business, and the American Public Health Association (http://www.apha.org) represents public health professionals.

SITES ON SPECIFIC FOOD-SAFETY TOPICS

Along with finding resources from broad—and perhaps overwhelming—general searches, it helps to begin a search within particular sites. Here are some recommendations organized by the major threats to food illness:

How to Research Threats to Food Safety

- **Food Additives:** Web pages offer wide diversity of viewpoints on this topic. A middle-of-the-road position comes from the Food and Drug Administration, which lists background information for consumers on food ingredients and packaging (http://www.cfsan.fda.gov/~dms/opa-bckg.html). The web pages of advocacy organizations take stronger positions. The Center for Science and the Public Interest argues that many approved food additives are in fact not safe (http://www.cspinet.org/reports/chemcuisine.htm), while the International Food Information Council represents the views of the food industry and disputes many of the claims about the dangers of food additives (http://ific.org/publications/brochures/additivesbroch.cfm).
- **Food Allergens:** The American Academy of Allergy, Asthma, and Immunology sponsors a web site for both researchers and victims (http://www.aaaai.org/patients/resources/fastfacts/food_allergy.stm). The page gives a careful overview of the demonstrated harm of food allergies and intolerances.
- **Foodborne Illness:** Researchers should consult the Gateway to Government Food Safety Information web page (http://www.foodsafety.gov). They can find long lists of documents on food safety under topics such as news and events, consumer advice, foodborne pathogens, industry assistance, and federal and state agencies. Combining links to highly technical information with those to general information for the public, this site presents a wealth of resources on foodborne illnesses.
- **Food Irradiation and GM Foods:** Web pages take divergent viewpoints on these food technologies. For the positive side, see the web pages from the FDA on "Food Irradiation: A Safe Measure" (http://www.fda.gov/opacom/catalog/irradbro.html) and "Biotechnology" (http://www.cfsan.fda.gov/~lrd/biotechm.html#label). For the negative side, click on the web page on food irradiation from the Center for Food Safety (http://www.centerforfoodsafety.org/food_irrad.cfm) and the web page on GM foods from the Center for Science in the Public Interest (http://www.cspinet.org/nah/11_01). For a balanced overview of GM foods, go to the Pew Initiative page on food and biotechnology (http://pewagbiotech.org).
- **Mad Cow Disease:** A site with links to information on BSE and CJD sponsored by the Centers for Disease Control and Prevention (CDC) (http://www.cdc.gov/ncidod/diseases/cjd/cjd.htm) contains descriptions of and materials on BSE, CJD, VCID, and prion diseases.
- **Pesticides, Metals, Chemicals, and Natural Toxins:** The FDA offers a comprehensive set of documents (http://vm.cfsan.fda.gov/~lrd/pestadd.html) that include much technical material, but the wide coverage of the web page makes it a good place to start.

149

- **Terrorist Threats:** The federal government provides helpful links at "Countering Bioterrorism and Other Threats to the Food Supply" (http://www.foodsafety.gov/~fsg/bioterr.html). As with other government sites, this one contains documents that present a more positive view of government efforts than others might. Still, the dozens of documents listed on the page cover essential information on the topic.

PRINT SOURCES

Despite the ease of obtaining a wealth of Internet information, books and articles available from libraries and bookstores remain crucial to researchers. Good books integrate material that is otherwise scattered, present information in a logical and understandable format, and allow for a comprehensive approach to the issues. Edited volumes with pieces from many authors help place multiple perspectives on a topic within a meaningful framework, and books with a single author or few coauthors present an integrated and in-depth viewpoint. Shorter articles cannot explore topics in as much depth as books but present ideas in a condensed format. All have advantages and can be found by using catalogs, indexes, bibliographies, and other guides.

BIBLIOGRAPHIC RESOURCES

To supplement catalogs at a city, school, or university library, which most researchers should also use, a comprehensive bibliographic resource can be found in the Library of Congress catalog online (http://catalog. loc.gov). To browse holdings by subject, users can enter the library home page, click "Basic Search," type in "food safety," and highlight "Subject Browse." A variety of subject headings will be listed. Alternatively, a keyword search of "food safety" (used in quotation marks to search for the exact phrase) returns a list of 325 references. The list can be narrowed by searching for more specific topics on food safety or using a guided search.

A listing of catalogs for specific libraries can be found through Yahoo! (http://dir.Yahoo.com/Reference/Libraries). Users can discover new references by browsing catalogs both within and outside their community. Each library will have its own search procedures, but the general rule of searching for specific keywords will most efficiently produce listings of relevant materials.

Bookstore catalogs not only allow searches of books currently in print on any variety of food-safety topics but also often have the advantage of providing summaries and reader reviews of books, which can help determine their relevance and value. In some cases, parts of a book can be viewed electronically. These advantages make electronic bookstores such as Amazon.com (http://www.amazon.com) and Barnes and Noble (http://www.barnesandnoble.com) valuable bibliographic aids. Unlike libraries, however, their searches exclude many books no longer in print.

Periodical indexes for searching for print articles are available at most libraries. *OCLC First Search* contains an electronic version of *Reader's Guide Abstracts* that will list articles in a large number of magazines. However, users generally need access to a subscribing library for this database. *InfoTrac* also compiles articles for general-interest audiences and sometimes includes an abstract with the citation, or an abstract and a full-text article. It again requires library privileges. *Ingenta Library Gateway* (http://www.ingenta.com) includes 11 million citations from more than 20,000 journals and allows searches within specific subject areas such as medicine and social science. Searching *Ingenta* is free, but delivery of an article requires a fee. Often specific magazines such as *Time* (http://www.time.com) will have a web site that allows users to search for articles, but sometimes they charge fees to access older articles.

Libraries usually subscribe to catalogs of newspaper articles, which can be particularly useful in obtaining information on current events. In addition, many newspapers maintain a web page with an archive of past articles. The *New York Times*, for example, allows searches of past articles (as well as the day's major stories) at its home page (http://www.nytimes.com). Articles from the last seven days are free, but accessing earlier articles requires a fee. A search on food safety will, as is typical, return too many stories to sort through, and narrower searches will work better. The *Washington Post* also provides a web page to search for articles (http://www.washingtonpost.com) but again requires purchase of older articles. Otherwise, Yahoo! (http://dir.yahoo.com/News_and_Media/Newspapers/) lists links to many newspapers that can be accessed via the web. However, local libraries will offer ways to access newspaper articles without a fee. Consult a librarian on how to use these and the other library resources mentioned in this section.

SPECIFIC BOOKS AND ARTICLES ON FOOD SAFETY TOPICS

Along with general bibliographic resources for print materials and the annotated bibliography in chapter 7, it helps to have a few books and articles to get started. The appendices to this volume include government documents on each of the food-safety topics; the overview they give of policies, regulations, and recommendations provides a good starting point. The documents represent the views of government agencies, primarily the Food and Drug Administration, and tend to present a more positive view of food safety than would critics. Still, given the central role of the government in protecting the public from harm, agency views are crucial in understanding the issues. Thus, the appendices present

- recommendations for consumers in using HACCP procedures for food safety at home;
- the actions taken by the Department of Health and Human Services to protect beef from mad cow disease;
- the actions taken by the Department of Health and Human Services to protect food from bioterrorism;
- the views of the Food and Drug Administration (FDA) on food additives;
- the procedures used by the Environmental Protection Agency to test and approve pesticides;
- a summary from the FDA of the nature and risks of food allergies;
- a defense of food irradiation from the FDA; and
- the polices of the FDA of GM foods.

In addition to these documents, a short list of recommended books and articles organized by the major threats to food illness follows:

- **Food Additives, Chemical, Toxins, and Allergens:** Several articles address these controversial topics evenhandedly. Sheila Globus ("Pros and Cons of Food Additives" *Current Health 2*, vol. 28, no. 2, October 2001, pp. 17–19) nicely summarizes the debates on food additives. Jennifer Wolcott ("An End to Organic Confusion?" *Christian Science Monitor*, October 16, 2002, p. 15) does much the same in discussing the dangers of pesticide residue on food and the possible benefits of organic food. Raymond Formanek, Jr., ("Food Allergies: When Food Becomes the Enemy." *FDA Consumer*, vol. 35, no. 4, July/August 2001, pp. 10–16) describes the causes of food allergies and intolerances, offers useful statistics on the occurrence and growth of the problem, and provides an excellent starting point for those wanting an overview of the topic.
- **Foodborne Illness:** A few recent books provide good starting points for those doing research on threats from food-based diseases. Morton Satin in *Food Alert! The Ultimate Sourcebook for Food Safety* (New York: Facts On File, 1999) offers a comprehensive overview of issues of foodborne illness. An article entitled "Food" by Jennifer Ackerman in *National Geographic* (vol. 201, no. 5, May 2002, pp. 2–51) likewise discusses the dangers of

foodborne pathogens but also gives attention to some of the underlying sources of today's safety problems, particularly the spread of pathogens that are immune to traditional methods of heating and cooling food. More practical issues are discussed in a *New York Times* article by Amanda Hesser ("Squeaky Clean? Not Even Close." January 28, 2004, p. F1), which lists a number of ways cooks at home promote the spread of bacteria in the food they eat and actions they need to take to minimize the risks of food prepared in the home kitchen.

- **Food Irradiation and GM Foods:** Print sources in the area of food technology sometimes include too much technical information for most users. One book authored by Richard L. Frank and Robert A. Hahn, *A Primer on Food Irradiation* (Elmwood Park, N.J.: Food Institute Information and Research Center, 2001) gives a short overview of essential information on food irradiation for nonexperts and considers both the pros and cons of the practice. On GM food, Bill Lambrecht's *Dinner at the New Gene Café* (New York: St. Martin's Press, 2000) describes the people and events behind the development of GM foods and the controversy the food has created. In "Will Frankenfood Save the Planet" (*Atlantic Monthly*, vol. 292, no. 3, October 2003, pp. 103–108), Jonathan Rauch discusses both the potential risks and benefits of bioengineered food.

- **Mad Cow Disease:** Philip Yam in *The Pathological Protein: Mad Cow, Chronic Wasting, and Other Deadly Prion Diseases* (New York: Copernicus Books, 2003) provides a fascinating history of mad cow and other prion diseases. For a shorter piece, a *Newsweek* article by Jerry Adler ("What's Safe Now" vol. 143, no. 2, January 12, 2004, pp. 42–28) reviews the efforts of the government to recall beef that may have come in contact with BSE-infected tissue and identifies several problems in the food-safety system. A more scientifically oriented article by Bruce Chesebro ("A Fresh Look at BSE," Science, vol. 305, September 24, 2004, pp. 1918–19, 1921) provides an up-to-date review of the evidence on the potential for the spread of BSE in the United States and suggests that the disease could take new and unexpected forms.

- **Terrorist Threats:** Most published books on this topic take the form of government reports, and one based on congressional testimony serves as an introduction to the issues: Lawrence J. Dyckman, *Bioterrorism: A Threat to Agriculture and the Food Supply* (Washington, D.C.: U.S. General Accounting Office, 2004). A more accessible article by Amanda Spake in *U.S. News & World Report* ("Food Fright: Preventing Food Terrorism," vol. 131, no. 26, December 24, 2001, pp. 48–50) describes concerns about terrorist attacks on the food supply, efforts to deal with the problem, and the importance of coordinating the actions of various agencies that regulate food.

LEGAL RESEARCH

Research on federal food-safety laws is relatively straightforward. The most important ones—the 1906 Pure Food and Drug Act; the 1906 Meat Inspection Act; the 1938 Federal Food, Drug, and Cosmetic Act; and the 1996 Food Quality Protection Act—can be found through a web search. More detail—and more complexity—on a variety of specific laws can be found through a search of the U.S. Code. Go to the Cornell Law School's U.S. Code web page (http://www4.law.cornell.edu/uscode), and click "Title 21 on Food and Drugs" to search for laws on food safety. For state laws, the National Association of State Departments of Agriculture (http://www.nasda-hq.org/nasda/nasda/Foundation/foodsafety) provides links to food regulations of every state.

Few court decisions directly address the issue of food safety (see the discussion in chapter 2 for those that do). However, several groups have sued the government to try to force a change in policies or enforcement. Information on the suits, jury decisions, awards, appeals, and final judgments can be found through searches of newspapers (*New York Times*) and general search engines (Google, Yahoo!). To obtain the written decisions in food-safety cases, consult electronic law libraries such as Westlaw and Lexis-Nexis. Opinions of the Supreme Court relevant to some food issues can be obtained from the Legal Information Institute (http://www.law.cornell.edu). With knowledge of the specific case, a web search that lists the names of the parties involved (with the plaintiff listed first, then "v." to represent versus, and the defendant listed last, such as in *Alliance for Bio-Integrity, et al. v. Donna Shalala*) and the case number will turn up the text of many rulings.

A WORD OF ADVICE

Along with its relevance to issues of diet and health, the diversity of topics, viewpoints, and information on threats to food safety make it a fascinating area of research. Although this diversity requires carefully defined questions to limit the material to cover, it also offers several opportunities. Use the research to find out more about science and disease, confront viewpoints that differ from your own, and discover fascinating topics that on first blush appear uninteresting. Do more than search out evidence to justify your own opinions on meat consumption, vegetarianism, processed foods, organic foods, government policies, and the food industry. In short, take this opportunity to learn as much as you can about new topics and ideas.

CHAPTER 7

ANNOTATED BIBLIOGRAPHY

The following annotated bibliography contains nine sections:

- general treatments of food safety
- foodborne illness
- mad cow disease (BSE)
- terrorism
- food additives
- chemical and natural toxins
- food allergens
- food irradiation
- genetically modified (GM) food

The sections correspond roughly to those in chapter 1 but begin with citations that cover multiple food-safety topics. Within each of these sections, the citations are divided into subsections on books, articles, and web documents. The topics and citations include technical and nontechnical works, in-depth and short treatments, and research and opinion pieces (see chapter 6 for an overview on how to most effectively use the diverse materials).

GENERAL TREATMENTS

BOOKS

Ashton, John, and Ron Laura. *The Perils of Progress: The Health and Environment Hazards of Modern Technology, and What You Can Do about Them.* London: Zed Books, 1999. Part 3 of the book includes five chapters on the dangers of food technology. The authors discuss food processing, food irradiation, and contamination of food by aluminum, cadmium, and pesticides. The theme of the book extends beyond food to argue that technological advances often threaten human health.

Beier, Ross C., Suresh D. Pillai, Timothy D. Phillips, and Richard L. Ziprin, eds. *Preharvest and Postharvest Food Safety: Contemporary Issues and Future Directions.* Ames, Iowa: Blackwell Publishing, 2004. This volume originates from the Center for Food Safety, Institute of Food Science and Engineering, at Texas A&M University—a nationally recognized research organization. Aimed at experts and food scientists, the articles in the volume cover topics of pathogen/host interaction, the ecology of foodborne hazards, microbe resistance to treatment, testing for contamination, means to decontaminate food, and risk analysis. Although the scientific material makes for difficult reading, the diverse topics covered in a single volume (nearly 450 pages) make it a useful resource. It also illustrates the vast amount of ongoing research related to food safety.

D'Mello, J. P. F., ed. *Food Safety: Contaminants and Toxins.* Cambridge, Mass.: CABI Publishing, 2003. Readers wanting up-to-date technical information will find this 452-page book useful. Each chapter, authored by an academic expert, describes a particular contaminant, toxin, or controversial practice in food production (e.g., genetically modified crops, food irradiation) and the latest scientific research on the topic. The book does not make for easy reading and is targeted to graduate students in the food sciences who have background knowledge in chemistry, nutrition, agriculture, and microbiology. However, nonexperts can also learn from the careful and objective view of food-safety risks provided by the book.

Dyckman, Lawrence J. *Federal Food Safety and Security System: Fundamental Restructuring Is Needed to Address Fragmentation and Overlap.* Washington, D.C.: U.S. General Accounting Office, 2004. Noting that the food supply of the United States is governed by more than 30 laws and 12 agencies, this report describes the problems with the fragmented system and possible ways to consolidate government oversight. A review of existing food programs reveals duplication and inconsistency of standards in food inspection and laws that prevent agencies from focusing efforts on points of highest risk. Based on its evaluation, the report then recommends that federal legislation establish a single, independent food-safety agency. Alternatively, it recommends that one current agency take the lead in food-safety inspection.

Hilts, Philip J. *Protecting America's Health: The FDA, Business, and One Hundred Years of Regulation.* New York: Alfred A. Knopf, 2003. The FDA has responsibility for ensuring the safety of about 80 percent of the nation's food. This history of the agency gives much attention to its other major duty—approving pharmaceutical drugs—and focuses largely on organizational changes and problems. However, it also highlights the politics of

Annotated Bibliography

protecting the public from unsafe food and how the FDA has been influenced by political debates.

Levy, Elinor, and Mark Fischetti. *The New Killer Diseases: How the Alarming Evolution of Mutant Germs Threatens Us All.* New York: Crown Publishers, 2003. Linking new foodborne illnesses such as *E. coli* and mad cow disease to other new diseases such as SARS, West Nile, and Ebola, this book asks if these diseases are the beginning of a future epidemic of mutant germs. In answering yes, the authors take a more alarmist view than most others. The first paragraph of chapter 1 states, "The human race is in the midst of a biological war against an army of microscopic foes that we have seriously underestimated. . . .The threat they pose is as formidable as any that the human race has ever faced." The deadly new strain of *E. coli* and prion-based mad cow disease are a crucial part of this threat, largely because the natures of the diseases are so different and so new. The information provided on food-based illness makes up only a few chapters of the book but offers a special perspective by linking it to other new diseases.

Millichap, J. Gordon. *Environmental Poisons in Our Food.* Chicago: PNB Publishers, 1992. While examining foodborne illness, food additives, food irradiation, pesticides in food, and food allergies in separate chapters, the book presents more information than most other treatments on contamination of food with trace metals. The book was written for family physicians who might need to know more about food toxins and is accessible to nonspecialists.

Nestle, Marion. *Food Politics: How the Food Industry Influences Nutrition and Health.* Berkeley: University of California Press, 2002. Professor and Chair of Nutrition and Food Studies at New York University, Dr. Nestle argues in this highly praised book that the food industry fails to meet the health needs of the population with the products it produces, processes, markets, and sells. Rather than focusing on nutrition and health, the industry spends money on marketing and advertising and uses political lobbying to influence public policy. According to the author, the end result, however unfortunate for consumers, is that food choices are determined by economic interests. The book does not concentrate on issues of food safety but provides one perspective on the persistence of food-safety problems and the minimal efforts of the industry to end them.

———. *Safe Food: Bacteria, Biotechnology, and Bioterrorism.* Berkeley: University of California Press, 2003. Building on her previous book on food politics, the author examines issues of food safety in this one and gives the same attention to detail and thorough research as before. *Safe Food* focuses mostly on genetically modified crops (i.e., biotechnology) and on foodborne illness (i.e., bacteria), while discussing food bioterrorism more briefly. In all areas, it provides much information on how food policies

157

emerged from the conflict between business goals of profit and consumer needs of safety. In the end, Nestle calls for new laws and agencies that do more to protect consumers.

Organization for Economic Cooperation and Development. *Emerging Risks in the 21st Century: An Agenda for Action.* Paris: Organization for Economic Cooperation and Development, 2003. Food safety makes up only part of this volume on the variety of risks faced by citizens of high-income nations. These nations need to address new and serious threats in five broad clusters: natural disasters, technological accidents, infectious diseases, food safety, and terrorism. The report recommends ways for governments to assess the risks and to develop ways to minimize them. Of special interest is the discussion on how food safety has similarities with other apparently different emerging risks.

Pennington, T. Hugh. *When Food Kills: BSE, E. Coli, and Disaster Science.* Oxford: Oxford University Press, 2003. Britain has suffered more than any other nation from mad cow disease (BSE) and its human counterpart (vCJD), but, as this book points out, it has also experienced problems with *E. coli* O157:H7, another type of deadly foodborne illness. The story of how a family owned butchering and bakery business in Scotland sickened dozens of people and killed several illustrates the risks. Workers who cut raw meat and then used the same knives to cut cooked meat infected people who thought that eating the cooked meat was safe. The book describes the failure of inspectors, government policies, and scientists to prevent such disasters. A bacteriologist who has advised the government about food crises, the author tells a discouraging story about food safety in Britain that offers lessons to the United States.

Rowell, Andrew. *Don't Worry, It's Safe to Eat: The True Story of GM Food, BSE, and Foot and Mouth.* London: Earthscan, 2003. In discussing the British epidemic of foot-and-mouth disease among cattle, the deaths of cattle and humans from BSE, and the controversy over genetically modified foods, the author criticizes political authorities and their response to each crisis. Interviews with scientists who warned of problems but were ignored illustrate the failure of the British government to protect the public from food dangers.

Schlosser, Eric. *Fast Food Nation: The Dark Side of the All-American Meal.* New York: Houghton Mifflin, 2001. This popular and critically acclaimed exposé of the fast-food industry gives considerable attention to the factory farms and meat-production facilities needed to supply the huge demand for fast food. Visits to farms and meatpacking plants by the author reveal ineffective federal oversight and contamination of food. He calls eating in the United States "a high-risk behavior." The book addresses many other problems beside food safety but treats unsafe food as the inevitable result of the growth of the fast-food industry and its efforts to attract people with low prices and large portions. Since the publication of this book, Schlosser has continued to advocate safer food policies and criticize the food industry.

Schmidt, Ronald H., and Gary E. Rodrick, eds. *Food Safety Handbook.* New York: Wiley, 2002. Advertised as a single comprehensive reference source on all food-safety issues, this massive 864-page book does indeed contain much information. Topics include risk assessment, food hazards, safety interventions, diet and health issues, and worldwide issues. The editors, professors of Food Science and Human Nutrition at the University of Florida, have generally selected articles written for experts.

Schumann, Michael S., Thomas D. Schneid, B. R. Schumann, and Michael J. Fagel. *Food Safety Law.* New York: Wiley, 1997. Although a bit dated, this book is one of the few to focus on legal aspects of food safety. It examines laws and regulations, describes changes in food inspection procedures, and offers numerous case studies of food disease outbreaks and the legal issues they raise. The authors include a practicing lawyer, law professor, and food industry businessman.

Spriggs, John, and Grant Isaac. *Food Safety and International Competitiveness: The Case of Beef.* New York: CABI Publishing, 2001. Food safety has clear implications for goals of competitiveness in international trade. Even if citizens remain satisfied with the safety standards in their country, the food industry may have to improve its standards to export its products to other countries. Taking the case of beef, a food vulnerable to several safety threats, this book examines the arrangements that four nations—the United States, Canada, the United Kingdom, and Australia—have established to ensure food safety. The comparisons across nations in the book shed light on policies in the United States.

U.S. Department of Agriculture, Food Safety and Inspection Service. *Protecting America's Meat, Poultry and Egg Products: A Report to the Secretary on the Food Security Initiatives of the Food Safety and Inspection Service.* Washington, D.C.: U.S. Department of Agriculture, Food Safety and Inspection Service, 2003. This short and clearly written report highlights key efforts of the Food Safety and Inspection Service. Largely a public relations document, it emphasizes the accomplishments and goals of the agency rather than its limitations. Still, with many helpful maps and charts, it provides a nice introduction to the agency.

U.S. Senate. *Food Safety and Security: Can Our Fractured Food Safety System Rise to the Challenge? Hearing before the Oversight of Government Management, Restructuring, and the District of Columbia Subcommittee of the Committee on Governmental Affairs, United States Senate, One Hundred Seventh Congress, First Session, October 10, 2001.* Washington, D.C.: U.S. Government Printing

159

Office, 2001. Held shortly after the September 11 terrorist attacks, this hearing gave new urgency to calls for a single food-safety agency. According to many senators and witnesses, the government would protect the public better from the threat of terrorist food tampering if a single agency for food safety existed. However, the criticisms of the existing complex system of divided responsibility apply more generally: All aspects of food safety would benefit from a single agency according to most at the hearing. Like other hearings on the topic, this one failed to generate sufficient support for legislation to change the nature of food responsibilities in the government.

———. *Nomination Hearing for Elsa A. Murano and Edward R. McPherson: Hearing before the Committee on Agriculture, Nutrition, and Forestry, United States Senate, One Hundred Seventh Congress, First Session, September 26, 2001.* Washington, D.C.: U.S. Government Printing Office, 2001. Dr. Elsa A. Murano, formerly a professor at Texas A&M University and director of the Center for Food Safety, became the undersecretary for food safety at the Department of Agriculture in the Bush administration. Given concerns about foodborne illness and mad cow disease, this position has come to take on considerable importance. The hearing raises issues of concern to the senators and offers insights into the views of Dr. Murano on addressing problems of food safety.

ARTICLES

Ackerman, Jennifer. "Food."*National Geographic*, vol. 201, no. 5, May 2002, pp. 2–51. In discussing the dangers of foodborne pathogens, this article gives attention to some of the underlying sources of today's safety problems, particularly the spread of pathogens that are immune to traditional methods of heating and cooling food. The article suggests that the public's desire for larger quantities of out-of-season, prepackaged, and low-cost meals contributes to the problem. This thorough and well-written treatment also examines topics such as how chickens become contaminated with bacteria, how the use of pesticides, hormones, and antibiotics affect food, how other countries regulate food safety, and how fish producers meet government standards to ensure safety and freshness.

Bryan, Frank L. "Reflections on a Career in Public Health: Evolving Foodborne Pathogens, Environmental Health, and Food Safety Programs."*Journal of Environmental Health*, vol. 65, no. 5, December 2002, pp. 14–25. The author reviews trends in foodborne disease and government policy since the 1940s. Based on his own experiences working on food-safety issues for the government, he hopes that future decisions about food safety will be based on science and practical needs rather than by the panic of the moment or pressures from uninformed groups.

Annotated Bibliography

Gardyn, Rebecca. "What's Cooking?" *American Demographics*, vol. 24, no. 3, March 2002, pp. 29–35. The food business has responded to recent demographic and lifestyle trends. Increased concern with food safety has accompanied other changes in food preferences for convenience, healthiness, emphasis on flavor, and customized products. Producers, retailers, and restaurants will need to attend to all these preferences, including food safety, to attract consumers in the future.

Nierenberg, Danielle. "The Commercialization of Farming: Producing Meat for a Hungry World." *USA Today (Periodical)*, vol. 132, January 2004, pp. 22–24. Developing nations such as the Philippines have become centers of large-scale livestock farms. This article describes concerns that intense production and slaughtering of animals for meat in nations that do not have the same regulations for disease prevention and testing as the United States can spread foodborne diseases. Yet the demand across the world for beef and other meats make this type of farming economically profitable.

Schlosser, Eric. "Bad Meat: The Scandal of Our Food Safety System." *The Nation*, vol. 275, no. 8, September 16, 2002, pp. 6–7. The author, a well-known critic of food production in the United States, argues that the meatpacking industry has gained undue influence with the Bush administration and Republican allies in Congress. Much of the influence comes from the large contributions made by the industry to political campaigns. Schlosser argues that as a result of the contributions, federal agencies have not done more to require testing or shut down plants with contaminated meats.

Spake, Amanda. "How McNuggets Changed the World." *U.S. News & World Report*, vol. 130, no. 3, January 22, 2001, p. 54. A brief history of McDonald's and its application of assembly line methods to food preparation can provide some background for understanding the growth of foodborne illnesses. This article argues that the huge demand for processed meat such as the reconstituted chicken in McNuggets and for cheap eggs in Egg McMuffins increases the spread of foodborne disease. It gives little direct attention to foodborne illness but places the disease trends in the context of the revolutionary growth of fast-food restaurants.

Taylor, Michael R., and Sandra A. Hoffman. "Redesigning Food Safety." *Issues in Science and Technology*, vol. 17, no. 4, Summer 2001, pp. 26–30. In reviewing recommendations from a report of the Institute of Medicine/National Research Council, the article identifies the need for a single, unified federal agency that would use science-based methods and knowledge to regulate food. It notes that Congress has been unable to pass such legislation but may be reconsidering its resistance given the recent appearance of new and increasingly dangerous microbes. However, some four years after publication of the article, the organization of food-safety regulation—and the problems it creates—remains much as it has for decades.

"Tell the Truth about Food: Food Prices Will Have to Rise." *New Statesman,* vol. 130, March 5, 2001, pp. 6–7. The point of this article is a simple one that is nonetheless seldom stated: Doing more to improve food safety will require higher food prices. Since many problems of food safety stem from intensive and efficient production methods, correcting those problems will slow production and raise prices. This piece argues that the government should take the lead in requiring these changes. The growing popularity of natural and organic food stores, despite generally higher prices than conventional grocery stores, suggests that many will accept higher prices for safer food.

Verfaillie, Hendrik A. "Securing Our Commitments to Agriculture: A Safe and Healthy Food Supply: Address, November 27, 2001." *Vital Speeches of the Day,* vol. 68, no. 7, January 15, 2002, pp. 216–219. In speaking to the Farm Journal Conference in Washington, D.C., the CEO of the Monsanto Company argues for the importance of plentiful and safe food for health, peace, and prosperity. He believes that improved agricultural products, including bioengineered foods, are a first step toward these goals.

Walters, Jonathan. "Spoiled-Food Federalism: Governments at All Levels Should Be Involved with Food Safety Issues." *Governing,* vol. 14, no. 8, May 2001, p. 12. Although the importance of food safety issues suggests that state and local governments should take action to deal with the problem, this article notes that they have left most regulation to the federal government. State and local governments may believe that food-safety issues are too complex for them to become more involved in enforcement. Yet the author argues that they have an important role to play in protecting citizens from threats to food safety.

WEB DOCUMENTS

"About Us." Center for Food Safety. Available online. URL: http://www.centerforfoodsafety.org/about_us.cfm. Downloaded in April 2006. The Center for Food Safety opposes what it views as harmful food-production technologies and advocates alternative approaches to safe food. Its web site includes discussion of genetically engineered food, irradiation of food, mad cow disease, and other new food technologies. The discussion presents only one side of the debate but relies on scientific studies to bolster the case it makes against modern techniques of food production.

"Fact Sheets: Foodborne Illness and Disease: Bovine Spongiform Encephalopathy." Food Safety and Inspection Service. Available online.

Annotated Bibliography

URL: http://www.fsis.usda.gov/Fact_Sheets/Bovine_Spongiform_Encephalopathy_BSE/index.asp. Downloaded in April 2006. The agency with the responsibility for testing cattle for the presence of foodborne disease and BSE offers links to the latest news, notices and directives, frequently asked questions, and research information. The site is especially useful for gathering information on current testing procedures.

"Food Safety." Center for Science in the Public Interest. Available online. URL: http://www.cspinet.org/foodsafety. Downloaded in April 2006. With the latest news on food safety, alerts about food-based disease outbreaks, legislative efforts, and consumer action, this page advocates greater government regulation and business effort to protect consumers from food contamination. Critics view the center as part of a puritanical, antipleasure crusade that promotes exaggerated claims, while defenders view the center as an honest voice for food safety that counters government inaction and the undue influence of the food industry on food choices.

"Food Safety." U.S. National Library of Medicine and National Institutes of Health, Medline Plus. Available online. URL: http://www.nlm.nih.gov/medlineplus/foodsafety.html. Updated on March 23, 2006. Medline, a prestigious source of information, articles, and research on medical topics, lists links to a variety of documents on food safety. The documents are for the public rather than specialists.

"General Food Safety Information." Center for Infectious Disease Research and Policy, Academic Health Center, University of Minnesota. Available online. URL: http://www.cidrap.umn.edu/cidrap/content/fs/food. Downloaded in April 2006. The lists of recent news stories and published articles on food safety make this web page a useful reference source. It also has other sections on bioterrorism, food security, foodborne diseases, BSE, vCJD, and irradiation.

"Kids, Teens, and Educators." FoodSafety.gov. Available online. URL: http://www.foodsafety.gov/~fsg/fsgkids.html. Updated on February 7, 2006. The links on this page lead to documents that will appeal to young readers—a group that needs to learn about food safety. It also includes games, puzzles, quizzes, career information, and tips on food safety when camping, babysitting, and taking a lunch to school.

"Resources." Food Safety Training and Education Alliance. Available online. URL: http://www.fstea.org/resources.html. Updated in April 2006. This alliance of government agencies and private trade associations provides information to help retail food outlets, foodservice workers, vending businesses, institutions, and regulators with education and training. The page includes training materials, regulations, funding opportunities, and survey results.

163

"Safe Food, From Farm to Fork." University of Guelph and Department of Plant Agriculture. Available online. URL: http://www.foodsafetynetwork. ca. Downloaded in April 2006. Much like in America, Canadian health authorities have expressed much concern about food safety. This web page presents links to numerous Canadian documents on the topic.

FOODBORNE ILLNESS

BOOKS

Barnes, Gary, ed. *Quick Reference to the 2001 FDA Model Food Code.* Upper Saddle River, N.J.: Prentice Hall, 2002. This abridged version of the FDA food code highlights crucial information on food safety for all persons involved in the food industry. It covers topics such as managing food personnel; treatment of food, equipment, and utensils; and handling waste, poison, and toxic materials. The shortened text and usefully formatted reference material proves easier and more efficient to use than the full FDA manual.

Buzby, Jean C., Paul D. Frenzen, and Barbara Rasco. *Product Liability and Microbial Foodborne Illness.* Washington, D.C.: U.S. Department of Agriculture, Economic Research Service, 2001. Available online. URL: http://www.ers.usda.gov/publications/aer799/aer799.pdf. Downloaded in April 2006. The threat of civil suits faced by food producers that sell contaminated products should encourage greater efforts at food safety. This study examines the outcomes of 175 jury trials involving foodborne illnesses. The results indicate, perhaps surprisingly, that legal actions against companies are rare and that awards to plaintiffs tend to be modest.

Cary, Jeffrey W., John E. Linz, and Deepak Bhatnagar, eds. *Microbial Foodborne Diseases: Mechanisms of Pathogenesis and Toxin Synthesis.* Boca Raton, Fla.: CRC Press, 1999. This edited volume focuses on advances in the molecular and cellular understanding of microbes that infect food. It includes 142 contributions that will appeal most to scientists and government officials.

Committee on the Review of the Use of Scientific Criteria and Performance Standards for Safe Food. *Scientific Criteria to Ensure Safe Food.* Washington, D.C.: National Academies Press, 2003. This report from the National Academy of Sciences finds use of Hazard Analysis and Critical Control Point (HACCP) procedures to have improved the safety of food. Still, the committee appointed to consider the scientific evidence on this improvement offers some suggestions for future change. It finds, for example, that companies and government agencies lack understanding of the latest scientific findings and the ability to fully exploit the data they collect to change procedures. The report offers a long list of recommendations that would help address these and other problems. Overall, the report offers insights into the current system of food-safety control but may prove most useful for scientists and those closely involved in food production and safety.

Davis, Karen. *Prisoned Chickens Poisoned Eggs: An Inside Look at the Modern Poultry Industry.* Summertown, Tenn.: Book Publishing Company, 1996. While concern about beef dominates food-safety discussion, critics of the food industry express similar concerns about poultry and eggs. In advocating animal rights and vegetarianism, the author describes the inhuman and unsanitary conditions of hens laying eggs and being slaughtered for meat. The passionately made claims for animal rights will not satisfy those looking for a more objective analysis, but the book expresses common criticism of modern poultry production.

Fox, Nichols. *It Was Probably Something You Ate: A Practical Guide to Avoiding and Surviving Foodborne Illness.* New York: Penguin Books, 1999. While the author's first book on the topic focused on the sources of the crisis in foodborne illness, this book does more to acquaint readers with the diseases themselves and the ways to avoid them. The first part of the book clearly—and entertainingly, given the technical and sometimes gruesome nature of the topic—describes some 20 microorganisms that can cause foodborne illness. The second part lists a set of steps people should take to minimize the risk of getting sick from food. Although a sourcebook for reference more than for entertaining reading, Fox writes well, presenting both technical material and daily advice with clarity and style.

―――. *Spoiled: Why Our Food Is Making Us Sick and What We Can Do about It.* New York: Basic Books, 1997. A journalist stimulated into action by the deaths from a new strain of the *E. coli* bacteria, Fox describes dozens of incidents of foodborne illness that have occurred in the United States through the mid-1990s. The book concludes that the wide variety of infected foods and the lethality of the infections point to fundamental problems with how food is produced, processed, and distributed. Intensive production of crops and animals, production of food in giant factories, shipment of products across long distances, and trade with foreign nations all contribute to the growing problem of foodborne illness.

Heady, Dotty. *Fifty Ways to Lose Your Lunch or 'Not THAT Restaurant, Robert': Stories of a Food Safety Consultant That Could Save Your Relationship, Your Restaurant (If You Own One) and Maybe Your Life.* Louisville, Ky.: Transformata Publishing, 2002. The author, who teaches at Sullivan University and consults across the nation on food sanitation and contamination prevention, provides advice to restaurant owners and employees on maintaining food safety. In making the case for the importance of the recommendations, the author argues that cleanliness and sanitation in food preparation can make or break a restaurant.

Labbé, Ronald G., and Santos García, eds. *Guide to Foodborne Pathogens.* New York: Wiley, 2001. The 22 contributions to this edited volume came from a conference on food safety held in Mexico in 1998. Written in language appropriate for general audiences, the book discusses the nature, distribution, prevention, and treatment of foodborne illnesses. Various chapters cover common pathogens and efforts to control them.

Latta, Sara L. *Food Poisoning and Foodborne Diseases.* Berkeley Heights, N.J.: Enslow Publishers, 1999. For those wanting readable introductions to technical topics, books for juveniles often offer a useful starting point. This book, part of the Diseases and People Series for grades 7 and up, is one such example. It includes useful references, a glossary, and some technical information but also explains the issues clearly in 120 pages and includes plenty of anecdotes to make the subject more personal. A good starting point for those new to the topic and wanting a quick overview.

Loken, Joan K. *The HACCP Food Safety Manual. New York:* Wiley, 1995. Since the 1990s, the Hazard Analysis and Critical Control Point (HACCP) system has become the key component of national efforts to maintain food safety in production. The scientific basis of HACCP can be difficult to comprehend, but this book tries to explain the basic points in ways that users rather than scientists can understand. It reviews the seven steps in the HACCP system, illustrating each with diagrams and text.

Matthews, Dawn D., ed. *Food Safety Sourcebook.* Detroit: Omnigraphics, 1999. The contents of this book include: basic consumer health information about the safe handling of meat, poultry, seafood, eggs, fruit juices, and other food items; facts about pesticides, drinking water, food safety overseas, and the onset, duration, and symptoms of foodborne illnesses; types of pathogenic bacteria, parasitic protozoa, worms, viruses, and natural toxins; the role of the consumer, the food handler, and the government in food safety; a glossary; and resources for additional help and information.

McSwane, David, Nancy Rue, Richard Linton, and Anna Graf Williams. *The Essentials of Food Safety and Sanitation. Third Edition.* Upper Saddle River, N.J.: Prentice Hall, 2002. This textbook, written for those taking classes on food safety and working in the food-service industry, provides more depth than the quick reference guide written by two of the authors (see Nancy Rue and Anna Graf Williams below). With chapter objectives, case studies, discussion questions, and quizzes, it better suits coursework than personal reading. Instructors using the text speak highly of it.

Miliotis, Marianne D., and Jeffrey Bier, eds. *International Handbook of Foodborne Pathogens.* New York: Marcel Dekker, 2003. The articles in this edited volume are targeted at food microbiologists, government officials dealing with food safety, and members of the food industry. More than many other similar volumes, this one gives special attention to the global distribution of foodborne disease and the need for international bodies to enforce worldwide standards of food safety.

National Research Council. *The Use of Drugs in Food Animals: Benefits and Risks.* Washington, D.C.: National Academies Press, 1999. This comprehensive review of scientific studies investigates claims that use of antibiotics and other drugs in food animals contributes to the development of foodborne microbes that are resistant to antibiotics. It concludes that the risks are real. Despite the benefits it may bring for killing normal bacteria and making food safer from some pathogens, the use of drugs in food animals also has the potential to increase the lethality of foodborne diseases.

Organization for Economic Cooperation and Development (OECD). *Foodborne Disease in OECD Countries: Present State and Economic Costs.* Paris: Organization for Economic Cooperation and Development, 2003. This organization includes high-income countries in Europe, North America, and Asia. The public in these countries expresses particular concern about their risks from foodborne diseases, while officials are also concerned with the economic and social costs of the diseases. The report describes incidents of foodborne illness across the OECD nations and strategies that can both improve public health and limit economic costs.

Parker, James N., and Philip M. Parker, eds. *The 2002 Official Patient's Sourcebook on Foodborne Diseases: A Revised and Updated Directory for the Internet Age.* San Diego: Icon Health Publications, 2002. Edited by a physician and Ph.D., this sourcebook aims to provide more detailed information about foodborne disease than victims might be able to get otherwise. It also directs patients to Internet sources of data, exploiting the wealth of medical information freely available on web pages (at the same time, it aims to censor Internet sites that endorse unsound claims). Access to information on current research, treatments, and tests should help patients with foodborne diseases deal better with their illness and treatment.

———. *Food Poisoning: A Medical Dictionary, Bibliography, and Annotated Research Guide to Internet References.* San Diego: Icon Health Publications, 2003. Like its companion medical dictionary on foodborne diseases, this medical dictionary on food poisoning offers detailed information for medical professionals, students, researchers, and patients. Besides definitions of terms, it also contains bibliographic references and a listing of Internet sources of information.

Ralston, Katherine, C. Philip Brent, YoLanda Starke, Toija Riggins, and C.-T. Jordan Lin. *Consumer Food Safety Behavior: A Case Study in Hamburger*

Cooking and Ordering. Washington, D.C.: U.S. Department of Agriculture, Economic Research Service, 2001. Based on evidence from a survey summarized in this report, Americans are eating hamburgers more well done than in the past. This change reduces the risk of getting *E. coli* O157:H7 by 4.6 percent and the cost of foodborne illnesses by $7.4 million a year. The change appears to reflect increased consumer concern about the dangers of foodborne illness in undercooked ground beef.

Robinson, Robert A. *Food Safety and Security: Fundamental Changes Needed to Ensure Safe Food.* Washington, D.C.: U.S. General Accounting Office, 2001. In this testimony made before a committee hearing of the U.S. Senate, the director of the Natural Resources and Environment section of the General Accounting Office summarizes problems with the food-safety system. He describes the patchwork of policies and agencies that currently govern food safety and argues for a more comprehensive approach that addresses problems from farm to table. To do so, a single independent agency needs to be established or diverse activities need to be consolidated under a single existing agency.

Rue, Nancy, and Anna Graf Williams. *Quick Reference to Food Safety and Sanitation.* Upper Saddle River, N.J.: Prentice Hall, 2002. Written in an easy-to-understand style and illustrated with pictures, diagrams, and cartoons, this book can serve as an introduction and guide for food-service workers. Since many states require managers to obtain food-service certification, the book can help them prepare. For those who have mastered the requirements of safe food handling and cooking, the book also provides a quick reference, listing for example the safe holding and cooking times for a variety of products. Although not targeted at general readers, those interested in food safety can learn about the procedures recommended for restaurants and other food businesses.

Satin, Morton. *Food Alert! The Ultimate Sourcebook for Food Safety.* New York: Facts On File, 1999. The distinguished author, a molecular biologist and internationally known expert on food safety and processing, offers an encyclopedic overview of foodborne illness. The book organizes the section on the sources of foodborne disease by type of product: poultry, meat, dairy and egg, fruits and vegetables, grains, and restaurants. It organizes the section on foodborne pathogens into categories relating to bacteria, toxins, parasites, fungi, and viruses. It also offers material on consumer protection and a bit on government policy. Containing densely packed information, the book works best as a reference source.

Scott, Elizabeth, and Paul Sockett. *How to Prevent Food Poisoning: A Practical Guide to Safe Cooking, Eating, and Food Handling.* New York: Wiley, 1998. This how-to book aimed at the general public discusses steps needed to select safe food, prevent food contamination at home, transport and store food properly, eat safely in restaurants, and reduce germs in the kitchen.

Technology Team. *Your Self-Study Guide to Understanding How to Develop a HACCP Plan.* Washington, D.C.: U.S. Department of Agriculture, Food Safety and Inspection Service, 1999. This guide offers clear instructions for businesses that need to implement the HACCP (Hazard Analysis and Critical Control Point) system for their business. It provides examples of how to apply the seven HACCP steps and ensure safer food production.

U.S. Department of Agriculture, Food Safety and Inspection Service. *Cooking for Groups: A Volunteer's Guide to Food Safety.* Washington, D.C.: U.S. Department of Agriculture, Food Safety and Inspection Service, 2001. Volunteers cooking for large groups can cause much damage through carelessness and ignorance. If volunteers are motivated, the guidance provided by the USDA can help educate them about food safety much as other programs help educate professional cooks.

U.S. Food and Drug Administration, Center for Food Safety and Applied Nutrition. *Bad Bug Book: Foodborne Pathogenic Microorganisms and Natural Toxins Handbook.* McLean, Va.: International Medical Publishing, 2004. Although the slang terminology used in the first part of the title might suggest otherwise, this book is designed for health-care professionals who diagnose and treat foodborne illness. Given its goal of protecting the safety of most of the nation's food, the Food and Drug Administration relies here on the expertise of its employees in making recommendations.

———. *Report of the FDA Retail Food Program Database of Foodborne Illness Risk Factors.* Washington, D.C.: U.S. Food and Drug Administration, 2000. To establish a national baseline on the occurrence of foodborne disease in retail establishments, the FDA Retail Food Program Steering Committee sent inspectors to a sample of hospitals, nursing homes, elementary schools, fast-food restaurants, full-service restaurants, and retail store departments selling meat, produce, deli foods, and seafood. With data from 17,477 observations, the report describes compliance in 1997 and goals for improvement by 2010. Although most readers will want to ignore the details on methodology, the tables on compliance disclose interesting information. For example, institutions and meat and seafood departments of retail outlets showed compliance over 80 percent of the time, while full-service restaurants showed compliance of only 60 percent. The restaurants performed poorly in maintaining proper temperatures of food and in ensuring personal hygiene of employees.

U.S. General Accounting Office. *The Agricultural Use of Antibiotics and Its Implications for Human Health.* Washington, D.C.: U.S. General Accounting Office, 1999. This report provided to Senator Tom Harkin (D-Iowa) reviews the evidence on whether antibiotics in animal feed produce antibiotic-resistant bacteria that can harm humans through foodborne disease. It notes that evidence exists for such a risk but that other sources of resistant bacteria—such as the overuse of antibiotics among humans—are more important. Still, the agricultural use of antibiotics contributes to the problem and led the General Accounting Office to recommend that the Departments of Agriculture and Health and Human Services set up a plan to determine how to more safely use antibiotics in agriculture.

————. *Food Safety: FDA's Imported Seafood Safety Program Shows Some Progress, but Further Improvements Are Needed: Report to Congressional Requesters.* Washington, D.C.: U.S. General Accounting Office, 2004. With 80 percent of seafood consumed in the United States being imported from other countries, the FDA has to make special efforts to ensure seafood safety. A previous evaluation by the General Accounting Office found flaws in FDA procedures, and in this report the office evaluates improvements made over the last several years. The title of the report summarizes its findings: Things are better but not yet good enough. For example, the report recommends that the FDA work more closely with other nations to establish food-safety standards for imported seafood, concentrate inspections on imports of highest risk, and consider employing third-party inspectors.

————. *Meat and Poultry: Better USDA Oversight and Enforcement of Safety Rules Needed to Reduce Risk of Foodborne Illnesses.* Washington, D.C.: U.S. General Accounting Office, 2002. This report on meat-inspection services finds many weaknesses. Of most importance, it argues that the Food Safety Inspection Service of the USDA does not accurately identify violations, in part because the criteria lack precision and clarity. The FSIS has responded to the report by implementing the specific recommendations for improving meat inspection.

————. *School Meal Programs: Few Instances of Foodborne Outbreaks Reported, but Opportunities Exist to Enhance Outbreak Data and Food Safety Practices: Report to Congressional Requesters.* Washington, D.C.: U.S. General Accounting Office, 2003. Since 28 million children receive daily meals through the federal school-meal program, Congress has taken a keen interest in the safety of the food that the government provides. This report to Congress from the General Accounting Office finds that 195 outbreaks of foodborne disease occurred in U.S. schools between 1990 and 1999—about 3 percent of the 7,390 outbreaks reported during that time period. Nearly half the school outbreaks came from improper food handling and preparation. Existing safeguards have helped limit the problem, but the report makes three recommendations: develop more accurate reporting, follow more stringent rules for purchasing safe food, and better train employees in safe food handling and cooking practices.

U.S. Senate. *Food Safety Recall Procedures. Hearings before a Subcommittee of the Committee on Appropriations, United States Senate, One Hundred Seventh Congress, Second Session, December 11, 2002.* Washington, D.C.: U.S. Government Printing Office, 2002. Although preventing outbreaks of foodborne illness is the first goal of the government and industry, recalling infected foods has importance as well. This hearing led by Senator Conrad Burns (R-Montana) addresses both of these topics. Witnesses from business and government discuss problems with the enforcement of food policies, the inspection of meat, and recall procedures. Some express concern that officials unfairly select products from small businesses for recall while doing less to monitor and control larger firms.

World Health Organization. *Hazard Characterization for Pathogens in Food and Water: Guidelines.* Geneva, Switzerland: World Health Organization, 2003. Illness spread through food and water represents a worldwide problem. Unsanitary living conditions and poverty in developing nations make such illness a major source of premature death. This volume from the World Health Organization offers guidelines to nations throughout the world on how to assess the seriousness of threats from food and water pathogens.

ARTICLES

Becker, Elizabeth. "Salmonella Survivor Endorses Push for Food Safety Agency." *New York Times,* February 12, 2003, p. A22. This story about the efforts of Representative Rosa L. DeLauro (D-Connecticut) to pass the Safe Food Act notes her personal interest in the legislation. As a two-year-old, DeLauro nearly died from *Salmonella* poisoning. More recently, deaths from *E. coli* contained in food have strengthened her resolve to require better food-safety enforcement by federal agencies.

———. "3 Lawmakers on Meat Rules Tour a Plant Doing It Right." *New York Times,* August 1, 2003, p. A14. After the disastrous spread of *E. coli* in its hamburgers, Jack in the Box restaurants chose to get its meat from a plant that had food-safety standards higher than required by the law. Members of the Congressional Food Safety Caucus visited the plant, which is run by Texas American Foodservice. The high standards in the plant raise debates in Congress over whether it is sufficient to enforce existing regulations or whether new, stricter regulations, such as those followed in this plant, are needed. Although Congress seems unwilling to pass any changes in the current law, the caucus continues to advocate new standards for meat production.

Threats to Food Safety

Bren, Linda. "Homemade Ice Cream: A Safe Summertime Treat" *FDA Consumer*, vol. 38, no. 4, July/August 2004, pp. 28–29. Because recipes for homemade ice cream often call for the use of raw eggs that can contain *Salmonella* bacteria, several outbreaks of food poisoning occur each year from this food. The article suggests using a cooked egg base as a way to enjoy homemade ice cream without the risk of getting foodborne disease.

Brody, Jane E. "A Recipe for Disaster on Your Kitchen Counter." *New York Times*, April 13, 2004, p. F7. The well-known health reporter and columnist for the *New York Times* describes a study that videotaped cooks working at home. The results were not encouraging. Subjects spent less than the recommended 20 seconds washing their hands, and only one-third used soap. In addition, "Surface cleaning was inadequate, with only one-third of surfaces thoroughly cleaned. Moreover, one-third of the subjects did not attempt to clean surfaces during food preparation. Nearly all subjects cross-contaminated raw meat, poultry, seafood, eggs, or unwashed vegetables with ready-to-eat foods multiple times during food preparation. Unwashed hands were the most common cross-contamination agent. Many subjects undercooked the meat and poultry entrées. Very few subjects used a food thermometer." After presenting this evidence, the author offers guidelines for safer food handling.

Buntain, B. J. "Emerging Challenges in Public Health Protection, Food Safety and Security: Veterinary Needs in the USDA's Food Safety and Inspection Service." *Journal of Veterinary Medical Education*, vol. 31, no. 4, Winter 2004, pp. 333–339. With the introduction of HACCP procedures, food-safety policy has shifted to prevention. One component of prevention involves the work of veterinarians in the field who can identify and treat sick livestock before they go to the slaughterhouse. The author of this article, the chief public health veterinarian of the Food Safety and Inspection Service, calls for more education of a new generation of veterinarians to deal with food-safety issues on the farm.

Burros, Marian. "F.D.A. Seeks Rule for Farms to Increase Egg Safety." *New York Times*, September 21, 2004, p. A21. Responding to demands of food-safety groups, the FDA proposed new regulations that would require farmers to reduce *Salmonella* in eggs. Farmers with more than 3,000 hens would need to buy from *Salmonella*-free stocks, improve cleanliness, do more testing, and keep better records. The egg industry expresses concern about the cost, while consumer groups praise the effort to hold producers rather than consumers responsible for food safety.

Buzby, Jean C. "Older Adults at Risk of Complications from Microbial Foodborne Illness." *Food Review*, vol. 25, no. 2, Summer/Fall 2002, pp. 30–35. As pointed out in this article, older persons are less likely to be infected by foodborne diseases, but when affected they are more likely to face serious illness and death. Given this fact, the aging of the population will likely increase food-related mortality risks. The larger number of persons in nursing homes, where unsanitary meal preparation can affect all residents, also heightens the risk.

Callaway, T. R., R. C. Anderson, T. S. Edrington, K. J. Genovese, R. B. Harvey, T. L. Poole, and D. J. Nisbet. "Recent Pre-Harvest Supplementation Strategies to Reduce Carriage and Shedding of Zoonotic Enteric Bacterial Pathogens in Food Animals." *Animal Health Research Review*, vol. 5, no. 1, June 2004, pp. 35–47. In this article, scientists at Texas A&M University, a nationally known center for the study of food safety, praise the efforts of slaughterhouses and food-processing plants to reduce bacterial contamination of food. They also identify the best methods to reduce the presence of dangerous bacteria in animals before they reach the slaughterhouse. The article uses many technical terms but offers strategies that farmers and ranchers can use to help reduce the threats to food safety in the early stages of the food chain.

Drew, Christopher, and Bud Hazelkorn. "U.S. Inquiry into Meat Safety in New York and New Jersey." *New York Times*, March 22, 2001, pp. A1, B8. Accusations of unsanitary conditions in meatpacking plants on the east coast and the failure of the USDA to properly regulate these plants received considerable attention in New York City. As described in this newspaper article, it led the agency to send inspectors from other parts of the country to check on the conditions and require changes.

Drexler, Madeline. "GH Investigates: The New Food Threat." *Good Housekeeping*, vol. 231, no. 1, July 2000, pp. 116–117, 174–176. Although not considered an investigative or scientific magazine, *Good Housekeeping* has an audience concerned with foodborne illness that is spread in home kitchens. The article describes the problems and offers advice on maintaining a healthy kitchen.

Gorbach, Sherwood L. "Antimicrobial Use in Animal Feed—Time to Stop." *New England Journal of Medicine*, vol. 345, no. 16, October 18, 2001, pp. 1202–1203. Reviewing several recent articles that demonstrate the presence of antibiotic-resistant bacteria in meat, the author of this editorial in one of the nation's most prestigious medical journals concludes that low-dose antibiotics in animal feed present a threat to human health. The animal antibiotics encourage the emergence of bacteria that, when infecting humans through food, do not respond to antibiotics and increase the risk of serious illness or death. The editorial concludes: "Antimicrobials should be used only when indicated in individual infected animals."

Grant, Diane. "Tracking a Killer: Listeriosis Outbreak in Montgomery County, Md." *Washingtonian*, vol. 35, no. 10, July 2000, pp. 39–45. Identifying the source of an outbreak of foodborne illness requires scientific detective work. This article tells of the efforts to uncover the cause of one outbreak of listeriosis—the most deadly of the foodborne diseases. It turns out the disease was spread by gourmet pate. Readers may find the work of public health officials in identifying the culprit as interesting as the work of police officials in identifying criminal offenders.

Hesser, Amanda. "Squeaky Clean? Not Even Close." *New York Times,* January 28, 2004, p. F1. The article lists a number of ways cooks at home promote the spread of bacteria in the food they eat. Common mistakes include failing to wash their hands before starting to cook, cleaning with bacteria-laden sponges, and reusing cutting boards before dishwashing at high temperatures. One expert cited in the article notes, surprisingly, that many cooks with clean kitchens actually spread disease by using towels and sponges with bacteria to wipe counters and dry hands. The article ends with a list of actions needed to promote safety in the home kitchen.

Hunter, Beatrice Trum. "How Safe Is Imported Produce." *Consumers' Research Magazine,* vol. 81, no, 9, September 1998, pp. 10–15. Describing some of the recent outbreaks of illness due to imported produce that was contaminated with foodborne disease, the article reviews the concerns about the health hazard. It also reports the response of the Fresh Produce Association of the Americas to claims that imported produce is more dangerous than domestically grown produce.

———. "The Risky Nature of the Norwalk Virus." *Consumers' Research Magazine,* vol. 84, no. 7, July 2001, pp. 21–24. Identified in 1972 after an earlier outbreak of food poisoning in an elementary school in Norwalk, Ohio, this virus is a major source of worldwide foodborne viral diseases. In describing the virus and the risks it presents, the article notes that the only prevention method is to use safe food-handling practices and thoroughly cook food.

Kamps, Louisa. "Poisoned Apples: Hidden Health Threat—Tainted Fruits and Vegetables." *Prevention,* vol. 56, no. 9, September 2004, pp. 142–149, 151. Although meat most often contains foodborne diseases, the problem has begun to appear increasingly in fruits and vegetables. This article cites statistics that one-third of the 76 million cases of food poisoning each year could be caused by contaminated produce. It also provides advice on how to avoid foodborne disease in produce and how to cope with food poisoning.

Mead, Paul S., Laurence Slutsker, Vance Dietz, Linda F. McCaig, Joseph S. Bresee, Craig Shapiro, Patricia M. Griffin, and Robert V. Tauxe. "Food-Related Illness and Death in the United States." *Emerging Infectious Diseases,* vol. 5, no. 5, September–October 1999, pp. 607–625. Also available online. URL:http://www.cdc.gov/ncidod/eid/vol5no5/mead.htm. Down-

Annotated Bibliography

loaded in April 2006. This article explains how researchers estimated the often-quoted figures on foodborne illness: 76 million persons become sick, 325,000 are hospitalized, and 5,000 die. Most readers will have difficulty following the calculations but may still get a sense of how scientists come up with these numbers.

Morales, S., P. A. Kendall, L. C. Medeiros, V. Hillers, and M. Schroeder. "Health Care Providers' Attitudes toward Current Food Safety Recommendations for Pregnant Women." *Applied Nursing Research*, vol. 17, no. 3, August 2004, pp. 178–186. Pregnant women represent a group particularly vulnerable to foodborne illness, and nurses have the opportunity to advise pregnant women about the importance of food safety. This article examines the knowledge of nurses about food safety and their efforts to convey that knowledge to pregnant women. It finds limitations in both knowledge and the time to discuss the issue among nurses and urges more education on food-safety issues.

Murphy, Dee. "Killer Bacteria: What You Need to Know about Food Safety." *Current Health 2*, vol. 26, no. 7, March 2000, pp. 6–12. The perhaps overdramatic reference to killer bacteria in the title of this article highlights worries about the emergence of new forms of foodborne disease that are both dangerous and resistant to antibiotics. The article notes that, despite efforts of manufacturers and the government to minimize the risk from foodborne bacteria, consumers need to do what they can to protect themselves by using food-safety precautions.

"Of Birds and Bacteria." *Consumer Reports*, vol. 68, no. 1, January 2003, pp. 24–28. Tests of store-bought chicken described in this article identify the presence of strains of *salmonella* and *campylobacter* that are resistant to antibiotics. The article calls for better laws and more stringent inspections to protect consumers from serious diseases carried by raw chicken and offers advice on preparing chicken in order to kill bacteria.

Redmond, E. C., and C. J. Griffith. "Consumer Food Handling in the Home: A Review of Food Safety Studies." *Journal of Food Protection*, vol. 66, no. 1, January 2003, pp. 130–161. A review of published studies on food handling at home finds that substantial numbers of consumers, even those who appear knowledgeable about food safety, frequently use unsafe food-handling practices. Given the inability to eliminate foodborne disease from the food consumers eat, new strategies of education will need to better train consumers.

Roach, Mary. "Germs, Germs Everywhere. Are You Worried? Get Over It." *New York Times*, November 9, 2004, p. F6. Noting that bacteria are everywhere and that antibacterial products for the home are useless, the author argues that people shouldn't worry so much about germs. The most serious risk comes from foodborne bacteria, but even here the risk can be exaggerated: Bacteria "need to multiply into the thousands or millions before they can overwhelm your immune system and cause symptoms. The only way common food-poisoning bacteria can manage this is to spend four or five hours reproducing at room temperature in something moist that you then eat . . . The best defense is the refrigerator. If you don't make a habit of eating perishable food that has been left out too long, don't worry about bacteria."

Rooney, Roisin M., Elaine H. Cramer, Stacey Mantha, Gordon Nichols, Jamie K. Bartram, Jeffrey M. Farber, and Peter K. Benembarek. "A Review of Outbreaks of Foodborne Disease Associated with Passenger Ships: Evidence for Risk Management." *Public Health Reports*, vol. 119, no. 4, July–August 2004, pp. 427–435. With the growth of the cruise ship industry and the risks to thousands of people on board who share the same food supply, outbreaks of food poisoning on ships have become increasing problematic. The study measures the extent of outbreaks over the period from 1970 to 2003 and finds that most of the 50 outbreaks could have been controlled by following safe food-handling and cooking techniques.

Scherer, Michael. "Meatpacking Maverick." *Mother Jones*, vol. 28, no. 6, November/December, 2003, pp. 26–27. This story about John Munsell, the owner of a small meatpacking plant in Montana, is critical of the USDA and large meatpacking corporations. Munsell discovered that meat he received from a plant owned by ConAgra in Greeley, Colorado, tested positive for *E. coli*, although the meat had been approved by the USDA. In response, the USDA closed down Munsell's small plant rather than try to locate the source of the problem. The story describes efforts of the USDA to silence Munsell's criticisms of the agency that has responsibility for the safety of meat.

Sharkey, Joe. "Aggressive Precaution in the Food You Eat." *New York Times*, October 12, 2004, p. C12. The author advises business travelers on how to avoid food poisoning. Of special advice: Avoid convention buffets. Even food properly handled by employees and kept at proper temperatures can become contaminated after dozens or hundreds of people have moved through the buffet line.

Sugarman, Carole. "STOP Report Assails Government for Persistent Threat of Foodborne Disease." *Food Chemical News*, vol. 45, no. 1, February 17, 2003, pp. 25–27. This article summarizes a report from the food-safety group Safe Tables Our Priority that is highly critical of the government's food-safety policies. The report, which came out on the 10-year anniversary of the deadly Jack in the Box food poisonings, identifies failures in safeguards on the farm and in slaughterhouses, the overreliance on consumers to protect themselves, the lack of knowledge of doctors about food pathogens, and inadequate government policies. The group met with the Department of Agriculture undersecretary for food safety, Elsa Murano, who expressed sympathy with the goals of the group but also noted that deaths from food poisoning have declined and that the agencies had made progress in dealing with the problem.

Wagner, Cynthia G. "Poisons on Our Plates." *The Futurist*, vol. 35, no. 4, July/August 2001, p. 6. Even if policies and good cooking practices help reduce the risk of foodborne disease, other changes in society may counter such progress. Population aging and weakening of the immune systems of the population, for example, may increase deaths from foodborne illness.

Wallace, Kathryn. "A Plateful of Trouble." *Reader's Digest*, vol. 165, August 2004, pp. 110–117. This article lays out basic concerns about food safety. It reviews the figures on incidents of foodborne diseases, the risks of contamination of nearly all types of foods, and the increase in recalls of food products. The article does not offer much in the way of original insight but does summarize the central facts.

Yeoman, Barry. "Dangerous Food: The Shocking Truth That Puts Your Family at Risk. N. Donley Lobbys for Meat Inspection in Wake of Son's Death from Contaminated Hamburgers." *Redbook*, vol. 195, no. 2, August 2000, pp. 110–111, 123–124. Along with the tragic story of the death from food poisoning of six-year-old Alex Donley, this article describes the efforts of S.T.O.P. (Safe Tables Our Priority)—a group founded by victims and family members of victims of food poisoning—to improve inspection procedures for meat.

WEB DOCUMENTS

"Antibiotic Resistance Project." Center for Science in the Public Interest. Available online. URL: http://www.cspinet.org/ar. Downloaded in April 2006. Concerned about the increasing ability of bacteria to evade antibiotics, this public interest group blames the overuse of antibiotics in both humans and animals. The page provides links to more information on the problem, describes legislative and regulatory actions to deal with it, and offers resources to consumers and health-care providers in minimizing use of antibiotics.

"Antibiotics and Safe Food." Animal Health Institute, Keep Animals Healthy. Available online. URL: http://www.ahi.org/antibioticsDebate/antibioticsandsafefood.asp. Downloaded in April 2006. The Animal Health Institute represents manufacturers of animal health-care products, including antibiotic feed additives. This web page defends the use of low-dose antibiotics in animal feed against increasingly strong criticisms made by scientists and physicians. The web page argues that antibiotics keep food animals healthy and, when used carefully, do not present a threat to human health.

"Bacteria and Foodborne Illness." National Digestive Diseases Information Clearinghouse, National Institute of Diabetes and Digestive and Kidney Diseases. Available online. URL: http://digestive.niddk.nih.gov/ddiseases/pubs/bacteria. Downloaded in April 2006. Many federal government agencies offer information on foodborne illness, and this web page authored by an agency of the National Institutes of Health provides a clear summary of important issues and a list of other organizations with special interest in the topic.

"Diagnosis and Management of Foodborne Illnesses: A Primer for Physicians and Other Health Care Professionals." American Medical Association. Available online. URL: http://www.ama-assn.org/ama/pub/category/3629.html. Updated on January 12, 2005. Although designed for physicians, this web page is written at an introductory level that the general public can understand. Along with introductory materials, it contains links to several booklets, each of which examines a different aspect of foodborne diseases.

"Fight BAC: Keep Food Safe from Bacteria." Partnership for Food Safety Education. Available online. URL: http://www.fightbac.org. Downloaded in April 2006. This program to promote food safety follows the recommendations of the Consumer Research Resources Center on how to develop an effective publicity campaign. In terms of content, the web page emphasizes the four steps—clean, separate, cook, and chill—for home food safety; in terms of presentation, it includes attractive visuals.

"Foodborne Diseases." Health Matters, National Institute of Allergy and Infectious Diseases. Available online. URL: http://www.niaid.nih.gov/factsheets/foodbornedis.htm. Posted in April 2002. This fact sheet describes five foodborne diseases caused by bacteria: botulism, campylobacteriosis, *E. coli* infection, salmonellosis, and shigellosis. The question-and-answer format of the page makes for clear explanations and easy understanding.

"Foodborne Diseases." World Health Organization. Available online. URL: http://www.who.int/topics/foodborne_diseases/en. Downloaded in April 2006. Compiles studies and data on global aspects of foodborne disease.

"Foodborne Illness." Centers for Disease Control and Prevention, Division of Bacterial and Mycotic Disease, Disease Information. Available online. URL: http://www.cdc.gov/ncidod/dbmd/diseaseinfo/foodborneinfections_g.htm. Updated on October 25, 2005. Presented in the form of questions and answers, this web page offers a useful introduction to the topic of foodborne illness. It describes the major types of diseases, the methods used by the CDC to investigate outbreaks, the causes of outbreaks, the treatment of the disease, and actions consumers can take to minimize risk. This is a good place to start in gathering information on the topic.

Annotated Bibliography

"Foodborne Illness Cost Calculator." Economic Research Service, U.S. Department of Agriculture. Available online. URL: http://www.ers.usda. gov/data/foodborneillness. Updated on March 31, 2006. This page allows users to estimate the economic costs of foodborne illness by changing the assumptions made about the loss of income from sickness.

"Foodborne Illness Education Center." U.S. Department of Agriculture/ Food and Drug Administration. Available online. URL: http://www. nal.usda.gov/foodborne. Updated in April 2006. Agencies in different departments of the government have collaborated to educate the public about foodborne illness. The web page provides food-safety education and training materials, HACCP training materials, discussion groups, and stories of strategies and solutions to food-safety problems.

"Foodborne Illnesses." Yahoo! Search Directory. Available online. URL: http://dir.yahoo.com/Health/Diseases_and_Conditions/Foodborne_ Illnesses. Downloaded in April 2006. This web page lists other web pages that provide information on foodborne illnesses. Internet users can scan possible sites from this page and select the ones of most value to them.

"Foodborne Illness: Prevention Strategies." Clemson Extension Home and Garden Information Center. Available online. URL: http://hgic.clemson. edu/factsheets/HGIC3620.htm. Downloaded in April 2006. Although brief in its coverage, this web page summarizes key points about the sources, consequences, and prevention strategies for foodborne illness. A good place to start for those wanting an introduction.

"Foodborne Pathogens." FoodSafety.gov. Available online. URL: http:// www.foodsafety.gov/~fsg/fsgpath.html. Updated on November 22, 2005. Like other pages within the FoodSafety site, this one offers dozens of links to government publications and information sheets. The links on this topic are listed without commentary or recommendations, making it hard to know which ones would prove most helpful. Still, this page can help in exploring the variety of resources available from the government.

"Food Safety and Nutrition." National Restaurant Association. Available online. URL: http://www.restaurant.org/foodsafety. Downloaded in April 2006. Concerned about negative publicity and harm to customers from outbreaks of food poisoning caused by restaurant food, the National Restaurant Association offers information to its members and the public on food safety. The link to foodborne illnesses lists the most common pathogens, and the how-to library presents information on keeping salad bars safe and working with health inspectors.

"HCWH Policy Statement on Antibiotics in Food." Health Care without Harm. Available online. URL: http://www.noharm.org/details.cfm?ID= 894&type=document. Downloaded in April 2006. This group opposes

179

the use of antibiotics in food animals and offers a useful listing of references that support its views.

"Home Food Safety: It's in Your Hands." American Dietetic Association and ConAgra Foods. Available online. URL: http://www.homefoodsafety.org. Downloaded in April 2006. The web page focuses on home-safety tips as a means of highlighting the importance to consumers of food safety. Some might view the sponsorship by ConAgra Foods, a large meatpacking company, as a ploy to shift attention away from the problems of food plants in providing safe products. In any case, the page has links to brochures, videos, and tips for safely dealing with a variety of foods.

"Top Ten Fast Food Chains: How Clean Are They?" Dateline NBC. Available online. URL: http://www.msnbc.msn.com/id/7150482. Updated on March 11, 2005. The television show *Dateline NBC* gathered information on critical health violations in 100 fast-food restaurants in each of 10 chains. This web page summarizes the results of the investigation. Critical health violations such as the presence of insects or rodents, lack of cleanliness, improper food temperatures, or failure of employees to wash hands occurred surprisingly often. Jack in the Box had the fewest critical violations—45 per 100 inspections—while McDonald's had the most, with 126 critical violations per 100 inspections.

MAD COW DISEASE (BSE)

BOOKS

Harris, D., ed. *Mad Cow Disease and Related Spongiform Encephalopathies.* New York: Springer, 2004. Part of a series of books on current topics in microbiology and immunology, this book describes current research on BSE, CJD, and prions. Most appropriate for biologists and medical researchers.

Icon Health Publications. *Mad Cow Disease—A Medical Dictionary, Bibliography, and Annotated Research Guide to Internet References.* San Diego: Icon Health Publications, 2004. Although designed for physicians and medical students, this volume offers a detailed reference source on BSE that others may find useful.

Kelleher, Colm A. *Brain Trust: The Hidden Connection between Mad Cow and Misdiagnosed Alzheimer's Disease.* New York: Paraview Pocket Books, 2004. This exposé by a biochemist argues that BSE in the United States may already have affected humans but has been hidden by the increase in Alzheimer's disease. If true, the threat of BSE would prove much more serious than experts claim. This allegation receives little support in the scientific community and gives much weight to conspiracies to hide the truth. Although exaggerated, the presentation of worst-case scenarios about mad cow disease is intriguing.

Klitzman, Robert. *The Trembling Mountain: A Personal Account of Kuru, Cannibals, and Mad Cow Disease.* Cambridge, Mass.: Perseus, 1998. Having spent a year doing research in Papua New Guinea in 1981 before starting medical school, the author describes his experiences working with the Fore—the formerly cannibalistic tribe that had suffered from the deadly disease kuru. He describes the people he met and his life with the tribe along with some detail on the disease and its relationship to mad cow disease. The stories give a personal face to the disease and the devastation it brought to this small and isolated society.

Margulies, Phillip. *Creutzfeldt-Jakob Disease.* New York: The Rosen Group, 2004. This short, 61-page book examines the history, current issues, and future of CJD, the more general form of the disease transmitted to humans from BSE. It is written at a level appropriate for young adults and aims to dramatize the discoveries made about this mysterious illness.

Nunnally, Brian K., and Ira S. Krull, eds. *Prions and Mad Cow Disease.* New York: Marcel Dekker, 2004. This edited volume of articles by scientists for scientists and government officials comes from a 2001 conference. It covers topics such as the diagnosis, causes, and prevention of bovine spongiform encephalopathy, and it describes current understandings of prions and efforts to develop a vaccine or cure. However, it may be too technical for many readers.

Powell, Douglas. "Mad Cow Disease and the Stigmatization of British Beef." In James Flynn, Paul Slovic, and Howard Kunreuther, eds., *Risk, Media, and Stigma: Understanding Public Challenges to Modern Science and Technology.* London: Earthscan Publications, 2001, pp. 219–228. In reviewing the mad cow crisis in Britain, the author strongly criticizes government claims made from 1986–1996 that BSE created no risk for humans. He argues that hiding the potential risk for the purpose of protecting the short-term economic interests of the cattle industry ultimately worsened the long-term harm. Had officials admitted their uncertainty about the possible harm of BSE to humans early on and developed ways to minimize the risk, the public might have been better protected from vCJD. They might also have avoided the collapse of the market for British beef that followed the 1996 announcement of the transmission of BSE to humans.

Rampton, Sheldon, and John Stauber. *Mad Cow U.S.A.: Could the Nightmare Happen Here?* Monroe, Maine: Common Courage Press, 2004. Highly critical of the British and American governments that, according to the authors, conspired with the food industry to hide the facts about mad cow disease from the public, this book warns of the risks of meat eating. The book correctly criticizes the denials of risk made by the British government to protect the beef industry but takes a more extreme view in claiming that the government is waging a war on free speech by passing laws that criminalize critics of food safety.

Ratzan, Scott C., ed. *The Mad Cow Crisis: Health and the Public Good.* New York: New York University Press, 1998. Articles in this edited volume address issues such as the transmission of BSE across species, the ability to predict the spread of BSE and vCJD, the media's coverage of the mad cow disease crisis, problems with public health policy, and needed changes in farming to avoid future food-disease problems. Although directed toward scholars rather than the general public and a bit dated, the volume includes articles on a wide range of topics.

Rhodes, Richard. *Deadly Feasts: The "Prion" Controversy and the Public's Health.* New York: Touchstone, 1998. The author, a Pulitzer Prize winner for his book, *The Making of the Atomic Bomb*, turns his writing skills to tracing the discovery of the deformed protein responsible for various forms of transmissible spongiform encephalopathy. Beginning with the puzzle of kuru among New Guinea tribes and ending with research on the future course of the disease, Rhodes concentrates on the scientific research but brings the technical details to life by describing the personalities of the scientists. Although the 1998 edition updates the original 1997 publication with some new information, the major weakness of the book is that much has happened in the six years since its publication. Still, it makes for fascinating reading and is filled with clear explanations of sometimes complex topics.

Ridgway, Tom. *Mad Cow Disease: Bovine Spongiform Encephalopathy.* New York: Rosen Publishing Group, 2002. Aimed at young adults and only 64 pages long, this short book complements Phillip Margulies's *Cruetzfeld-Jakob Disease.* It describes in simple terms how prions affect brain cells in mad cow disease and how the disease affects the behavior of cows before death. In answer to the question, "Are we safe?" the author admits that our limited scientific knowledge and difficulty in testing for prions in animals and food make it impossible to say.

Schwartz, Maxime, and Edward Schneider. *How the Cows Turned Mad.* Berkeley: University of California Press, 2003. Described as a scientific thriller and written in nontechnical prose, this book traces the discovery of the causes of scrapie, kuru, mad cow disease, CJD, and prions and discusses related scientific discoveries over the last 100 years. Maxime Schwartz, a microbiologist and former head of the Pasteur Institute, originally published the book in France and gives more attention to continental Europe than other books.

Annotated Bibliography

U.S. General Accounting Office. *Mad Cow Disease: Improvements in the Animal Feed Ban and Other Regulatory Areas Would Strengthen U.S. Prevention Efforts: Report to Congressional Requesters.* Washington, D.C.: U.S. General Accounting Office, 2002. Also available online. URL: http://www.gao.gov/new.items/d02183.pdf. Posted in November 2002. An audit by the U.S. General Accounting Office of USDA and FDA procedures to prevent an outbreak of BSE finds room for improvements. The report notes that inspection efforts have failed to keep pace with the increases in meat imports, do enough to ensure compliance of private firms with rules to keep animal protein out of cattle feed, and maintain sufficiently detailed records. The agencies responded to these criticisms by improving their inspection and record-keeping activities, but another audit is needed to determine if these changes have been effective.

U.S. Senate. *Mad Cow Disease: Are Our Precautions Adequate? Hearing before the Subcommittee on Consumer Affairs, Foreign Commerce, and Tourism of the Committee on Commerce, Science, and Transportation, United States Senate, One Hundred Seventh Congress, First Session.* Washington, D.C.: U.S. Government Printing Office, April 4, 2001. Predating the discovery of the first instance of mad cow disease in the United States, this hearing presents views of senators and witnesses on actions needed to protect the nation from the kind of human and bovine disaster that occurred in Britain. Discussion often centers on the need to protect cattle and the safety of food without generating undue concern among the public and harming the sale of U.S. beef. Senators want to protect the beef industry as well as the public. Witnesses include both critics of present policy who believe actions to protect the safety of food are insufficient and representatives of the meat and feed industry who defend the actions taken thus far.

————. *To Examine the Current Situation Regarding the Discovery of a Case of Bovine Spongiform Encephalopathy in a Dairy Cow in Washington State as it Relates to Food Safety, Livestock Marketing and International Trade. Hearing before the Committee on Agriculture, Nutrition, and Forestry, United States Senate, One Hundred Eighth Congress, Second Session.* Washington, D.C.: U.S. Government Printing Office, January 27, 2004. The long title describes the contents of this volume. Senators on the committee express their views about the risks to food and, in many cases, to the international livestock trade and the financial well-being of ranchers. They also contain the testimony of three witnesses: Ann Veneman, secretary of agriculture; Lester Crawford, deputy commissioner, Food and Drug Administration; and Alfonso Torres, associate dean for veterinary public policy, College of Veterinary Medicine, Cornell University. The testimony summarizes the actions of the USDA and FDA to deal with the discovery of BSE in the United States and provides some background on the disease and its potential effects. However, the nature of the Senate hearing sometimes makes it hard to follow the details of the discussion.

Van Zwanenberg, Patrick, and Erik Millstone. "'Mad Cow Disease' 1980s–2000: How Reassurances Undermined Precaution." In Poul Harremoëes, David Gee, Malcolm MacGarvin, Andy Stirling, Jane Keys, Brian Wynne, and Sofia Guedes Vaz, eds., *The Precautionary Principle in the 20th Century: Late Lessons from Early Warnings.* London: Earthscan Publications, 2002, pp. 170–184. Based on numerous case studies of health and environmental problems, this book develops the theme that inaction by governments in response to early warnings have made the consequences of the problems all the more serious. The precautionary principle advocates action to deal with potentially serious problems before studies demonstrate strong or certain proof of harm. The principle applies clearly to the mad cow crisis, as discussed in this particular chapter. By waiting for indisputable proof of the link between BSE and human disease, officials in the United Kingdom put its population at risk and contributed to the collapse of its beef industry.

Walters, Mark Jerome. *Six Modern Plagues and How We Are Causing Them.* Washington, D.C.: Island Press/Shearwater Books, 2003. The plagues referenced in the title involve diseases that have jumped across species. Along with mad cow disease, the veterinarian author examines a variety of other diseases that have been spread in part by animals and food products. He argues that, in one sense, humans have contributed to these plagues by changing the environments in which animals live and the kinds of interactions that take place between humans and animals.

Yam, Philip. *The Pathological Protein: Mad Cow, Chronic Wasting, and Other Deadly Prion Diseases.* New York: Copernicus Books, 2003. Although only two of the 14 chapters focus on mad cow disease, this highly recommended book offers an exceptionally well-written, up-to-date, and science-based history of the disease and others stemming from prions. The author interviewed several families of the victims of vCJD and BSE, who tell sad stories of the devastating deaths of their children and loved ones. He also highlights scientific developments up to 2003 and efforts to develop a cure for the disease.

ARTICLES

Adler, Jerry. "Mad Cow: What's Safe Now?" *Newsweek*, vol. 143, no. 2, January 12, 2004, pp. 42–48. Describing the efforts of the government to recall beef that may have come in contact with BSE-infected tissue, this article identifies several problems in the food-safety system. Multiple government agencies with overlapping jurisdictions and laws that in some

184

Annotated Bibliography

cases date back nearly a century contribute to difficulties in protecting the public from unsafe food.

Amsden, David. "Let Us Eat Steak! Unfazed Beef Eaters Bite Back." *New York*, vol. 37, no. 1, January 12, 2004, p. 10. Interviews with New Yorkers reveal that steaks and beef remain popular with the public despite the discovery of mad cow disease in the United States. The article also interviews several food-industry representatives about the continued popularity of beef.

Balter, Michael. "Uncertainties Plague Projections of vCJD Toll." *Science*, vol. 294, no. 5543, October 26, 2001, pp. 770–771. This article reveals the difficulties in predicting the consequences of BSE for human health. Some scientists suggest that worldwide deaths from vCJD have already peaked, while others expect the trend to continue upward. A key obstacle in estimating future trends comes from the unknown genetic susceptibility of the population to the disease.

Bren, Linda. "Agencies Work to Corral Mad Cow Disease." *FDA Consumer*, vol. 38, no. 3, May/June 2004, pp. 28–35. Reviews the response of the FDA and USDA to the discovery of a cow with BSE in Washington State in December 2003 and the new procedures developed by the agencies to protect beef from this disease.

Breu, Giovanna. "Is Our Beef Safe? Interview with G. Legname." *People*, vol. 61, no. 1, January 12, 2004, pp. 113–114. Although *People* magazine is generally not a source of scientific information, this issue interviews a molecular biologist at the University of California on the health risks of BSE.

Brink, Susan, and Nancy Shute. "Is It Safe?" *U.S. News & World Report*, vol. 136, no. 1, January 12, 2004, pp. 16–21. Those looking for a simple answer to this question will have trouble finding it. The article reviews the reassurances offered by the government and the cattle industry as well as claims from industry critics that more needs to be done to ensure the safety of beef products. In the end, the article explains why settling the debate is so difficult: Scientists understand so little about prions that it is hard to know how and if BSE might emerge and spread.

Chesebro, Bruce. "A Fresh Look at BSE." *Science*, vol. 305, September 24, 2004, pp. 1,918–1,919, 1,921. This up-to-date review of the evidence on the potential for the spread of BSE in the United States suggests that the disease could take new and unexpected forms. Cross-infection from other species or spontaneous development may lead to BSE-like diseases despite efforts to eliminate the use of animal protein in cattle feed. Efforts to protect humans from these risks must focus on careful testing and care in use of cows for human food.

Forbes, Ian. "Making a Crisis out of a Drama: The Political Analysis of BSE Policy-Making in the UK." *Political Studies*, vol. 52, no. 2, June 2004,

185

pp. 342–357. The safety of food from BSE depends on government policies and regulations, and the British government received severe criticism for not doing more to protect its citizens from contaminated beef and vCJD. This article uses the mad cow disease episode to analyze policy making in the United Kingdom. It offers a balanced view of the difficulties faced by the government in making its decisions.

Freese, Betsy. "Miles to Go on Mad Cow." *Successful Farming*, vol. 102, no. 3, Mid-February 2004, p. 57. The author urges farmers not to be reassured by the continued steady demand for beef despite the discovery of BSE in the United States. She argues that, to protect against future problems, farmers should overhaul their feeding system to ensure cattle do not get animal protein. Only with this kind of change will consumers remain confident in the long run of the safety of beef.

Freinkel, Susan. "Could You Get Mad Cow from a Pill?" *Health*, vol. 15, no. 5, June 2001, pp. 66–70. Although the greatest threat of contracting BSE comes from eating contaminated beef, this article identifies another possible source. Some pills that promise increased energy, intelligence, and sexual vitality use dried tissue from animal glands, which could contain prions from infected animals. The government does not regulate these supplements the same way it regulates the distribution of beef.

Helps, C. R., A. V. Fisher, D. A. Harbour, D. H. O'Neill, and A. C. Knight. "Transfer of Spinal Cord Material to Subsequent Bovine Carcasses at Splitting." *Journal of Food Protection*, vol. 67, no. 9, September 2004, pp. 1,921–1,926. The veterinarian authors demonstrate that sawing cattle carcasses along the spine transfers tissue from this part of the cow to other parts. Such transfer could contaminate otherwise healthy meat with BSE-infected tissue from the spinal cord of an infected cow. To protect against contamination, food processors may need to do more to clean saws and cutting instruments.

Hodel, Lindsey. "Mad Cow Disease Hits Home." *Mother Earth News*, no. 203, April/May 2004, p. 22. This article views the discovery of a cow with BSE in the United States much more negatively than the government agencies. It argues that regulations remain insufficient to protect the public. The continued use of animal protein in feed for some livestock and the lack of testing of live animals reveal the limitations of current policies.

Hurst, Blake. "Mad Cow Sanity." *The American Enterprise*, vol. 15, no. 3, April/May 2004, p. 11. Arguing that the beef supply in the country is safe, the author criticizes the media for exaggerating the threat and calls for more rational reporting on the issue.

Jalonick, Mary Clare. "Embattled Meat and Cattle Industry Finds Potent Ally in White House." *CQ Weekly*, vol. 62, no. 5, January 31, 2004, pp. 291–292.

Critics of government food policies hope that the discovery of BSE in the United States will put pressure on the White House to do more to ensure the safety of beef. They believe that the National Cattlemen's Beef Association, which has opposed more stringent regulations on beef safety, has had undue influence on President George W. Bush. The article describes the political dealings among the multiple parties involved with this issue.

Levine, Ed. "Where's the Beef From?" *Business Week*, no. 3869, February 9, 2004, p. 96. The article in this business magazine describes the desires of many consumers to pay higher prices for beef raised on family farms with organic feed and careful processing. They believe that this would help protect them from mad cow and other diseases spread by eating beef.

McCombie, Brian. "Mysterious Disease Spreads in Deer, Elk: Wasting Illness May Travel via Game Farms." *Mother Earth News*, no. 204, June/July 2004, pp. 44–49. Although it has not spread to humans, chronic wasting disease among deer and elk has similarities to mad cow disease and could jump species much as mad cow disease did. This article describes the spread of the disease in Colorado, Nebraska, and Wyoming and suggests that the disease emerged in game farm animals before spreading to deer and elk in the wild. The disease warrants care in eating game meat that might be affected by the disease.

McNeil, Donald G., Jr. "Inspector General Details Flaws in Mad Cow Testing." *New York Times*, July 15, 2004, p. A20. A report from the inspector general in the Department of Agriculture criticized the voluntary nature of the testing program for BSE and cited two incidents in which testing regulations had been violated. The mistakes involved the failure to identify a cow as a downer, which would have required more detailed testing, and the slaughter of an animal suspected of having BSE. The incidents did not lead to an outbreak of BSE but indicated the need for improving testing procedures.

Moss, Michael, Richard A. Oppel, Jr., and Simon Romero. "Mad Cow Forces Beef Industry to Change Course." *New York Times*, January 5, 2004, pp. A1, A14. The article describes controversy over the use of downer cows—those unable to stand or walk—in meat for human consumption. The beef industry has long resisted efforts to prohibit the use of these animals in human food, claiming that their meat is healthy. However, the higher rate of BSE in downer cows contradicts this claim and would lead to banning of downer cows for human food.

Normile, Dennis. "First U.S. Case of Mad Cow Sharpens Debate over Testing." *Science*, vol. 303, no. 5655, January 9, 2004, pp. 156–157. Although most agree that some form of testing is necessary to prevent BSE from spreading to food products, determining the best means of doing the testing provokes debate. While the public favors testing of all slaughtered cattle, some scientists and the USDA favor an approach that concentrates on animals at highest risk and relies more on sampling procedures.

Sterling, Bruce. "Why Europe Has No Taste for the Future." *Wired*, vol. 12, no. 2, February 2004, p. 82. The author suggests that deaths in Europe from eating beef with mad cow disease have made the public overly suspicious of technological breakthroughs in agriculture that could end hunger and malnutrition. Concerns about the purity of food raised by BSE incidents make Europeans unwilling to take advantage of these breakthroughs.

Talbot, David. "Where's the Beef From? Tracking Systems." *Technology Review*, vol. 107, no. 5, June 2004, pp. 48–53, 55–56. The government aims to improve the safety of beef by developing a national identification system that would allow quick recall of meat found to contain mad cow disease. This article describes the benefits of a digital record-keeping system. Improved tracking might, for example, help ensure that animals have been raised on organic feed and are free of certain diseases.

Thomas, Cathy Booth. "How Now, Mad Cow? Effects of Mad Cow Scare on Beef Industry." *Time*, vol. 163, no. 2, January 12, 2004, pp. 46–48. Describing the economic impact of the first confirmed instance of mad cow disease in the United States, the article notes that 30 countries banned the import of U.S. beef. The beef industry has improved its performance since then, but continued concerns of consumers across the world about food safety could lead to future problems.

Van Zwanenberg, Patrick, and Erik Millstone. "BSE: A Paradigm of Policy Failure." *The Political Quarterly*, vol. 74, no. 1, January/March 2003, pp. 27–37. Using the mad cow disease crisis as a means to understand the use of science in public policy, this article provides a detailed review of government decision making on the issue.

Zaun, Todd. "World Business Briefing Asia: Japan: Beef Ban Reconsidered." *New York Times*, September 10, 2004, p. W1. Japan banned the import of U.S. beef after a case of BSE was discovered in the United States. Having already suffered from an outbreak of BSE, Japan wanted the United States to test all its cattle for the disease. The United States has resisted testing cattle less than 20 months old because tests cannot detect the disease, and Japan seemed ready to accept the exceptions.

WEB DOCUMENTS

"Bovine Spongiform Encephalopathy (BSE)." Department of Environment, Food, and Rural Affairs. Available online. URL: http://www. defra.gov.uk/animalh/bse. Downloaded in April 2006. This agency of the U.K. government offers information and links specific to BSE issues in Britain.

"Bovine Spongiform Encephalopathy: 'Mad Cow Disease.'" FoodSafety. gov. Available online. URL: http://www.foodsafety.gov/~fsg/bse.html. Downloaded in April 2006. Although not itself a direct source of information, this web page offers links to documents on BSE from four federal agencies: the Centers for Disease Control and Prevention, the Foreign Agricultural Service, the Food and Drug Administration, and the Food Safety Inspection Service. It also offers links to international documents from the World Health Organization.

"The Brain Eater." Nova Online, PBS Online. Available online. URL: http://www.pbs.org/wgbh/nova/madcow. Downloaded in November 2004. This online companion site to the popular PBS television show *Nova* focuses on the scientific background of BSE. It addresses several intriguing questions: Could experts have discovered the link between mad cow disease in cattle and humans sooner, do prions really exist, and how does the mad cow crisis illustrate the vital relationship between science and society? The television show first ran on August 17, 1999, and the web page has not been updated to include more recent information. Still, *Nova* is known for dramatizing scientific discoveries and making fundamental science accessible to the public. This web page does much the same for selected issues about mad cow disease.

BSE (Bovine Spongiform Encephalopathy, or Mad Cow Disease). Centers for Disease Control and Prevention. Available online. URL: http://www.cdc. gov/ncidod/dvrd/bse. Updated March 15, 2006. The CDC web page describes BSE and the extent of its presence in the United States. It also has links to similar pages on CJD disease, a news archive, and references and resources. The page nicely summarizes key facts about the disease and directs readers to helpful sources of related information.

"BSE—Bovine Spongiform Encephalopathy." Google. Available online. URL: http://directory.google.com/Top/Science/Technology/Food_Science/ Consumer_Concerns/BSE_-_Bovine_Spongiform_Encephalopathy. Downloaded in April 2006. This compilation of web pages falls within the Science, Technology, Food, and Consumer categories (and highlights additional information on BSE within the health and Europe categories). The links give special attention to news and information about the disease in other nations. The page proves a useful starting place for reviewing web documents.

"BSEinfo.org." Cattlemen's Beef Board & National Cattlemen's Beef Association. Available online. URL: http://www.bseinfo.org. Downloaded in April 2006. Contrasting with the many web pages critical of government-inspection policies, this web page from beef producer groups defends the safety of beef and the effectiveness of current policies.

"BSE Information Source." Iowa State University Iowa Beef Center. Available online. URL: http://www.iowabeefcenter.org/content/bsemain.htm. Downloaded in April 2006. Designed primarily to help Iowa Beef producers and related industries, this web page contains articles by Iowa State University experts, cattle ranchers, and food-processing companies on a variety of topics ranging from rapid testing for BSE to meat recovery procedures. It also includes reports on the beef market implications of BSE testing results.

"BSE Test Results." U.S. Department of Agriculture. Available online. URL: http://www.aphis.usda.gov/lpa/issues/bse_testing/test_results.html. Downloaded in April 2006. This web page reports daily results from BSE testing and a weekly summary of the test results since June 1, 2004. For each week, a table lists the number of negative tests, the number of inconclusive tests, the final results of the inconclusive tests, and the number of positive tests. Based on testing 682,552 cows through April 2006, the table on the web page shows two positive results and two inconclusive results that upon further testing proved negative.

"Choosing Safer Beef to Eat." Center for Science in the Public Interest. Available online. URL: http://www.cspinet.org/foodsafety/saferbeef. html. Downloaded in April 2006. This organization devoted to eliminating hazards from food and improving healthful eating notes that the risk of getting vCJD from eating infected beef are incredibly small. Still, it suggests ways to lower the risk even more. The page also lists links to recent new articles on BSE and food safety.

"Commonly Asked Questions about BSE in Products Regulated by FDA's Center for Food Safety and Applied Nutrition (CFSAN)." U.S. Food and Drug Administration. Available online. URL: http://vm.cfsan.fda.gov/ ~comm/bsefaq.html. Downloaded in April 2006. This web page reviews the facts about BSE and offers assurances from the agency in charge of preventing the human exposure to the disease. It argues that, given the regulations and safeguards that are in place, BSE is extremely unlikely to become established in the United States. It notes that the FDA prohibits the use of the following cattle material in human food: parts of nonambulatory, disabled (downer) cattle; organs of cattle 30 months of age or older; tonsils and small intestines; mechanically separated beef; and uninspected and unapproved cattle—all most likely to contain infectious prions.

"Cow Madness." University of Wisconsin. Available online. URL: http:// whyfiles.org/012mad_cow. Downloaded in April 2006. With funding from the National Science Foundation, the University of Wisconsin has created a number of web pages on scientific issues that it calls the "Why Files." This "Why File" web page on mad cow disease provides a clear summary of the issues and glossary of the terms that serves as a short and helpful introduction to the topic.

"Creutzfeld-Jakob Disease." Medline Plus. Available online. URL: http:// www.nlm.nih.gov/medlineplus/creutzfeldtjakobdisease.html. Downloaded in April 2006. Funded by the National Institutes of Health, this web page offers up-to-date information on the human form of mad cow disease. Various links describe the disease, answer questions consumers might have about it, and review some of the ongoing research to prevent and cure the disease.

Gregor, Michael. "Could Mad Cow Disease Already be Killing Thousands of Americans Every Year?" Common Dreams News Center. Available online. URL: http://www.commondreams.org/views04/0107-07.htm. Posted on January 7, 2004. Common Dreams describes itself as a progressive organization. This article takes a decidedly minority viewpoint in suggesting that classic CJD might stem from BSE. Although vCJD, which has a proven link to BSE and has not appeared in America (except for one person who came to the United States after living most of her life in Britain), the classic CJD appears in hundreds of cases each year. No one knows what causes classic CJD, but most experts do not attribute the cause to BSE. This article suggests that the possible link between BSE and CJD needs to be examined more carefully.

"Mad Cow Disease." Center for Food Safety. Available online. URL: http://www.centerforfoodsafety.org/mad_cow_di3.cfm. Downloaded in April 2006. Generally critical of government food policy and supportive of more stringent efforts to protect food safety, this organization provides a balanced summary of the risks of mad cow disease. It also, however, suggests several additional steps it believes government agencies should take to protect the public from the disease.

"Mad Cow Disease: Mad Cow Q & A." Center for Consumer Freedom. Available online. URL: http://www.consumerfreedom.com/issuepage. cfm/topic/5. Downloaded in April 2006. This center promotes consumer responsibility for food choices and opposes efforts of activists, government officials, and others to limit freedom of food choices. The articles it includes on the web page aim to combat exaggerated claims made about the risks of mad cow disease.

"Mad Cow Disease, Mad Deer Disease: Chronic Wasting Disease, Bovine Spongiform Encephalopathy." Organic Consumers Association. Available online. URL: http://www.organicconsumers.org/madcow.htm. Downloaded in April 2006. This group opposes most modern agricultural practices used in the United States today and argues that existing safety measures do not do enough to protect consumers from BSE and related diseases. The web page includes a large number of news stories and reports, many of which suggest that BSE may be more of a hazard than the government is willing to admit.

"Mad Cow Update: How to Limit Your Risk." ConsumerReports.org. Available online. URL: http://www.consumerreports.org/cro/health-fitness/mad-cow-disease-update-705.htm. Posted in July 2005. This respected organization gives specific advice to consumers about ways to avoid mad cow disease. Recognizing that the risk of human infection from BSE in the United States appears small but is really unknown, the web page suggests that, if giving up beef altogether is not an option, consumers should eat organic or grass-feed beef and avoid hamburgers, hotdogs, and sausages that are most likely to contain nervous-system tissue and infectious prions.

"Number of Reported Cases of Bovine Spongiform Encephalopathy (BSE) in Farmed Cattle Worldwide (Excluding the United Kingdom)." World Organization for Animal Health. Available online. URL: http://www.oie.int/eng/info/en_esbmonde.htm. Updated on April 6, 2006. This organization presents a table with the number of BSE cases in 22 countries and another table for the United Kingdom. Spain, Portugal, Ireland, and Germany have had more than 50 confirmed cases of BSE in 2004, while Britain had the most confirmed cases, with 169.

"The Official Mad Cow Disease Home Page." Sperling Biomedical Foundation. Available online. URL: http://www.mad-cow.org. Updated on April 17, 2001. Although a few years old, this web page contains more than 7,561 links to articles, news stories, and web pages on mad cow disease, vCJD, prions, and related diseases.

"Oprah Winfrey: Mad Cow Disease." Ecomall. Available online. URL: http://www.ecomall.com/greenshopping/eioprah.htm. Downloaded in April 2006. Those wanting to see the transcript of the controversial Oprah show on mad cow disease can find it on this page.

Scalise, Frederick W. "Mad Cow Disease: The Myths, the Facts, and a Prescription for Food Safety." Omnicom Research and Information Systems. Available online. URL: http://www.angelfire.com/biz7/oris/commentary/ORIScomment/Mad_Cow_Diseax.html. Updated on September 28, 2004. The author argues that people are less safe from BSE than is commonly assumed and recommends several additional steps they should take to better protect themselves. He criticizes the beef industry and the government for opposing more stringent rules about cattle testing and beef processing and for putting short-term economic interests ahead of public safety.

TERRORIST THREATS

BOOKS

Chalk, Peter. *Hitting America's Soft Underbelly: The Potential Threat of Deliberate Biological Attacks against the U.S. Agricultural and Food Industry.* Santa

Monica, Calif.: RAND Corporation, 2004. In this 68-page volume, Chalk describes the vulnerability of the nation to agriculture bio-attacks, the potential impact of a major act of agricultural terrorism, and the new policies needed to prevent or mitigate the consequences of an attack.

Committee on Biological Threats to Agricultural Plants and Animals, National Research Council. *Countering Agricultural Bioterrorism*. Washington, D.C.: National Academies Press, 2002. Noting that attacks could come from foreign or domestic groups and target preharvest plants and animals or postharvest production and distribution, this book identifies many points of vulnerability of U.S. agriculture. It gives special attention to policy changes needed to defend against attacks on agriculture.

Dyckman, Lawrence J. *Bioterrorism: A Threat to Agriculture and the Food Supply*. Washington, D.C.: U.S. General Accounting Office, 2004. Based on the testimony of the director of natural resources and the environment at the General Accounting Office, this report identifies several gaps in the federal government's controls for protecting the food supply. The government needs to improve protection against tampering with agricultural products, the release of deadly animal diseases, the import of contaminated food, and the security lapses at animal disease labs.

Food Safety and Inspection Service. *FSIS Safety and Security Guidelines for the Transportation and Distribution of Meat, Poultry, and Egg Products*. Washington, D.C.: U.S. Department of Agriculture, 2003. Meat, poultry, and egg products can be contaminated by disease agents through deliberate acts of terrorism as well as through unsanitary conditions and poor refrigeration. This booklet describes procedures to ensure the safety of food from such contamination, including special suggestions to prevent terrorist attacks on food. In offering guidance, the pamphlet clearly presents the steps needed to protect food being transported through air, road, sea, or rail.

Frazier, Thomas W., and Drew C. Richardson. *Food and Agricultural Security: Guarding against Natural Threats and Terrorist Attacks Affecting Health, National Food Supplies, and Agricultural Economics*. New York: New York Academy of Sciences, 2000. This book includes both industry and government experts discussing potential bioterrorism against agricultural crops and domestic animals. The chapters come from papers presented at the International Conference on Food and Agricultural Security and sponsored by the U.S. Department of Agriculture, FBI Scientific Laboratory, the Department of Defense Veterinary Service Activity, the American Veterinary Medical Association, the Louisiana State University, and the National Consortium for Genomic Resources Management.

Homeland Agro-Security Task Force. *Initiatives in Agricultural Security*. New York: Experiment Station Committee on Organization and Policy of the Board of Agricultural Assembly, National Association of State Universities and Land-Grant Colleges, 2002. Also available online. URL: http://www.escop.msstate.edu/committee/agro-security-initiative.pdf. Downloaded in April 2006. Experts from universities across the nation plan to provide up-to-date information and services to government and private organizations, with the goal of preventing domestic and foreign threats to U.S. food-production and agricultural systems. The volume describes the strategies to be used in reaching this goal.

Kohnen, Anne. *Responding to the Threat of Agroterrorism: Specific Recommendations for the United States Department of Agriculture.* Cambridge, Mass.: Belfer Center for Science and International Affairs, Harvard University, 2000. Also available online. URL: http://bcsia.ksg.harvard.edu/BCSIA_ content/documents/Responding_to_the_Threat_of_Agro terrorism.pdf. Downloaded in April 2006. Showing that concerns about a terrorist attack on agriculture predate the September 11 attacks, this report describes the potential harm of such an attack and the ways to prevent it. Such concerns have, of course, only been heightened by the September 11 attacks.

Pate, Jason, and Gavin Cameron. "Covert Biological Weapons Attacks against Agricultural Targets: Assessing the Impact against U.S. Agriculture." In Arnold M. Howitt and Robyn L. Pangi, eds., *Countering Terrorism: Dimensions of Preparedness.* Cambridge: MIT Press, 2003, pp. 195–218. In contrast to many works on agroterrorism, this one relies on a unique evidence base—the Weapons of Mass Destruction Terrorism Incidents Database at the Center for Nonproliferation Studies, Monterey Institute. Selecting those incidents from the database involving agriculture, the authors find that the greatest threat has come from terrorists who have tampered with agricultural products during shipment rather than from destruction of crops and animals in the field. Scholarly in nature and filled with footnotes, this chapter provides a careful and insightful evaluation of the potential for terrorists to harm the food supply.

U.S. Food and Drug Administration. *Retail Food Stores and Food Service Establishments: Food Security Prevention Guidance.* Washington, D.C.: U.S. Food and Drug Administration, 2004. This short booklet written in simple language provides a list of the actions managers can take to minimize the opportunity for terrorists or criminals to tamper with the food in stores. Recommendations to investigate suspicious activity, screen staff, train workers in food security procedures, check incoming shipments, and maintain the security of the store translate general goals into specific actions.

———. *Strategic Action Plan, Food and Drug Administration: Protecting and Advancing America's Health.* Washington, D.C.: Food and Drug Administration, 2003. Also available online. URL: http://www.fda.gov/oc/mcclellan/

Annotated Bibliography

FDAStrategicPlan.pdf. Downloaded in April 2006. In providing a roadmap of the actions the FDA needs to take in the next century, this volume includes a chapter on protecting Americans from terrorism.

U.S. Senate. *Federal Biodefense Readiness, Hearing of the Committee on Health, Education, Labor, and Pensions, United States Senate, One Hundred Eighth Congress, First Session.* Washington, D.C.: U.S. Government Printing Office, July 24, 2003. The hearings provide statements and testimony of three experts dealing with the threat of biological terrorism: Julie Louise Gerberding, director of the Centers for Disease Control and Prevention; Mark B. McClellan, commissioner of the Food and Drug Administration, Department of Health and Human Services; and Elias A. Zerhouni, director of the National Institutes of Health. While the prepared statements offer background on the efforts of the agencies, the questions of the senators and response of the experts do more to reveal the political disagreements over the effectiveness of the approaches. Senator Edward Kennedy of Massachusetts, for example, criticizes White House efforts to protect the nation from biological attacks.

World Health Organization. *Terrorist Threats to Food: Guidance for Establishing and Strengthening Prevention and Response Systems.* Geneva, Switzerland: Food Safety Department, World Health Organization, 2002. Also available online. URL: http://www.who.int/foodsafety/publications/general/en/terrorist.pdf. Downloaded in April 2006. Terrorist contamination of food has global implications: It can affect trade in food products and harm countries other than those attacked by terrorists. In this volume, the World Health Organization aims to educate and coordinate worldwide prevention measures.

ARTICLES

Cameron, Gavin, Jason Pate, and Kathleen Vogel. "Planting Fear: Agroterrorism." *The Bulletin of the Atomic Scientists,* vol. 57, no. 5, September/October 2001, pp. 38–44. The authors review the threats to agriculture from terrorism but also suggest that the threat may be less serious than alarmists claim. They further argue that increased vigilance and some institutional reforms could effectively reduce the consequences of bioterrorism. More than most writings on the topic, this article takes an optimistic view.

Casagrande, Rocco. "Biological Terrorism Targeted at Agriculture: The Threat to National Security." *The Nonproliferation Review,* vol. 7, no. 3, Fall/Winter 2000, pp. 92–105. Published before the 2001 terrorist attacks, this article offers an early statement of concern about agroterrorism. While highlighting the potential for Islamic militants to damage the

195

country through terrorist attacks on agriculture, it also notes the potential for extremist environmental groups to do the same. Several of the recommendations it makes for protecting the country from biological terrorism targeted at agriculture have been adopted since the September 11 attacks.

Daniels, Catherine, and Sally O'Neal Coates. "Focus on Agriculture and Food Terrorism." *Agrichemical and Environmental News,* Issue 187, November 2001, pp. 1–20. Also available online. URL: http://www.aenews. wsu.edu/Nov01AENews/NovAENews01.pdf. Downloaded in April 2006. Normally focused on issues of pesticide use and the environment, this magazine presented a special issue soon after September 11 on agriculture and food terrorism. Articles describe the possible use of pesticides and crop dusters as weapons and the basics of an antiterrorism plan. Some articles offer examples of previous terrorist attacks on food that have had small effects, but others suggest the potential for something more serious.

Dupont, Daniel G. "Food Fears." *Scientific American,* vol. 289, October 2003, pp. 20, 22. Stating that al Qaeda has put the food supply on its list of potential targets in the United States, the author reviews efforts to identify the potential harm of a terrorist attack on our agriculture. For example, a simulation run by the National Defense University on the introduction of foot-and-mouth disease by a terrorist suggests that the disease would spread to one-third of the nation's cattle before it could be stopped. The serious consequences of such an event require greater action by the government, industry, and farmers to prevent it.

Khan, Ali S., David L. Swerdlow, and Dennis D. Juranek. "Precautions against Biological and Chemical Terrorism Directed at Food and Water Supplies." *Public Health Reports,* vol. 116, no. 1, January/February 2001, pp. 3–14. This article reviews instances of the deliberate contamination of food and water supplies and assesses the vulnerability of the country to such attacks.

Looker, Dan. "Sustaining a Nation: Agriculture after Sept. 11 Attacks." *Successful Farming,* vol. 99, no. 14, December 2001, pp. 22–24. An article for farmers highlights concerns not only about Mideastern terrorists but also groups in the United States opposed to modern agricultural practices. Extremist groups might wish to destroy fields that use genetically modified crops or try to kill animals they believe are subject to immoral treatment. The article provides advice to farmers to deal with the threat of these sorts of attacks.

Meadows, Michelle. "The FDA and the Fight against Terrorism." *FDA Consumer,* vol. 38, no. 1, January/February 2004, pp. 20–22. The article describes the new Office of Counterterrorism Policy at the Food and

Annotated Bibliography

Drug Administration. The agency aims to safeguard food and medical supplies from a terrorist attack and to make drugs, vaccines, and information available in case of an attack.

"One Year Later." *Consumer Reports*, vol. 68, no. 9, September 2002, pp. 12–13. The article summarizes the Public Health Security and Bioterrorism Preparedness and Response Act of 2002 and the efforts made by the country to protect itself from biological attacks on humans and agriculture. It also describes additional efforts that need to be taken by both the government and by individuals to reach this goal.

"Operation Liberty Shield: New Food Security Guidance." *FDA Consumer*, vol. 37, no. 3, May/June 2003, pp. 18–19. Operation Liberty Shield is a multiagency plan to protect the nation from terrorism, and the FDA plays an important role in the operation. This article describes many of the actions taken by the agency: collaborating with the food industry to reduce threats, increasing surveillance of the domestic food industry, upgrading the monitoring of imported foods, enhancing collaboration with other government agencies, and helping manufacturers reduce the risk of food tampering.

Risen, James, with Don Van Natta, Jr. "Threats and Responses: Terror Network; Plot to Poison Food of British Troops Is Suspected." *New York Times*, January 24, 2003, p. A1. British police arrested Islamic militants planning to lace the food supply of British soldiers with the poison ricin. The militants allegedly hoped to gain access to a military base in the United Kingdom. One member of the group who worked for a food-preparation company had been in contact with someone working on a military base. Although evidence of the plot is limited, the potential for such actions demonstrates the importance of issues of food safety.

Spake, Amanda. "Food Fright: Preventing Food Terrorism." *U.S. News & World Report*, vol. 131, no. 26, December 24, 2001, pp. 48–50. Written shortly after the September 11 attacks, this article describes concerns about terrorist attacks on the food supply and early congressional efforts to deal with the problem. It identifies the daunting nature of any effort to regulate the food supply and highlights the importance of coordinating the actions of various agencies that regulate food.

Spillman, Diana-Marie. "Do American Citizens Consider Their Food Supply at Risk for Terrorism Attack?" *Psychological Reports*, vol. 93, no. 3, December 2003, pp. 1159–60. A survey of Americans about the risks of a terrorist attack on food supplies finds that few have changed their eating and purchasing habits since September 11, 2001. However, many also believe that the food supply is at risk.

WEB DOCUMENTS

Apatow, Stephen M. "Agricultural Security: Veterinary and Scientific Experts Outline Priority Issues." Humanitarian Resource Institute. Available online. URL: http://www.humanitarian.net/biodefense/ap11602.html. Posted on January 16, 2002. Concerned that the introduction of foreign animal diseases into multiple locations and with multiple pathogens could cause major damage to American agriculture, the author summarizes the views of experts on how to address this potential problem.

"Countering Bioterrorism and Other Threats to the Food Supply." FoodSafety.gov. Available online. URL: http://www.foodsafety.gov/~fsg/bioterr.html. Downloaded in April 2006. This web resource collects articles and statements from a variety of government agencies—the Food and Drug Administration, Department of Agriculture, Food Safety and Inspection Service, Environmental Protection Agency, Centers for Disease Control and Prevention, and the Department of Homeland Security—on protecting the food supply from terrorism. Many of the articles offer tips to the public.

"Criminal Justice Resources: Agro-Security." Michigan State University Libraries. Available online. URL: http://www.lib.msu.edu/harris23/crimjust/agrosec.htm. Downloaded in April 2006. This web site compiles a list of other web sites related to the protection of the nation's food supply from terrorism. It also provides links to related topics of bioterrorism, weapons of mass destruction, and terrorist groups.

"Fact Sheet: Strengthening the Security of Our Nation's Food Supply." Department of Homeland Security. Available online. URL: http://www.dhs.gov/dhspublic/display?theme=43&content=3802. Posted on July 6, 2004. Like the Department of Agriculture and the Food and Drug Administration, the U.S. Department of Homeland Security has described the actions it has taken to protect the food supply from terrorism. This document lists many such actions, including the development of new technology, establishment of partnerships with universities and businesses, and coordination of interagency actions.

"Food Defense and Terrorism." U.S. Food and Drug Administration, Center for Food Safety and Applied Nutrition. Available online. URL: http://www.cfsan.fda.gov/~dms/fsterr.html. Updated on April 7, 2006. This web page lists dozens of links to FDA documents on topics such as detention of food, registration of food facilities, prior notice of food shipments, and bioterrorism. The up-to-date information on how the agency intends to protect food from terrorists and the considerable choice in the documents readers can examine provides an essential resource for those interested in government policies against food terrorism.

Annotated Bibliography

"Homeland Security Presidential Directive/HSPD-9. Subject: Defense of United States Agriculture and Food." White House. Available online. URL: http://www.whitehouse.gov/news/releases/2004/02/20040203-2.html. Posted on January 30, 2004. The directive makes the secretary of the Department of Homeland Security responsible for working with the Department of Agriculture, Department of Health and Human Services, the Environmental Protection Agency, and multiple intelligence agencies to implement plans for protecting the food supply. The plans deal with awareness and warning, assessment of vulnerability, responding to attacks, outreach and professional development, and research and development.

Mintz, John, and Joby Warrick. "U.S. Remains Unprepared for Bioterror Attack." WashingtonPost.com. Available online. URL: http://www.washingtonpost.com/wp-dyn/articles/A32738-2004Nov7.html. Posted on November 8, 2004. Despite new homeland security programs and substantial increases in funding, the United States remains, according to this article, largely unprepared to defend itself against a biological attack. The article does not focus specifically on food terrorism, but the problems it describes in preventing bioterrorism certainly affect the food supply.

"New Rules Require Better Food Records." CNN.com. Available online. URL: http://blog.lib.umn.edu/gruwell/publichealthliaison/012117.html. Downloaded in April 2006. In a press conference to announce his resignation as secretary of the Department of Health and Human Services, Tommy Thompson said he worried every single night about a terrorist attack on food. He said, "For the life of me, I cannot understand why the terrorists have not attacked our food supply because it is so easy to do." A few days later, he said that new record-keeping rules would do much to help with deliberate contamination of food.

"Risk Assessment for Food Terrorism and Other Food Safety Concerns." U.S. Food and Drug Administration, Center for Food Safety and Applied Nutrition. Available online. URL: http://vm.cfsan.fda.gov/~dms/rabtact.html. Posted on October 13, 2003. In compiling information from experts and dozens of scholarly references, this document describes the methods used to calculate the likely consequences of a terrorist attack on the food supply. It gives examples of terrorist and non-terrorist tampering with food that have occurred in the past and uses instances of accidental food contamination to estimate the harm of intentional tampering. The risk assessment concludes "that there is a high likelihood, over the course of a year, that a significant number of people will be affected by an act of food terrorism or by an incident of unintentional food contamination that results in serious foodborne illness."

"USDA Homeland Security Efforts." U.S. Department of Agriculture. Available online. URL: http://www.usda.gov/homelandsecurity/factsheet58.pdf.

Posted in May 2003. In response to the September 11 attacks, the USDA appointed a Homeland Security Council to focus on the safety of the food supply, agriculture production, and USDA facilities. This four-page statement summarizes the efforts recommended by the council and the actions taken by the agency in response to the recommendations. The department has increased its efforts to prevent foreign pests and diseases from being brought across U.S. borders, worked to create a surveillance system to identify diseases before they can spread, and developed new ways to test for the presence of biological and chemical agents in food.

FOOD ADDITIVES

BOOKS

Blaylock, Russell L. *Health and Nutrition Secrets That Can Save Your Life.* Albuquerque: Health Press, 2002. Blaylock, who in an earlier book coined the term *exotoxins* to refer to how additives such as MSG and aspartame damage nerve cells, offers a wide-ranging critique (520 pages) of additives in food, the danger of heavy metals and fluoride to health, and the risks to families from biohazards. The section on food additives makes up only one part but differs from other books in treating the topic as part of larger issues of food health. Like many other books warning of the dangers of food additives, readers will need to treat the claims of this one with caution.

Branen, Alfred Larry, P. Michael Davidson, and Seppo Salminen. *Food Additives.* 2nd ed. New York: Marcel Dekker, 2001. At 952 pages, this book contains much information on the chemical makeup of food additives and the evaluation of their safety. The text contains more technical detail than all but specialists in the area will want. However, with numerous published books that are highly critical of food additives, the academic scientists present a valuable perspective on the issue.

Farlow, Christine Hoza. *Food Additives: A Shopper's Guide to What's Safe and What's Not.* 5th ed. Denver: Kiss for Health Publishing, 2004. Shoppers can carry and consult this short book of 72 pages as they make purchases. Rather than defining and describing each item (as the *Dictionary of Food Additives* by Ruth Winter does), the book lists more than 1,300 food additives with codes to indicate their safety and purpose. For example, it lists acesulfame-K as an unsafe artificial sweetener in processed foods that may cause low blood sugar attacks in humans and cancer and elevated cholesterol in lab animals. Implying that shoppers should not depend on the FDA approval, the book is stringent in its evaluation of additives.

Annotated Bibliography

Sarjeant, Doris, and Karen S. Evans. *Hard to Swallow: The Truth about Food Additives.* 2nd ed. Burnay, B.C., Canada: Alive Books, 2003. Accusing health officials of acting in the interests of food manufacturers rather than consumers, this book advertises itself as a "wakeup call to the shocking state of our food laws and is a primer for those who want to know why the food supply is genetically manipulated, bombarded with radiation and laced with additives." Readers should view the accusations with caution, but this book represents one of the many available for purchase that condemns the use of food additives.

Winter, Ruth. *A Consumer's Dictionary of Food Additives: Descriptions in Plain English of More Than 12,000 Ingredients Both Harmful and Desirable Found in Foods.* 6th ed. New York: Three Rivers Press, 2004. Additives are listed alphabetically, each with a description of its purpose, risks, and benefits. The book also includes explanations of the meaning of terms such as *lite, fat-free,* and *all-natural,* and it describes methods of processing food. Most entries consist of a few sentences, but those on more controversial additives receive longer treatments. Readers can learn much about the nature of food additives from reading the book but can use it more effectively as a reference guide. Those concerned about food additives in their diet can look up the meaning of unfamiliar terms on food labels and even use the book to select food products while shopping.

ARTICLES

Bren, Linda. "FDA's Response to Food, Dietary Supplement, and Cosmetic Adverse Events." *FDA Consumer,* vol. 37, no. 4, July/August 2003, pp. 12–13. Articles in this journal reflect the views of the FDA, and this one reviews the agency's actions to protect the safety of the public from dangerous food additives. It describes one effort called the Adverse Event Reporting System (AERS) that goes beyond the usual approval process for food additives. The system is designed to identify adverse events related to food or color additives, obtain and analyze information on the events, and make recommendations for re-evaluating the safety of additives or coloring.

Globus, Sheila. "Pros and Cons of Food Additives." *Current Health 2*, vol. 28, no. 2, October 2001, pp. 17–19. In presenting a fair-minded summary of the debate, this article cites the views of Fergus Clydesdale, professor and head of the department of food science at the University of Massachusetts, in defense of food additives as well as those of more critical consumer groups.

Lewis, Carol. "The 'Poison Squad' and the Advent of Food and Drug Regulation." *FDA Consumer,* vol. 36, no. 6, November/December 2002, pp. 12–15. The history of the regulation of food additives in the United States begins with a study in 1902 that fed volunteers several poisons commonly used in small amounts as food preservatives. The volunteers, called the poison squad, did not appear to suffer long-term harm from the poisoning, but short-term sickness led the scientists in charge to conclude that accumulation of poisons, even when taken in small amounts, presented dangers to the public. The study led to banning of these preservatives and better government regulation of food additives.

Murphy, Kate. "Do Food Additives Subtract from Health?" *Business Week*, May 6, 1996, pp. 140–141. Also available online. URL: http://www.businessweek.com/archives/1996/b3474110.arc.htm. Posted on May 6, 1996. Although a bit dated, this article offers a balanced assessment of the benefits and risks of food additives, recommending that consumers eat a variety of foods to avoid overexposure to any one set of additives. It also notes that research on food additives, as on other topics, remains open to interpretation and cannot provide absolute assurance of safety.

Nestle, Marion. "The Selling of Olestra." *Public Health Reports*, vol. 113, no. 6, November–December 1998, pp. 508–520. This article makes the case that approval of the fat substitute olestra did not come from the scientific demonstration of its safety—questions still remain about how it may interfere with absorption of nutrients and affect long-term digestion. Rather, it came from pressure exerted on the FDA by politicians and Procter and Gamble, the inventor and maker of the product. It also came from marketing and publicity about the benefits to consumers who cut fat from their diets. The article does not review the scientific evidence on the additive but focuses instead on the politics of food additive approval.

Rados, Carol. "GRAS: Time-Tested, and Trusted, Food Ingredients." *FDA Consumer*, vol. 38, no. 2, March/April 2004, pp. 20–21. In its journal for consumers, the FDA often includes articles such as this one that reassure readers of the safety of food additives. The article lauds the proven track record of safety for GRAS (Generally Recognized as Safe) additives and the requirements needed for the FDA to approve other additives. It notes that additives not approved through these procedures cannot be used and that health claims made about additives must meet FDA standards.

Sullum, Jacob. "The Anti-Pleasure Principle: Center for Science in the Public Interest." *Reason*, vol. 35, no. 3, July 2003, pp. 24–32. With many books and web pages critical of certain food additives, readers may want to see the views of those critical of the critics. This article accuses the Center for Science and the Public Interest, which has been a leader in opposing approval by the FDA of many food additives, of grossly exaggerating the trivial risk of food additives and other dietary practices. Sullum

202

offers a minority viewpoint in the criticisms, one opposed to government policies that limit freedom of food choices by consumers.

WEB DOCUMENTS

"Additives and Ingredients for Healthy Eating." Food Additives and Ingredients Association. Available online. URL: http://www.faia.org.uk. Downloaded in April 2006. This organization representing businesses that manufacture and market food additives not surprisingly takes a positive view of the value of additives in improving the safety, taste, and texture of food. On this web page, the organization describes these benefits in more detail and defends the safety of food additives. Indeed, it claims that food additives go through more careful testing than the foods to which they are added: "It is often claimed that chemicals are added to food without adequate safety testing. In fact, the opposite is true: Chemicals whose composition and purity are known and which have been fully tested are added to foods about which we know comparatively little."

"CSPI's Guide to Food Additives." Food Safety Food Additives. Available online. URL: http://www.cspinet.org/reports/chemcuisine.htm. Downloaded in April 2006. Although not as long or as detailed as some of the books on food additives, this web page from the Center for Science in the Public Interest nonetheless provides essential information. It classifies nearly 100 common food additives in five categories: safe, unsafe in large amounts, caution (try to avoid), unsafe for some people, and unsafe in normal amounts. The CSPI views food additives more critically than the FDA, and many experts will not agree with their classification, but it offers a perspective that many consumers will find helpful.

"FDA Backgrounder: Milestones in U.S. Food and Drug Law History." U.S. Food and Drug Administration. Available online. URL: http://www.fda.gov/opacom/backgrounders/miles.html. Updated in August 2005. This list of events, policy changes, and accomplishments nicely reviews milestones in the history of U.S. food and drug laws from 1820 to 2005. The listed items are brief but cover historical background information not easily obtained elsewhere.

"FDA/IFIC Brochure: Food Additives." U.S. Food and Drug Administration. Available online. URL: http://vm.cfsan.fda.gov/~lrd/foodaddi.html. Posted in January 1992. Although written nearly 15 years ago, the information this web page presents on the benefits of additives for food consistency, nutritional value, wholesomeness, texture, and flavor has stayed relevant. The clearly written text gives many examples of these benefits, explains testing procedures, and defends additives without overstating the case. Its summary concludes that food and color additives are more strictly regulated today than any other time in history and require demonstrated safety at intended levels before they can be used in food.

"Food Ingredients and Colors." International Food Information Council. Available online. URL: http://ific.org/publications/brochures/foodingredandcolorsbroch.cfm. Posted in March 2005. Based on information from the FDA, this web page offers a favorable view of the benefits and safety of food additives. In addition, it briefly addresses some controversial issues by noting that many claims about the harm of food additives have been demonstrated false by scientific studies. With funding from food, beverage, and agricultural industries, this organization can be expected to view food additives positively.

"Food Additives Color Additives Q&A." U.S. Food and Drug Administration. Available online. URL: http://www.cfsan.fda.gov/~dms/qa-adfq.html. Downloaded in April 2006. The FDA provides answers to questions such as: "How are additives regulated?" "Is olestra safe?" and "Why are color additives used in food?" The short and clear answers allow readers to understand the views of the government on critical food-additive issues.

"Food Ingredients and Packaging: Background Information for Consumers." U.S. Food and Drug Administration. Available online. URL: http://www.cfsan.fda.gov/~dms/opa-bckg.html. Updated on March 28, 2006. This web site has links to dozens of FDA documents on food additives. Users can examine the views of the agency on specific additives such as olestra, MSG, and sugar substitutes or find out more about the Office of Food Additive Safety.

Vogt, Donna U. "Food Additive Regulations: A Chronology." CRS Report for Congress. Available online. URL: http://www.ncseonline.org/NLE/CRSreports/Pesticides/pest-5.cfm?&CFID=18010170&CFTOKEN=72878622. Updated on September 13, 1995. This history of food-additive regulations begins with a summary of debates ongoing in the 1990s over standards in evaluating the safety of food additives for cancer. It then traces changes in regulations since 1889 that have led to current policies. It also discusses the petition process required for approval of food additives.

CHEMICAL AND NATURAL TOXINS

BOOKS

Berkson, Lindsey. *Hormone Deception: How Everyday Foods and Products Are Disrupting Your Hormones—and How to Protect Yourself and Your Family.* Lincolnwood, Ill.: Contemporary Books, 2000. Arguing in general that the large number of artificial chemicals in the environment can cause health problems by disrupting hormone levels, this book discusses the specific consequences of hormone use in food animals.

Cabras, P. "Pesticides: Toxicology and Residues in Food." In D'Mello, J. P. F., ed., *Food Safety: Contaminants and Toxins.* Cambridge, Mass.: CABI Publishing, 2003, pp. 91–124. In reviewing the scientific evidence, this expert concludes that pesticide residues on food are so small as to produce little risk for humans.

Garland, Anne Witte. *The Way We Grow: Good-Sense Solutions for Protecting our Families from Pesticides in Food.* New York: Berkley Books, 1993. Critical of the government for not doing enough to prevent pesticides from contaminating food, the author suggests ways for consumers to protect themselves. The short book provides background information on shopping for safe foods but also on how to support groups fighting to change pesticide laws.

Gebo, Sue. *What's Left to Eat?* New York: McGraw-Hill, 1992. Chapter 3 presents a comprehensive discussion of some 30 natural toxins in food. Readers concerned about chemical additives may find the extent of natural toxins in food surprisingly high.

Hall, Darwin C., and L. Joe Moffitt, eds. *Economics of Pesticides, Sustainable Food Production, and Organic Food Markets.* New York: Elsevier, 2002. This edited volume on food production addresses issues of food safety only indirectly but nonetheless gives useful background information. It provides a brief history of pesticide use in agriculture, describes recent trends in pesticide management and organic food products, and examines the economic decisions farmers must make about pesticide use.

Hamilton, Denis, and Stephen Crossley, eds. *Pesticide Residues in Food and Drinking Water: Human Exposure and Risks.* New York: John Wiley, 2004. Articles by experts in this book address a variety of topics on how to assess the risks of pesticides for human health. The book makes the point that, given the continued use of pesticides to improve food production, the key question becomes how much residue can safely be allowed on food. The articles examine new methods and studies that address this question.

Lawson, Lynn. *Staying Well in a Toxic World: Understanding Environmental Illness, Multiple Chemical Sensitivities, Chemical Injuries, and Sick Building Syndrome.* Evanston, Ill.: Lynnword Press, 2000. Focused on the toxic effects of chemicals from a variety of sources—carpets, computers, and cosmetics—this book also discusses pesticides and chemical pollutants that can enter our bodies through food. The food-safety material represents only a small part of the book but fits logically with other sections on chemical threats to health.

U.S. House of Representatives. *The Status of Implementation of the Food Quality Protection Act of 1996: Hearing before the Subcommittee on Environment and Hazardous Materials of the Committee on Energy and Commerce, House of Representatives, One Hundred Seventh Congress, Second Session, March 25, 2002.* Washington, D.C.: U.S. Government Printing Office, 2002. The testimony in this hearing portrays the debates over enforcing new rules for allowable pesticide residue on food. Representatives from farm states criticize the EPA for basing decisions to ban pesticides on media publicity rather than sound science, consumer groups criticize the EPA for not doing enough to protect children from pesticides in food, and all groups criticize the delay in implementing actions required by legislation. Representatives from the EPA defend their actions but do not satisfy critics.

ARTICLES

Ames, Bruce N., Renae Magaw, and Lois Swirsky Gold. "Ranking Possible Carcinogenic Hazards." *Science,* vol. 236, no. 4799, April 17, 1987, pp. 271–280. This important article demonstrates that natural chemicals in food pose a bigger cancer risk than artificial chemicals and pesticides. Given that people eat food with natural toxins without concern, the findings imply that the lower levels of pesticides and artificial chemicals in food should also not cause great concern.

Baker, Brian P., Charles M. Benbrook, Edward Groth III, and Karen Lutz Benbrook. "Pesticide Residues in Conventional, IPM-Grown and Organic Foods: Insights from Three U.S. Data Sets." *Food Additives and Contaminants,* vol. 19, no. 5, May 2002, pp. 427–442. Also available online. URL: http://www.consumersunion.org/food/organicsumm.htm. Downloaded in April 2006. This study concludes that organically grown foods contain fewer pesticides than conventionally grown foods but, perhaps surprisingly, are not free altogether from pesticides. Although the article does not address whether pesticide levels in either types of food are high enough to cause health problems, it reassures those committed to purchasing organic foods that they do in fact reduce the amount of pesticide residue they consume.

Conan, Kerri. "Why the Meat Label is a Must-Read." *Health,* vol. 17, no. 4, May 2003, pp. 152, 154, 156. This article notes that the concerns of shoppers about the use of growth-stimulating hormones in animals have led many to buy organic meats. It describes changes made in the grocery industry to meet the demand for hormone-free and organic meat.

Annotated Bibliography

"How Safe Is Our Produce." *Consumer Reports*, vol. 64, no. 3, March 1999, pp. 28–31. Having examined pesticide levels in 27,000 fruit and vegetable samples, the Consumers Union concludes that many levels are too high and pose a health risk to children. Apples, grapes, green beans, peaches, pears, spinach, and winter squash showed the highest toxicity. Many scientists have criticized the claim that the pesticide levels are unsafe, but the article summarizes an enormous amount of work done to document the levels.

Järup, Lars. "Hazards of Heavy Metal Contamination." *British Medical Journal*, vol. 68, no. 1, 2003, pp. 167–182. As described in this article, four heavy metals present the greatest threat to human health—lead, cadmium, mercury, and arsenic. Foods represent only one way these metals can enter the body but often are a major source of potential harm. This article describes the physiological effects of these metals, how they can enter the food system, and the extent of the risk today.

Roosevelt, Margot. "Got Hormones?" *Time*, vol. 162, no. 25, December 22, 2003, p. 52. Monsanto, the maker of a genetically engineered growth hormone that increases milk production of dairy cows, sued a dairy for advertising that its milk contained no artificial hormones. As described in this article, the company argues that use of its hormone presents no safety dangers and disputes statements that hormone-free milk is healthier. The suit reflects more general debate about the potential harm for human health of the use of growth hormones in food animals.

Wolcott, Jennifer. "An End to Organic Confusion?" *Christian Science Monitor*, October 16, 2002, p. 15. Also available online. URL:http://www.csmonitor.com/2002/1016/p15s02-lifo.html. Downloaded in April 2006. Those concerned about pesticide and artificial chemicals in their food often want to buy organic products, but the definition of organic has made it difficult for shoppers to know just what they are getting. This article reviews the new government definition of *organic*, its allowable use on food labels, and background information on organic products.

WEB DOCUMENTS

"Consumer Concerns about Hormones in Food." Cornell University Program on Breast Cancer and Environmental Risk Factors in New York State. Available online. URL: http://envirocancer.cornell.edu/FactSheet/Diet/fs37.hormones.pdf. Posted in June 2000. This document presents a careful review of the evidence on the potential harm to humans of hormones given to food animals. It evenhandedly discusses the benefits of hormones for agricultural production and the charges made about the risks of the practice for people who consume meat. In the end, it concludes that the evidence does not demonstrate harm to human health from animal hormones.

"A Consumer's Guide to Pesticides and Food Safety." International Food Information Council. Available online. URL: http://ific.org/publications/brochures/pesticidebroch.cfm. Posted in November 1995. This web page describes the benefits of pesticides for food production, the government regulation of pesticides, and debates over the harm for human health of pesticides. It concludes that the benefits of a diet rich in fruits and vegetables outweigh the risks of pesticide residue in food.

Parnes, Robin Brett. "How Organic Food Works." HowStuffWorks.com. Available online. URL: http://home.howstuffworks.com/organic-food.htm. Downloaded in April 2006. The meaning of "organic" is less clear than it might seem. The author explains that organic food is defined by how it cannot be produced rather than by how it is produced and describes the prohibited practices. It also distinguishes between "organic" and "natural," compares organic and conventional food, and describes trends in organic farming.

"Pesticides." Environmental Protection Agency. Available online. URL: http://www.epa.gov/pesticides. Updated on April 11, 2006. The numerous links on this page describe the procedures used by the EPA to regulate pesticides, the health problems pesticides may pose, the means used to assess the risks of pesticides, and the meaning of organically grown food. The documents defend the agency's procedures to ensure the safety of food.

"Pesticides, Metals, Chemical Contaminants and Natural Toxins." U.S. Food and Drug Administration, Center for Food Safety and Applied Nutrition. Available online. URL: http://vm.cfsan.fda.gov/~lrd/pestadd.html. Updated on March 28, 2006. The FDA provides dozens of links to government reports on a variety of food contaminants such as pesticides, lead, mercury, chemical pollutants, and natural toxins. The reports vary in accessibility, with some written for the public but many others better suited for scientists. Still, the comprehensive nature of the topics listed makes this web page a valuable resource.

"rBGH." Center for Food Safety. Available online. URL: http://www.centerforfoodsafety.org/rbgh_hormo.cfm. Downloaded in April 2006. The title of this web page refers to the bovine growth hormone that helps dairy cows produce more milk. Opposed to the use of this hormone, the Center for Food Safety argues that its presence in milk can harm humans and seeks to force the FDA to remove the hormone from the market.

FOOD ALLERGENS

BOOKS

Barber, Marianne S., Maryanne Bartoszek Scott, Elinor Greenberg, and Hugh A. Sampson. *The Parent's Guide to Food Allergies: Clear and Complete Advice from the Experts on Raising Your Food-Allergic Child.* New York: Owl Books, 2001. Because children are more vulnerable to food allergies than adults, parents often need guidance in dealing with the problem. This book addresses not only the ways to avoid offending foods, including discovering the presence of hidden allergens in products, but also discusses ways to deal with the worry and stress brought on by childhood allergies. Written by a parent of a child with food allergies in collaboration with physicians and researchers, it aims to give practical yet scientifically valid advice.

Lessof, M. H. *Food Intolerance.* London: Chapman and Hall, 1992. Although dated, this book presents a careful discussion of food intolerance that avoids some of the more exaggerated claims of popular books. The author writes clearly, covers a variety of topics, and describes the physiological causes of food intolerance.

Metcalfe, Dean D., Hugh A. Sampson, and Ronald A. Simon, eds. *Food Allergy: Adverse Reactions to Food and Food Additives.* Third Revised Edition. Boston: Blackwell Publishers, 2003. Those wanting a comprehensive treatment of the topic with an emphasis on the scientific basis of food allergies will find this book useful. Along with material on the immune system and the physiology of allergies, the chapters contributed by experts discuss contemporary debates over food additives, food biotechnology, and psychiatric aspects of food intolerance.

Parker, James N., and Philip M. Parker, eds. *Food Allergies: A Medical Dictionary, Bibliography, and Annotated Research Guide to Internet References.* San Diego: ICON Health Publications, 2003. Although offering more detail than most readers will want, this electronic book does much to evaluate Internet sources of food allergy information. The annotations for web sites help in separating facts from exaggerations and reliable guidance from speculations.

Walsh, William E. *Food Allergies: The Complete Guide to Understanding and Relieving Your Food Allergies.* New York: John Wiley and Sons, 2000. The large number of books on food allergies suggests there is a good deal of concern about the problem among the public (a search for books on food allergies on Amazon.com lists 499 hits). This book by a physician who suffers from food allergies offers a readable yet accessible discussion of the varied sources of the problem. It also gives advice on how to avoid foods that tend to produce allergies and develop a diet that minimizes the effects of allergies.

Wedman-St. Louis, Betty. *Living with Food Allergies: A Complete Guide to a Healthy Lifestyle.* Chicago: Contemporary Books, 1999. Compared to the food allergy book by William Walsh, this book by a nutritional specialist gives more attention to allergy-free diets and recipes.

ARTICLES

Ezzell, Carol. "Fixing Food." *Scientific American*, vol. 288, no. 1, January 2003, pp. 24–25. One solution to the threat brought on by food allergies may have other drawbacks. This article describes how peanuts have been genetically modified to get rid of proteins that cause allergic reactions and how the procedures can be used for wheat, milk, shellfish, eggs, and tree nuts. However, genetically modified foods raise other safety issues and may not be accepted by those without allergies.

Flora, Carlin. "Widespread Reactions: More Kids—and Parents—Are Living with Food Allergies." *Psychology Today*, vol. 37, no. 3, May/June 2004, p. 34. The author reviews an interesting explanation for rising levels of food allergies—a trend that has occurred in developed countries but not developing countries. Perhaps the exposure of Americans to fewer germs means their immune systems produce antibodies that fight non-harmful food substances instead.

Formanek, Raymond, Jr. "Food Allergies: When Food Becomes the Enemy." *FDA Consumer*, vol. 35, no. 4, July/August 2001, pp. 10–16. Also available online. URL: http://www.fda.gov/fdac/features/2001/401_food. html. Revised in April 2004. The article describes the causes of food allergies and intolerances, offering useful statistics on the occurrence and growth of the problem. For those wanting an overview of the issue, it provides an excellent starting point.

Mead, Rebecca. "When Edibles Attack: Food Allergy Ball at the Plaza Hotel in Manhattan." *New Yorker*, vol. 79, no. 39, December 15, 2003, pp. 44–45. Widespread concern about food allergy problems extends to New York City elite. A ball at the ritzy Plaza Hotel raised more than $9 million for research and education on the dangers of food allergies. The article describes the ball and the problem of food allergies.

"The Peanut Problem—Solved?" *Reader's Digest*, vol. 162, June 2003, p. 59. Although a problem for only a small segment of the population, peanut allergies subject victims to the risk of severe reactions and even death. One solution to this food-safety danger may come from developing a compound that, by binding with antibodies, prevents them from responding to peanut exposure. Although experimental and not likely to receive approval for widespread use quickly, the procedure described in this article could help millions.

Annotated Bibliography

Roth, Kimberlee. "Food-Allergy Sufferers, Rejoice." *Health*, vol. 18, no. 9, November 2004, p. 168. This brief article describes the benefits of new federal legislation for those with food allergies. The Food Allergen Labeling and Consumer Protection Act will, effective January 1, 2006, require clear labels that identify the presence of major food allergens in products.

Shute, Nancy. "For Some, the Wrong Food Is Deadly." *U.S. News & World Report*, vol. 128, no. 18, May 8, 2000, p. 53. The value of this short sidebar comes from the connection it makes between food allergies and a cover story of the magazine on the allergy explosion. The article notes that food allergies are relatively uncommon but are also among the most dangerous. It describes the problems one mother of a son with food allergies faces in trying to find out if fries are cooked in peanut oil or what ingredients school lunches include.

WEB DOCUMENTS

"Food Allergies." Keep Kids Healthy. Available online. URL: http://www.keepkidshealthy.com/welcome/commonproblems/food_allergies.html. Downloaded in April 2006. A short and helpful guide for parents who have children with food allergies.

"Food Allergies." Yahoo! Search Directory. Available online. URL: http://dir.yahoo.com/Health/Diseases_and_Conditions/Food_Allergies. Downloaded in April 2006. This listing of dozens of food allergy sites highlights links on specific products—sulfites, wheat, peanuts, and milk—as well as to more general topics.

"Food Allergy and Anaphylaxis Network." Food Allergy and Anaphylaxis Network Home Page. Available online. URL: http://www.foodallergy.org. Downloaded in December 2004. This resource page lists information on dealing with food allergies but also aims to organize, raise funds, and advocate for the interests of those with food allergies. It contains allergy-free recipes, advice for teens, and recent news.

Kritz, Francesca. "Fighting Food Allergies: New Efforts Are Making Schools a Safer Place for Kids." MSNBC.com. Available online. URL: http://www.msnbc.msn.com/id/5594864. Updated on August 24, 2004. Although parents can do much to control the home diet of children with food allergies, dealing with school food can be more of a problem. This article describes changes made in school lunch programs to help children with food allergies and offers guidance on what parents can do to help their children deal with food allergies in school.

211

"Patient/Public Education: Fast Facts." American Academy of Allergy, Asthma, and Immunology. Available online. URL: http://www.aaaai.org/patients/resources/fastfacts/food_allergy.stm. Downloaded in April 2006. Supported by experts in the area, this page on food allergies provides facts, statistics, and links to obtain additional information.

Schardt, David. "Food Allergies." Nutrition Action Health Letter. Available online. URL: http://www.cspinet.org/nah/04_01. Posted in April 2001. Along with presenting facts and statistics on food allergies, this clearly written and helpful article tells stories of those who died or nearly died from food allergies. It also argues for new labeling requirements, a goal realized with 2004 legislation.

FOOD IRRADIATION

BOOKS

Frank, Richard L., and Robert A. Hahn. *A Primer on Food Irradiation*. Elmwood Park, N.J.: Food Institute Information and Research Center, 2001. At 17 pages, this short document highlights essential information on food irradiation for nonexperts and considers both the pros and cons of the practice.

International Consultant Group on Food Irradiation. *Facts about Food Irradiation*. Vienna: International Atomic Energy Agency, 1999. Also available online. URL: http://www.iaea.org/programmes/nafa/d5/public/foodirradiation.pdf. Downloaded in April 2006. In this thorough, 53-page statement of support for food irradiation, a group of experts appointed by agencies that have stood behind the technology for decades presents arguments in its favor.

Joint FAO/IAEA/WHO Study Group. *High-Dose Irradiation: Wholesomeness of Food Irradiated with Doses above 10kGy*. Geneva: World Health Organization, 1999. An earlier report from three agencies—the Food and Agricultural Organization of the United Nations, International Atomic Energy Agency, and World Health Organization—had concluded that doses of radiation under 10 kilograys (a special unit of measure for this type of energy) had no toxic effects on food. However, higher doses of radiation that kill pathogens with even greater certainty would guarantee the safety of food for people with suppressed immune systems or under medical treatment. The report concludes that the high-dose radiation, when used under approved practices, can be considered safe.

Komolprasert, Vanee, and Kim Matthew Morehouse, eds. *Irradiation of Food and Packaging: Recent Developments*. Oxford: Oxford University Press,

Annotated Bibliography

2004. Given the growing interest in using irradiation to improve food safety, the American Chemical Society sponsored a symposium to review the most recent research. The papers gathered in this book discuss improvements in technology; the effectiveness in eliminating pathogens from meats, fruits, and vegetables; the application to food packaging; and possible developments in the future. Like other volumes written by and for specialists, this one makes for difficult reading, but the summaries and overviews give an up-to-date view of food irradiation from scientists studying the procedures.

Meins, Erika. *Politics and Public Outrage: Explaining Transatlantic and Intra-European Diversity of Regulations on Food Irradiation and Genetically Modified Food.* Munich: Lit Verlag, 2003. Although European nations oppose U.S. food-safety practices in regard to use of hormones and antibiotics for food animals, most nations share the positive view of food irradiation. Despite this general support, nations have varied in how they regulate food irradiation, a topic explored in some detail by this study.

Satin, Morton. *Food Irradiation: A Guidebook.* 2nd ed. Boca Raton, Fla.: CRC Press, 1996. Satin served as the director of agricultural services in the United Nations division of the Food and Agricultural Organization. Although many developments have occurred since its publication in 1996, the book still offers a valuable overview of food irradiation that is written for popular as well as scientific audiences. In addressing controversy over the technology, Satin argues that the benefits justify its widespread use, but he also recognizes the importance of giving consumers choices in the kind of products they can buy.

U.S. General Accounting Office. *Food Irradiation: Available Research Indicates That Benefits Outweigh Risks: Report to Congressional Requesters.* Washington, D.C.: U.S. General Accounting Office, 2000. The GAO has often criticized food-safety procedures followed by government agencies but in this case affirms the policies adopted for food irradiation. In its report to Congress, the agency states that "Scientific studies conducted by public and private researchers worldwide over the past 50 years support the benefits of food irradiation while indicating minimal potential risks." In reaching this conclusion, the report answers concerns expressed about the safety of the process.

Wilkinson, V. M., and G. W. Gould. *Food Irradiation: A Reference Guide.* Oxford: Reed Educational and Professional Publishing, 1996. Organized as a dictionary, this reference guide includes comprehensive information and definitions of terms relating to food irradiation. It spans fields of biology, physics, politics, law, and chemistry in its review and includes numerous references.

ARTICLES

Fox, John A. "Influences on Purchase of Irradiated Foods." *Food Technology,* vol. 56, no. 11, November 2002, pp. 34–37. With scientists nearly all in support of food irradiation, the major obstacle to the widespread use of the technique comes from consumers. This article discussed ways to counter the negative publicity about irradiated food and convinced consumers of the safety of irradiated food.

Giles, Jim. "U.S. Chemist Attacks Consumer Magazine's Food Safety Work." *Nature,* vol. 431, September 9, 2004, p. 117. As reported in this article, a scientist at the meetings of the American Chemical Society criticized an influential study in *Consumer Reports* that cites evidence of contamination and poor taste of irradiated meat. Professor Joseph Rosen of Rutgers University claims that *Consumer Reports* ignored published studies that contradicted the magazine's views.

Gillette, Becky. "Try Our Nukeburgers." *E: The Environmental Magazine,* vol. 11, no. 4, July/August 2000, pp. 40–41. In making the case against irradiated meat—nukeburgers—poultry, and other products, the author cites an interesting fact: No new studies of the effects of eating irradiating food by lab animals have occurred since 1982. While the FDA says the evidence is strong enough to not require more studies, the article cites experts who disagree.

"Irradiation Revisited: As FDA Considers Expanded Use, New Health Concerns Arise." *Food Safety Review,* vol. 2, Winter 2002, pp. 1–8. The Center for Food Safety, an organization opposed to food irradiation, lays out its objections in this article. Along with identifying what it views as unacceptable risks to consumers from eating irradiated food, the article criticizes the FDA for past approval of irradiation and possible extensions to new products. It also offers advice on the political actions that those opposed to food irradiation can take.

Lortie, Brett. "Where's the (Irradiated) Beef?" *The Bulletin of the Atomic Scientists,* vol. 60, no. 6, November/December 2004, pp. 6–7. Although one might expect strong support among atomic scientists for applications of nuclear energy to food safety, this article written for such an audience views the practice with skepticism. It describes the bankruptcy of a firm that irradiates food, the unpleasant taste of irradiated meat, and the low sales of irradiated foods—all indications of problems faced by the technology.

Osterholm, Michael T., and Andrew P. Norgan. "The Role of Irradiation in Food Safety." *New England Journal of Medicine,* vol. 350, no. 18, April 29, 2004, pp. 1,898–1,901. The authors argue that physicians concerned about sickness and death from foodborne illness should support food irradiation. Despite improvements in food safety made by the meat and poultry industry and wider knowledge of the need to fully cook meat and poultry, foodborne illness remains a public health problem. Although the public has so far shown little interest in irradiated food, the authors believe that physicians and health-care professionals can use education to overcome this resistance and improve public health.

Parnes, Robin Brett, William C. Idell, and Audrey L. Anastasia Kanik. "Food Irradiation: An Overlooked Opportunity for Food Safety and Preservation." *Nutrition Today*, vol. 38, no. 5, September/October 2003, pp. 174–185. Reflecting a theme common in many favorable articles on food irradiation, this article suggests that the technology is underutilized. Fully developed and studied now for decades, irradiation needs to be used more on food. The article also provides a useful history of the technique.

Tauxe, Robert V. "Food Safety and Irradiation: Protecting the Public from Foodborne Infections." *Emerging Infectious Diseases* vol. 7, no. 3, Supplement, June 2001, pp. 516–521. Also available online. URL: http://www. cdc.gov/ncidod/eid/vol7no3_supp/tauxe.htm. Updated on April 21, 2003. The author places food irradiation in a line of techniques developed over the last century to improve food safety. Earlier techniques such as public sanitation and pasteurization of milk remain crucial to food safety but can be effectively supplemented by food irradiation. The article lists the foodborne diseases that irradiation can prevent and estimates the deaths that can be saved from its use.

"The Truth about Irradiated Meat." *Consumer Reports*, vol. 68, no. 8, August 2003, pp. 34–37. This article counters many claims made by proponents of food irradiation. Tests done for the article disclose, for example, that irradiated meat contains bacteria, causes subtle taste differences, and may produce harmful chemical by-products. The article recommends that producers do more to eliminate pathogens in meat and poultry before they are sold and consumers do more to make sure they cook food thoroughly. In the meantime, more research should be done on food irradiation before health officials recommend it for widespread use.

Wood, Olivia Bennett, and Christine M. Bruhn. "Position of the American Dietetic Association: Food Irradiation." *Journal of the American Dietetic Association*, vol. 100, no. 2, February 2000, pp. 246–253. The American Dietetic Association (ADA) favors the use of food irradiation: "It is the position of the ADA that food irradiation enhances the safety and quality of the food supply and helps protect consumers from foodborne illness.

The ADA encourages the government, food manufacturers, food commodity groups, and qualified food and nutrition professionals to work together to educate consumers about this additional food safety tool and make this choice available in the marketplace."

WEB DOCUMENTS

Epstein, Samuel. "Opinion: Food Irradiation Threatens Public Health, National Security." Organic Consumers Association. Available online. URL: http://www.organicconsumers.org/irrad/epsteinoped1.cfm. Downloaded in April 2006. Along with making the usual criticisms of the safety and wholesomeness of irradiated food, Epstein argues that irradiation threatens national security. He states: "Of particular current concern are terrorist attacks to steal radioactive cobalt pellets [used in food irradiation]. These could be mixed with conventional explosives to produce so-called dirty bombs, whose effects could be devastating."

"Food Irradiation." Center for Food Safety. Available online. URL: http://www.centerforfoodsafety.org/food_irrad.cfm. Downloaded in April 2006. One of the leading opponents of food irradiation summarizes the reasons for its opposition and provides links to other documents critical of the technology.

"Food Irradiation." Centers for Disease Control and Prevention. Available online. URL: http://www.cdc.gov/ncidod/dbmd/diseaseinfo/foodirradiation.htm. Updated on October 11, 2005. In answering 20 questions about food irradiation, the agency in charge of monitoring and preventing disease outbreaks offers a highly favorable view. The questions range from the basic ("What is food irradiation?") to the technical ("How do you measure the amount of radiation used?"), but in all cases they are answered clearly. The web page offers a helpful introduction to the topic.

"Food Irradiation: A Safe Measure." U.S. Food and Drug Administration. Available online. URL: http://www.fda.gov/opacom/catalog/irradbro.html. Posted in January 2000. The FDA favors the use of food irradiation and presents the arguments for that position on this web page.

"Food Irradiation Facts." University of California, Davis, Center for Consumer Research. Available online. URL: http://ccr.ucdavis.edu/irr. Updated on May 7, 2000. Relying on the generally positive evaluation of food irradiation by scientific researchers, this web page presents a similarly positive view. It attacks critics directly by including a section on myths about food irradiation and sponsors a message board to solicit public opinion on the topic.

Annotated Bibliography

Graham, Karen. "FAQs about Food Irradiation." Critical Mass Energy and Environment Program, Public Citizen. Available online. URL: http://www.citizen.org/cmep/foodsafety/international/canada/articles.cfm?ID=9532. Downloaded in January 2005. To see the diversity of opinion on food irradiation, compare the answers to frequently asked questions given on this web page by Public Citizen, perhaps the country's top critic of food irradiation, with the answers to frequently asked questions given by the CDC. The answers on this web page conclude, among other things, that no studies have proven food irradiation to be safe because they have not used the 100-fold safety factor applied to pesticides. Methods to deal with bacteria-contaminated food should therefore focus on improving procedures on the farm, in the slaughterhouse, and in the home rather than on food irradiation.

"Irradiation." FoodSafety.gov. Available online. URL: http://www.foodsafety.gov/~fsg/irradiat.html. Updated on December 23, 2005. Like other food-safety web pages, this one lists links to relevant government documents available from the Centers for Disease Control and Prevention, the Food Safety and Inspection Service, the Food and Drug Administration, and the Department of Agriculture—all agencies favoring food irradiation.

"What's in the Beef? Scientists Question the Safety of Irradiated Ground Beef." Public Citizen and Center for Food Safety. Available online. URL: http://www.citizen.org/documents/beeftesting.pdf. Posted in November 2003. Extending the criticisms offered by these two agencies in their earlier report, "Hidden Harm," this report focuses on proposals to allow irradiation of ground beef. In comparing irradiated and nonirradiated ground beef purchased in Washington, D.C., grocery stores, it finds that their radiated ground beef contained a chemical shown in some studies to cause cancer and birth defects in lab animals. The presence of the chemical does not by itself mean it will harm humans, but the finding contradicts other claims of complete safety of irradiated meat.

Worth, Mark, and Peter Jenkins. "Hidden Harm: How the FDA Is Ignoring the Potential Dangers of Unique Chemicals in Irradiated Food." Public Citizen and Center for Food Safety. Available online. URL: http://www.mindfully.org/Food/Irradiation-FDA-IgnoringDec01.htm. Downloaded in April 2006. Two leading organizations in the battle against food irradiation express concerns about the risks of the technology for food safety and accuse the FDA of ignoring evidence of these risks. In citing many scientific studies that support their view, the organizations dispute the scientific claims made by government officials on behalf of food irradiation.

GENETICALLY MODIFIED (GM) FOODS

BOOKS

Altieri, Miguel A. *Genetic Engineering in Agriculture: The Myths, Environmental Risks, and Alternatives.* 2nd ed. Oakland, Calif.: Food First, 2004. Food First is an organization devoted to ending world hunger, and this book published by the organization considers the potential benefits of genetic engineering for reaching this goal. The author, a professor at the University of California, Berkeley, argues against reliance on GM foods. Rather than an inexpensive source of food, genetic engineering creates products that are better suited for large industrial farms than small family farms common in much of the world.

Charles, Daniel. *Lords of the Harvest: Biotech, Big Money, and the Future of Food.* Cambridge, Mass.: Perseus Publishing, 2001. This readable history of GM foods gives special attention to battles between biotechnology corporations and protest groups. It presents debates fairly from the perspectives of both sides and only in the epilogue addresses the question of whether GM foods are safe. There, the author notes that answers to the question rely more on moral beliefs than scientific fact.

Cummins, Ronnie, and Ben Lilliston. *Genetically Engineered Food: A Self-Defense Guide for Consumers.* New York: Marlow and Company, 2000. Although most chapters describe the history and risks of GM foods, the book aims primarily to guide consumers in their food purchases. It lists the foods most likely to contain GM ingredients, the companies that produce or manufacture most GM food, and brands that supply food free of GM ingredients. Although the wide range of foods that contain GM ingredients make it seem nearly impossible to avoid GM food altogether, buying organic foods in natural food stores will minimize the risk.

Evenson, R. E., V. Santaniello, and Robert E. Evenson, eds. *Consumer Acceptance of Genetically Modified Foods.* Cambridge, Mass.: CABI Publishing, 2004. Papers from a 2002 conference of economists address issues such as consumer attitudes, willingness to pay for GM foods, and the finances of the food biotechnology industry. Of special interest are the comparisons across nations of attitudes toward GM food and the less positive views in Europe compared to the United States.

Fedoroff, Nina, and Nancy Marie Brown. *Mendel in the Kitchen: A Scientist's View of Genetically Modified Foods.* Washington, D.C.: National Academies Press, 2004. A leading expert in plant biotechnology and a science writer present a generally positive view of GM foods. They write that most concerns expressed about GM foods are overstated and that the products have the potential to do much good in the world. The book also offers a readable introduction to genetic engineering and its history.

Fumento, Michael. *BioEvolution: How Biotechnology Is Changing Our World.* San Francisco: Encounter Books, 2003. This book offers an optimistic, perhaps even utopian, view of the benefits of biotechnology. Although covering benefits more generally in areas of health and the environment, it also focuses on GM foods. A summary on the backcover states: "Biotech will make fields more fertile, producing crops that are more abundant; healthier; and more nutritious and flavorful. Plant diseases will be wiped out. Malnutrition will disappear as food is produced on less land, using less water, in colder climates, and using fewer chemicals."

Hart, Kathleen. *Eating in the Dark: America's Experiment with Genetically Engineered Food.* New York: Pantheon, 2002. Echoing a key complaint about GM foods, this book describes the hidden spread of GM products and their unknown safety. The result, according to the author, is a public health nightmare. The FDA must take much of the responsibility for this nightmare. It has failed to regulate GM foods and needs to improve the situation by informing the public about what is contained in their food. In making her case, the author interviews scientists, farmers, industry members, and activists and examines the workings of the EPA, FDA, and other government agencies that set policies for GM foods.

Institute of Medicine and National Research Council. *Safety of Genetically Engineered Foods: Approaches to Assessing Unintended Health Effects.* Washington, D.C.: National Academies Press, 2004. Also available online. URL: http://www.nap.edu/books/0309092094/html. Downloaded in April 2006. A scientific evaluation of the safety of GM foods concludes that they do not present unique risks and that special regulations are not needed. At the same time, however, the evaluation suggests that genetic engineering could produce some unintended and harmful toxins. This threat comes more from the toxin than the genetic engineering, and safety regulations should focus on testing for toxins rather than prohibiting genetic engineering.

Lambrecht, Bill. *Dinner at the New Gene Café.* New York: St. Martin's Press, 2000. The journalist author describes the people and events behind the development of genetically modified foods and the controversy the food has created. The portraits of the scientists at the Monsanto Corporation who made important discoveries about genetic engineering of food, farmers who have planted GM foods, and opponents in the United States and Europe who have prevented greater use of the products make for interesting reading. Less a reference source with details about GM foods than a compilation of stories, the book makes abstract debates more real and fairly presents the views of those on both sides.

Lurquin, Paul F. *High Tech Harvest: Understanding Genetically Modified Food Plants.* Boulder, Colo.: Westview Press, 2002. A biologist and geneticist aims in this book to explain the scientific basis of GM foods, hoping to inform the public about the ongoing controversies. Avoiding either extreme, he argues that GM foods are neither inherently dangerous nor safe. Rather, they offer potential benefits when used carefully and evaluated scientifically. Readers will learn much about genetics and its history from this book.

Martineau, Belinda. *First Fruit: The Creation of the Flavr Savr Tomato and the Birth of Biotech Foods.* New York: McGraw-Hill, 2001. A geneticist and member of the team that developed the Flavr Savr tomato, the author tells the story of the development, marketing, regulation battles, and ultimate failure of this product. Genetically modified to ripen longer on the vine without spoiling, this tomato was the first GM food marketed in the United States. The author offers a fair-minded history of the product and more generally describes both the potential and the risks of food biotechnology.

McHughen, Alan. *Pandora's Picnic Basket: The Potential and Hazards of Genetically Modified Foods.* Oxford: Oxford University Press, 2000. A Canadian scientist who developed a GM crop, McHughen presents both sides of the debate and offers facts to help readers reach their own conclusion. However, he remains skeptical of many criticisms made of GM foods because they lack rigorous scientific evidence or distort known facts. In the end, the book offers a generally positive view of GM foods.

Miller, Henry I., and Gregory Conko. *The Frankenfood Myth: How Protest and Politics Threaten the Biotech Revolution.* Westport, Conn.: Praeger Publishers, 2004. The book argues that unnecessary regulations have restricted research on biotechnology and limit the potential benefits for the food industry. Misinformation about the issue passed on by the press, government agencies, and businesses has also led to unwarranted public resistance to GM products. The authors suggest changes in policy that can unlock the potential of this new technology.

Smith, Jeffrey M. *Seeds of Deception: Exposing Industry and Government Lies about the Safety of the Genetically Engineered Foods You're Eating.* Fairfield, Iowa: Yes! Books, 2003. Highly critical of GM food and the agricultural industry, this book presents its arguments clearly and thoroughly and includes many stories about the efforts of GM food opponents to warn of its dangers. One chapter lays out the safety risks of GM foods, and other chapters describe efforts of GM food companies to mislead the public about the safety of their products. Those wanting to know more about the arguments against GM foods will find this a useful source.

Thompson, Paul B. *Food Technology in Ethical Perspective.* London: Blackie Academic and Professional, 1997. Thompson, a professor of applied ethics at Purdue University, considers a variety of ethical issues raised by genetic engineering of food. He first makes the case for the benefits of GM food but then considers several risks. Food biotechnology may have unintended consequences, customers may not be fully informed about the nature of the food, the environment may be harmed, and merging different species may violate social and religious principles. While addressing issues of widespread interest, the book includes much material of primary interest to academics and philosophers.

ARTICLES

Becker, Elizabeth. "Battle over Biotechnology Intensified Trade War." *New York Times*, May 29, 2003, p. C1. The United States and President George W. Bush have criticized the European Union's restrictions on imports of GM crops. Some view the restrictions as a way to avoid competing with American farmers and blocking sales of safe American agricultural products. A suit alleging unfair trade that has gone to the World Trade Organization illustrates the conflicting views of the United States and the European nations on GM crops.

Boyer, Paul. "Unwarranted Fear of GMOs Harms Us All." *New Perspectives Quarterly*, vol. 21, no. 4, Fall 2004, pp. 105–107. A Nobel Prize–winning chemist argues that the applications of genetic engineering have much potential to improve the well-being of humanity. He criticizes views common among environmentalists that genetic engineering is inherently dangerous and worries that the influence of such views will hamper progress.

Brody, Jane E. "Facing Biotech Foods without the Fear Factor." *New York Times*, January 11, 2005, p. F7. While recognizing that the public remains wary of GM food, the personal health columnist for the *New York Times* also describes widespread misconceptions. She notes, for example, that nearly all food has been genetically modified by centuries of crossbreeding and that new forms of genetic engineering so far have not presented a major risk to food safety.

Finucane, M. L., and J. L. Holup. "Psychosocial and Cultural Factors Affecting the Perceived Risk of Genetically Modified Food: An Overview of the Literature." *Social Science and Medicine*, vol 60, no. 7, April 2005, pp. 1603–1612. Rather than focusing on the actual risks of GM food, this article concentrates on the risks perceived by the public in the United States, Europe, and nations of the developing world.

"Genetically Modified Food: Understanding the Societal Dilemma." *American Behavioral Scientist*, vol. 44, no. 8, April 2001, pp. 1,225–1,437. A special issue of this journal contains a variety of articles that address the ethics, economics, and environmental impact of GM foods. Special attention is given to the underlying sources of public disagreements over the issues.

Keeler, Barbara. "A Nation of Lab Rats." *Sierra*, vol. 86, no. 4, July/August 2001, p. 45. The author suggests that since GM foods have not undergone extensive government testing, the real tests for safety come from consumption of the foods at the dinner table of Americans. Concerned about the possible harm of the foods, she criticizes the government for failing to properly regulate GM foods and protect the public.

Lewis, Carol. "A New Kind of Fish Story." *FDA Consumer*, vol. 35, no. 1, January/February 2001, pp. 14–20. New developments may extend genetic engineering from crops to fish by adding genes to speed the growth of a type of Atlantic salmon. However, transgenic animals raise new food-safety questions that may require special investigation by the FDA and some convincing of consumers of the safety of this food.

"A Look into the Biotech Laboratory." *FDA Consumer*, vol. 37, no. 6, November/December 2003, p. 31. This article reports on the work of a lab at Cornell University to add new genes to rice plants and make them more resistant to drought and cold, and also on the work at the USDA's Agricultural Research Station to remove a gene from soybeans thought to cause allergic reactions.

"The Men in White Coats Are Winning, Slowly." *The Economist*, vol. 373, October 9, 2004, pp. 63–66. This article describes the success of genetic engineering in nonfood uses, concluding that inroads made in other areas will make the continued application of the technology to food uses all the more likely in the future.

Nemecek, Sasha. "Does the World Need GM Foods? Yes." *Scientific American*, vol. 284, no. 4, April 2001, pp. 62–63. An interview with Robert B. Horsch, the vice president of product and technology cooperation at Monsanto Company, highlights the many potential benefits of GM foods. Monsanto is viewed as a villain by opponents to GM foods but also has the respect of many scientists for its groundbreaking work on genetic engineering. Readers of this interview can judge for themselves if Horsch makes a convincing case.

Newbury, Umut. "Anti-Frankenfood Movement Grows." *Mother Earth News*, no. 205, August/September 2004, p. 18. Mendocino County in California has banned growing of GM crops, an action that the author hopes will lead to similar bans elsewhere. The article also describes opposition to GM foods in many European nations.

Nichols, John. "The Three Mile Island of Biotech?" *The Nation*, vol. 275, no. 23, December 30, 2002, pp. 11, 13–16. Citing concerns expressed by some scientists that GM foods may harm the immune system of consumers, the author argues that efforts to create pharmaceutical plant products from genetic engineering are a serious public health threat.

Pollack, Andrew. "Narrow Path for New Biotech Food Crops." *New York Times*, May 20, 2004, p. C1. This article from the business section of the newspaper describes the problems businesses have had in marketing GM foods. The high cost of developing and testing the products and the resistance of consumers make many newly created GM foods unprofitable. As a result, GM foods have had success for only a few products and only in a few nations.

Ralli, Tania. "Modified-Food Labeling Begins in Europe." *New York Times*, April 21, 2004, p. F6. Unlike the United States, the European Union now requires that all food sold with GM ingredients must say so on the label. The strict rules and consumer resistance to GM foods have led European companies to avoid adding GM ingredients to their products.

Rauch, Jonathan. "Will Frankenfood Save the Planet"" *Atlantic Monthly*, vol. 292, no. 3, October 2003, pp. 103–108. While recognizing the potential risks of bioengineered food, the author also sees the benefits. With food production likely needing to double or triple over the next few decades, an increase of this size will require massive amounts of polluting pesticides and fertilizers. GM foods offer an alternative that might help meet the twin goals of greater food production and environmental protection.

Schapiro, Mark. "Sowing Disaster?" *The Nation*, vol. 275, no. 14, October 28, 2002, pp. 11–15, 17–19. Although Mexico banned GM corn in the late 1990s, it appears that genes from American GM corn have made their way into local varieties of Mexican corn. This outcome shows, according to the article, that GM organisms can spread beyond the control of governments and farmers. It could also mean that new varieties of GM corn will come to crowd out and ultimately destroy the natural varieties that now exist throughout the world.

"Sowing Seeds of Discord." *Environment*, vol. 45, no. 8, October 2003, pp. 6–7. This article reports on findings that farmers are routinely planting more insect-resistant corn than federal regulations allow. It criticizes government agencies for failing to properly control GM crops containing natural pesticides.

Strauss, Mark. "When Malthus Meets Mendel: Can Biotechnology End Hunger?" *Foreign Policy*, no. 119, Summer 2000, pp. 105–112. The potential for GM foods to address problems of world hunger makes the technology particularly relevant to foreign policy. Although attractive to developing nations, the technology is unlikely to end world hunger for several reasons. According to the article, multinational firms may use the technology to maximize profits rather than help the poor, and the risks of genetic pollution may threaten native species and the environments of poor nations.

Toke, Dave. "GM Crops: Science, Policy and Environmentalists." *Environmental Politics*, vol. 10, no. 4, Winter 2001, pp. 115–120. As described in this article, environmentalists have different views on GM foods. Some believe that the use of GM crops through careful research, trial and error, and slow adoption can help avoid the harm to the environment caused by modern farming practices. More radical environmentalists, however, oppose use of GM crops in any form and advocate organic farming.

Wheelwright, Jeff. "Don't Eat Again Until You Read This." *Discover*, vol. 22, no. 3, March 2001, pp. 36–43. A review of the StarLink corn scandal, in which GM corn meant only for animal feed worked its way into the human food supply.

WEB DOCUMENTS

"Are You Eating Genetically Modified Food" CNN.com. Available online. URL: http://www.ndmnutrition.com/rueating_gmo_foods.htm. Downloaded in April 2006. This recent news story answers yes, most people are eating genetically modified food—although few know they are doing so. It reports recent survey results that less than half of the people interviewed knew GM foods or ingredients of foods were sold in supermarkets. Yet about 75 percent of processed foods contain GM ingredients.

"Biotechnology." U.S. Food and Drug Administration. Available online. URL: http://www.cfsan.fda.gov/~lrd/biotechm.html#label. Updated on November 14, 2005. The FDA has links to dozens of documents on this web page. Sections on food labeling and information for consumers may be especially useful, but other sections on international standards and safety assessments may also be worth examining.

"The Campaign to Label Genetically Engineered Foods." The Campaign: Grassroots Political Action. Available online. URL: http://www.thecampaign.org. Downloaded in April 2006. Those wanting to learn what they can do to advocate for labeling requirements on GM foods can consult this web page. It lists three basic steps one can take to help reach this goal and a variety of other actions that can also help in the campaign.

Europa. "Biotechnology: Introduction." Food and Feed Safety. Available online. URL: http://europa.eu.int/comm/food/food/biotechnology/index_en.htm. Downloaded in April 2006. The European public has shown much more resistance to GM foods than the American public, and European governments have placed stringent restrictions on the import and sale of GM foods. This web page from the European Commission includes links to its directives on GM foods and provides a source of information on policy differences between the European Union and the United States.

"Food and Agriculture Highlights." BIO: Biotechnology Industry Organization. Available online. URL: http://www.bio.org/foodag. Downloaded in April 2006. A trade organization that supports and lobbies for member biotechnology companies has devoted this web page to food issues. The section on facts and fiction about plant and animal biotechnology defends the safety of GM foods against the claims of opponents. Other sections offer additional information on legislative action, nutrition, and labeling—all from a pro-GM food perspective.

"Food and Biotechnology." Pew Initiative. Available online. URL: http://pewagbiotech.org. Downloaded in April 2006. With funding from the Pew Charitable Trust, this initiative aims to provide an independent and objective source of credible information on GM foods. It succeeds in reaching its goal: This highly recommended web page contains much useful and unbiased information from news reports, public opinion polls, and fact sheets.

"Genetically Engineered Foods: Are They Safe?" Center for Science in the Public Interest, Nutrition Action. Available online. URL: http://www.cspinet.org/nah/11_01. Posted in November 2001. In an interview, the codirectors of the Biotechnology Project at the Center for Science and the Public Interest summarize concerns about GM foods but also recognize some of the potential benefits of the new technology.

"Genetically Modified Food." Yahoo! News. Available online. URL: http://story.news.yahoo.com/fc?cid=34&tmpl=fc&in=Science&cat=Genetically_Modified_Food. Downloaded in April 2006. Along with a sampling of recent news articles and opinion pieces on the topic, this Yahoo! Science page includes links to other GM food web sites.

"GM Organisms." NewScientist.com. Available online. URL: http://www.newscientist.com/channel/life/gm-food. Downloaded in April 2006. An archive of scientific articles on GM foods and related topics. With continual updating, the archive covers recent developments in GM food research and potential new products.

"List of Completed Consultations on Bioengineered Foods." U.S. Food and Drug Administration. Available online. URL: http://www.cfsan.fda.gov/~lrd/biocon.html. Posted in November 2005. FDA policy recommends that companies consult with the agency about GM foods under development. This page lists those GM foods that have been submitted for consultation and shows the wide variety of products that have been developed for sale.

Pusztai, Arpad. "Genetically Modified Foods: Are They a Risk to Human/Animal Health?" ActionBioscience.org. Available online. URL: http://www.actionbioscience.org/biotech/pusztai.html. Posted in June 2001. A well-known and early critic of the safety of GM foods presents the case against the new technology. The page also includes links to other articles on bioscience and genetic engineering.

"Say No to Genetic Engineering." Greenpeace. Available online. URL: http://www.greenpeace.org/international_en/campaigns/intro? campaign_id=3942. Downloaded in April 2006. This environmental organization opposes the release of GM organisms into the environment because they contaminate natural organisms and pollute the plant gene pool. This web page and the links it contains explain the organization's policy in more detail and provide information on what it views as a threat to food safety.

CHAPTER 8

ORGANIZATIONS AND AGENCIES

The food-safety organizations and agencies listed in this chapter fall into six categories:

- federal government agencies
- state government associations and agencies
- international organizations
- business organizations and trade associations
- consumer advocacy organizations
- research and education organizations

All organizations favor food safety and state their commitment to addressing threats to food safety, but each type of organization typically differs in the kinds of actions they believe need to be taken to deal with the problems.

For each organization, the listings include the web site and e-mail. Many organizations do not list their e-mail address but include a web page from which users can submit questions and comments via e-mail. In these cases, the text notes that e-mail is available via web form. The listings then include phone numbers (when available), postal addresses, and brief descriptions. The state government section does not include listings for each of the 50 states but does provide listings of a few organizations that have collected information on food-safety agencies in each of the states.

FEDERAL GOVERNMENT AGENCIES

Center for Food Safety and Applied Nutrition (CFSAN)
URL: http://vm.cfsan.fda.gov
Phone: (888) 723-3366
5100 Paint Branch Parkway

College Park, MD 20740-3835
A unit of the Food and Drug Administration that regulates food additives and domestic and imported foods. In recent years it has devoted

227

additional resources to protecting the food supply from acts of terrorism.

Centers for Disease Control and Prevention (CDC)
URL: http://www.cdc.gov
E-mail: web form
Phone: (800) 311-3435
1600 Clifton Road
Atlanta, GA 30333
Lead federal agency for protecting the health and safety of Americans both at home and abroad. To help promote the health of the public, it tracks the spread of foodborne illnesses.

Customs and Border Protection (CBP)
URL: http://www.customs.ustreas.gov
E-mail: web form
Phone: (202) 354-1000
1300 Pennsylvania Avenue, NW
Washington, DC 20229
Focuses on controlling movement of people across U.S. borders and on stopping the entrance of terrorists into the country. Since moving to the Department of Homeland Security, it has given increasing attention to inspection of food imports and stopping bioterrorism.

Food and Drug Administration (FDA)
URL: http://www.fda.gov
E-mail: web form
Phone: (888) 463-6332
5600 Fishers Lane
Rockville, MD 20857

Promotes public health by reviewing clinical research and regulating food and medical products to ensure they are safe. Its goals have come to include preventing terrorist contamination of food products as well as regulating food additives.

Foodborne Illness Education Information Center
URL: http://www.nal.usda.gov/foodborne
E-mail: foodborne@nal.usda.gov
Phone: (301) 504-6365
National Agricultural Library/USDA
Beltsville, MD 20705-2351
A unit of the Food and Drug Administration and the Food Safety and Inspection Service that provides special information for food-service workers, child-care providers, and children. It sponsors a food safety web page (http://www.foodsafety.gov) with hundreds of links to sources on food safety.

Food Safety and Inspection Service (FSIS)
URL: http://www.fsis.usda.gov
E-mail: fsis.outreach@usda.gov
Phone: (202) 720-7025
1400 Independence Avenue, SW
Room 331-E
Washington, DC 20250
The public health agency unit of the U.S. Department of Agriculture has responsibility for inspecting and approving the nation's commercial supply of meat, poultry, and egg products as safe, wholesome, and correctly labeled and packaged.

National Aeronautics and Space Administration (NASA)
URL: http://www.nasa.gov
E-mail: public-inquiries@hq.nasa.gov
Phone: (202) 358-0001
300 E Street, SW
Washington, DC 20546-0001
The nation's leading agency for space exploration played a small part in the history of food safety by adopting irradiated food for use by astronauts in space.

National Institutes of Health (NIH)
URL: http://www.nih.gov
E-mail: nihinfo@od.nih.gov
Phone: (301) 496-4000
900 Rockville Pike
Bethesda, MD 20892
Supports scientific research and the application of knowledge to extend healthy life and reduce the burdens of illness and disability. An important aspect of these research goals is protection from infectious diseases spread by food.

National Organic Program (NOP)
URL: http://www.ams.usda.gov/nop
Phone: (202) 720-3252
1400 Independence Avenue, SW
Room 4008-South Building
Washington, DC 20250-0020
A program within the USDA that develops national standards for organic agricultural products and certifies farms and food producers wanting to label their products as organic. It relies on assistance from a 15-member National Organic Standards Board made up of farmers, scientists, environmentalists, and consumer advocates.

Office of Food Additive Safety (OFAS)
URL: http://www.cfsan.fda.gov/~dms/opa-help.html
E-mail: premarkt@cfsan.fda.gov
Phone: (301) 436-1200
5100 Paint Branch Parkway
College Park, MD 20740-3835
A unit of the FDA with a separate Division of Petition Review that evaluates the safety of new food additives. It must give approval before companies can market products with the new additives.

Office of Food Security and Emergency Preparedness (OFSEP)
URL: http://www.fsis.usda.gov/about/OFSEP
E-mail: mphotline.fsis@usda.gov
Phone: (888) 674-6854
1400 Independence Avenue, SW
Room 331-E
Washington, DC 20250
Manages homeland security activities within the Food Safety and Inspection Service and makes sure that policy makers, scientists, field staff, and management are prepared to prevent and respond to any food security threat.

Office of Pesticide Programs
URL: http://www.epa.gov/pesticides

**E-mail: opp-web-comments@
epa.gov
Ariel Rios Building
1200 Pennsylvania Avenue, NW
Washington, DC 20460**
A unit of the EPA that works on pesticide issues relating to their proper use, environmental effects, and health and safety risks.

**U.S. Department of Agriculture
(USDA)
URL: http://www.usda.gov
E-mail: agsec@usda.gov
1400 Independence Avenue, SW
Washington, DC 20250**
Its mission includes ensuring the safety of the food supply. Although traditionally focused on the inspection of food to prevent the spread of natural disease, it has given special attention in recent years to threats from bioterrorism and mad cow disease.

**U.S. Department of Health and
Human Services (HSS)
URL: http://www.hhs.gov
Phone: (877) 696-6775
200 Independence Avenue, SW
Washington, DC 20201**
The major government agency for protecting the health of Americans and providing essential services. Through its agencies, the Food and Drug Administration, the Centers

for Disease Control and Prevention, and the National Institutes of Health, it plays a crucial role in protecting food safety.

**U.S. Department of Homeland
Security (DHS)
URL: http://www.dhs.gov/
dhspublic
E-mail: web form
Phone: (202) 282-8000
Washington, DC 20528**
An agency established after the September 11, 2001, attacks that centrally coordinates operations once part of several separate agencies. It plays a crucial role in preventing bioterrorism and has implemented a variety of actions to improve food security.

**U.S. Government Accountability
Office (GAO)
URL: http://www.gao.gov
Phone: (202) 512-3000
441 G Street, NW
Washington, DC 20548**
Formerly the General Accounting Office, it serves as the investigative arm of Congress by studying programs and expenditures of the federal government. It has examined many food safety programs and has offered advice on how the programs can improve their performance.

STATE GOVERNMENT ASSOCIATIONS AND AGENCIES

California Department of Food
and Agriculture (CDFA)
URL: http://www.cdfa.ca.gov/
ahfss/ah/food_safety.htm
E-mail: ahbfeedback@cdfa.ca.gov
Phone: (916) 654-0466
1220 N Street
Sacramento, CA 95814
California grows and exports much
of the nation's fruits and vegetables
and gives special attention to food-
safety issues.

National Association of State
Departments of Agriculture
(NASDA)
URL: http://www.nasda-hq.org/
nasda/nasda/Foundation/
foodsafety
E-mail: nasda@patriot.net
Phone: (202) 296-9680
1156 15th Street, NW
Suite 1020
Washington, DC 20005-1704
The association provides links to
the food regulations of every state.

INTERNATIONAL ORGANIZATIONS

European Union (EU)
URL: http://europa.eu.int/pol/
food/index_en.htm
E-mail: web form
Phone: (+32) 2 299 96 96
B-1049 Brussels
Belgium
An organization of European na-
tions that has set stringent regula-
tions for the use of hormones in
food animals and the selling of
GM food products. This has lead
to disagreement with the United
States, which views the policies as
a way to prevent imports of their
products.

Food and Agriculture
Organization of the United
Nations (FAO)
URL: http://www.fao.org

E-mail: FAO-HQ@fao.org
Phone: (+39) 6 570 53625
Viale delle Terme di Caracalla
00100 Rome
Italy
Has a mission of raising the levels
of nutrition, agricultural productivity, and quality of life of rural populations, particularly in developing
nations. It recommends the use of
food irradiation but has been more
cautious about use of GM foods.

World Health Organization
(WHO)
URL: http://www.who.int/en
E-mail: info@who.org
Phone: (+ 41) 22 791 21 11
Avenue Appia 20
1211 Geneva 27
Switzerland

An agency of the United Nations that deals with global health issues. In the area of food safety, it protects food from terrorism, provides guidelines to test for BSE in cattle, tracks the outbreaks of foodborne illness, and recommends procedures to ensure food is kept safe.

World Trade Organization (WTO)
URL: http://www.wto.org
E-mail: enquiries@wto.org

Phone: (+41) 22 739 51 11
Centre William Rappard
Rue de Lausanne 154
CH-1211 Geneva 21
Switzerland
A global organization that deals with international trade rules. It has been asked to rule on accusations made by the United States that restrictions of the European Union on meat from animals raised with hormones and on GM foods amount to unfair trading practices.

BUSINESS ORGANIZATIONS AND TRADE ASSOCIATIONS

American Farm Bureau (FB)
URL: http://www.fb.org
E-mail: webmaster@fb.org
Phone: (847) 969-2976
1501 East Woodfield Road
Suite 300W
Schaumburg, IL 60173-5422
An organization that represents the interests of and provides support to farmers and ranchers. It has been active in debates over pesticide use and food safety, becoming involved in a suit against the EPA over setting acceptable levels of pesticide residue on food.

American Meat Institute (AMI)
URL: http://www.meatami.com
E-mail: web form
Phone: (202) 587-4200
1150 Connecticut Avenue, NW
12th floor
Washington, DC 20036

The nation's oldest and largest meat and poultry trade association. It supports the efficiency, profitability, and safety of the worldwide meat and poultry trade. In this role, it gives much attention to government food-safety policies and how they affect producers.

Animal Health Institute (AHI)
URL: http://www.ahi.org
E-mail: rphillips@ahi.org
Phone: (202) 637-2440
1325 G Street, NW
Suite 700
Washington, DC 20005
This trade association of manufacturers of pharmaceutical products for animals supports the routine use of low-dose antibiotics to help food animals grow. It argues that this practice does not lead to the transfer of antibiotic-resistant bacteria to humans.

**Biotechnology Industry
  Organization (BIO)**
URL: http://www.bio.org/foodag
E-mail: info@bio.org
Phone: (202) 962-9200
1225 I Street, NW
Suite 400
Washington, DC 20005
A trade organization for the biotechnology industry. In representing many firms with an interest in developing GM crops and foods, it attempts to counter what it views as the many myths about plant and animal biotechnology.

Food Products Association (FPA)
URL: http://www.safefood.org
E-mail: web form
Phone: (202) 639-5900
1350 I Street, NW
Suite 300
Washington, DC 20005
A trade association serving the worldwide food and beverage industry. It provides scientific and technical assistance on food safety and food security to its members and represents their interests in the areas of public policy.

**Grocery Manufacturers of
  America (GMA)**
URL: http://www.gmabrands.
  com
E-mail: info@gmabrands.com
Phone: (202) 337-9400
2401 Pennsylvania Avenue, NW
2nd Floor
Washington, DC 20037
A trade group devoted mostly to advancing the policy interests of

those manufacturing brands for sale in grocery stores, but one also focused on helping members deal with emergency food recalls and terrorist threats.

Jack in the Box
URL: http://www.jackinthebox.
  com
E-mail: web form
Phone: (858) 571-2121
9330 Balboa Avenue
San Diego, CA 92123-1516
After several customers died and hundreds became sick from its hamburgers in 1993, this fast-food company made major changes in its food-safety efforts. It now has in place a comprehensive, "farm to fork" system of managing product quality and safety.

McDonald's Corporation
URL: http://www.mcdonalds.
  com/corp.html
E-mail: web form
Phone: (800) 244-6227
2111 McDonald's Drive
Oak Brook, IL 60523
In publicizing its commitment to food safety, McDonald's has required its meat producers to minimize use of antibiotics and has distributed a food-safety brochure called "A Parent's Guide to Playing It Safe at Home" with its Happy Meals for children.

Monsanto Company
URL: http://www.monsanto.com
E-mail: web form
Phone: (314) 694-1000

800 North Lindbergh Boulevard St. Louis, MO 63167
An agricultural products company best known for its plant seeds, Roundup herbicide, and GM crops. Although recognized scientifically for its advances in genomics, it has been criticized by opponents of GM foods for its aggressive promotion of the products.

National Cattlemen's Beef Association (NCBA)
URL: http://www.beef.org
Phone: (303) 694-0305
9110 East Nichols Avenue
Suite 300
Centennial, CO 80112
An association of cattle and beef producers that sponsors a web page on BSE. The web page notes the concerns cattlemen have with protecting the safety of beef and describes the efforts made by industry and the government to protect American beef from BSE.

National Restaurant Association
URL: http://www.restaurant.org
E-mail: media@dineout.org
Phone: (202) 331-5900
1200 17th Street, NW
Washington, DC 20036
A leading business association for the restaurant industry that gives special attention to issues of food safety by providing training resources for restaurant owners and employees.

Odwalla Products
URL: http://www.odwalla.com

E-mail:
consumers@odwalla.com
Phone: (800) 639-2552
120 Stone Pine Road
Half Moon Bay, CA 94019
A company that makes fresh, natural, and nutritious juices for health-conscious consumers. After a death caused by one of its unpasteurized juices, the company began to use a special form of pasteurization to kill bacteria in its products.

Procter & Gamble (P&G)
URL: http://www.pg.com
E-mail: web form
Phone: (800) 543-1745
One Procter & Gamble Plaza
Cincinnati, OH 45202
The company that developed and marketed olestra, a food that has the texture of fat but is not absorbed into the bloodstream. The FDA gave approval to the company to sell this product but also required a label warning of possible unhealthy side effects.

Sizzler Steakhouse
URL: http://www.sizzler.com
E-mail: web form
Phone: (818) 662-9900
15301 Ventura Blvd.
Garden Office Building
Building B
Suite 300
Sherman Oaks, CA 91403
A restaurant chain specializing in grilled foods. Patrons of a Milwaukee franchise became sick (and in a few cases died) from fruit in a salad bar that had become contaminated with dangerous bacteria.

CONSUMER ADVOCACY ORGANIZATIONS

Alliance for Biointegrity
URL: http://www.biointegrity.
  org
E-mail: info@biointegrity.org
Phone: (206) 888-4852
2040 Pearl Lane
Suite 2
Fairfield, IA 52556
A major partner in a suit against the FDA, it opposes the unlabeled sale of GM foods and accuses the FDA of failing to regulate the safety of these foods. The suit failed, but the organization continues to publicize the risks it sees in GM foods.

Center for Consumer Freedom (CCF)
URL: http://www.consumer
  freedom.com
E-mail: info@consumerfreedom.
  com
Phone: (202) 463-7112
P.O. Box 27414
Washington, DC 20038
An organization funded by restaurants and food companies. It favors the right of adults and parents to eat and drink what they want and opposes the efforts of food activists, government officials, and health-care professionals to limit the food choices of the public.

Center for Food Safety (CFS)
URL: http://www.centerforfood
  safety.org
E-mail: office@centerforfood
  safety.org

Phone: (202) 547-9359
660 Pennsylvania Avenue, SE
Suite 302
Washington, DC 20003
Opposes food-production technologies such as genetic engineering, irradiation, and animal hormones and advocates for safer alternatives such as organic farming and ranching methods. It has in particular led efforts to oppose the marketing of irradiated meat.

Center for Science in the Public Interest (CSPI)
URL: http://www.cspinet.org
E-mail: cspi@cspinet.org
Phone: (202) 332-9110
1875 Connecticut Avenue, NW
Suite 300
Washington, DC 20009
An organization that advocates for nutrition and health, food safety, and sound science. It has been critical of fast-food businesses and the failure, in its view, of the government to fully protect the public from unsafe foods.

Community Food Security Coalition (CFSC)
URL: http://www.foodsecurity.
  org
E-mail: mail@anncherin.com
Phone: (310) 822-5410
P.O. Box 209
Venice, CA 90294
An organization that advocates for self-reliance and sustainability

235

among communities in growing and obtaining their food. It has argued that problems of food safety and vulnerability to food terrorism are worsened by processing of food for shipment across long distances.

Consumer Federation of America (CFA)
URL: http://www.consumerfed.org
E-mail: cfa@consumerfed.org
Phone: (202) 387-6121
1424 16th Street, NW
Suite 604
Washington, DC 20036
A pro-consumer group and research organization that sponsors the Food Policy Institute. It does research and advocacy for a safer, healthier, and more affordable food supply and has criticized government meat-inspection policies and lack of testing for GM foods.

Consumers Union
URL: http://www.consumersunion.org
Phone: (914) 378-2000
101 Truman Avenue
Yonkers, NY 10703-1057
An independent agency that tests consumer products as a way to inform consumers, protect the public, and advocate for consumer interests. It publishes *Consumer Reports*, which has included several articles critical of government policies on food safety, pesticide use, and food irradiation.

Environmental Working Group (EWG)
URL: http://www.ewg.org

E-mail: web form
Phone: (202) 667-6982
1436 U Street, NW
Suite 100
Washington, DC 20009
An environmental group that sponsors research on threats to health and the environment. It publishes Food News, a web page designed to help consumers make healthier food choices and find pesticide-free and organic foods to purchase.

Food Allergy and Anaphylaxis Network (FAAN)
URL: http://www.foodallergy.org
E-mail: faan@foodallergy.org
Phone: (800) 929-4040
11781 Lee Jackson Highway
Suite 160
Fairfax, VA 22033-3309
A group that promotes awareness, education, and research related to food allergies and anaphylaxis and helps those affected by the disease. It works to improve safety from food allergens through labeling, emergency medical services, and food preparation in schools, restaurants, and airlines.

Friends of the Earth (FOE)
URL: http://www.foe.org
E-mail: foe@foe.org
Phone: (877) 843-8687
1717 Massachusetts Avenue, NW
Suite 600
Washington, DC 20036-2002
A network of environmental groups, it played a major role in the battle

over GM foods by demonstrating that GM corn had illegally made its way into corn taco shells sold in supermarkets. It advocates better testing and mandatory labeling for GM foods.

Greenpeace
URL: http://usactions.
greenpeace.org
E-mail: info@wdc.greenpeace.org
Phone: (202) 462-1177
702 H Street, NW
Washington, DC 20001
An international environmental organization involved in activities to protect the environment and endangered species. It opposes genetic engineering as unsafe for the environment and, when done to food, unsafe for consumption.

Natural Resources Defense Council (NRDC)
URL: http://www.nrdc.org
E-mail: nrdcinfo@nrdc.org
Phone: (212) 727-2700
40 West 20th Street
New York, NY 10011
An environmental action group with the goal of protecting the planet's wildlife and wild places. It has special concerns about the toxic effects of pesticides and has sued the EPA several times to restrict

the allowable residue of pesticides on food.

Organic Consumers Association (OCA)
URL: http://www.organic
consumers.org
E-mail: web form
Phone: (218) 226-4164
6101 Cliff Estate Road
Little Marais, MN 55614
This organization represents the interests of organic consumers by opposing GM foods and modern factory farms, supporting conversion of agriculture to organic methods, and advocating stricter USDA standards for labeling organic foods.

Safe Tables Our Priority (S.T.O.P.)
URL: http://www.safetables.org
E-mail: mail@safetables.org
Phone: (802) 863-0555
P.O. Box 4352
Burlington, VT 05406
An organization founded by victims and relatives of victims of the *E. coli* outbreak spread by Jack in the Box hamburgers. It has the mission of preventing unnecessary illness and loss of life from pathogenic foodborne illness and has promoted stronger food-safety laws and regulations.

RESEARCH AND EDUCATION ORGANIZATIONS

American Public Health Association (APHA)
URL: http://www.apha.org
E-mail: comments@apha.org
Phone: (202) 777-2742
800 I Street, NW
Washington, DC 20001-3710
An association of public health professionals devoted to preventing disease and promoting health. It has taken positions on food-safety issues by demanding that the government do more to minimize the risks of foodborne disease and end the routine use of antibiotics in food animals.

American Veterinary Medical Association (AVMA)
URL: http://www.avma.org/pubhlth/biosecurity
E-mail: avmainfo@avma.org
Phone: (847) 925-8070
1931 North Meacham Road
Suite 100
Schaumburg, IL 60173
This association of veterinarians offers links to pages on biosecurity updates, mad cow disease, and disaster preparedness. With expertise in diagnosing and treating large animal diseases, it can play an important role in food safety.

Center for Non-Proliferation Studies (CNS)
URL http://cns.miis.edu
E-mail: cns@miis.edu
Phone: (831) 647-4154
460 Pierce Street
Monterey, CA 93940
A research and information center that is part of the Monterey Institute of International Studies. It has the goal of preventing the spread of weapons of mass destruction and maintains a database on incidents of terrorism and bioterrorism.

Food Allergy Initiative (FAI)
URL: http://www.foodallergy initiative.org
E-mail: info@foodallergy initiative.org
Phone: (212) 527-5835
237 Park Avenue
21st Floor
New York, NY 10017
Helps victims of food allergies by supporting research to find a cure and to improve clinical treatment. It also helps to raise public awareness about the seriousness of the problem.

Foundation on Economic Trends (FOET)
URL: http://www.foet.org
Phone: (202) 466-2823
1660 L Street, NW
Suite 216
Washington, DC 20036
Examines how science and technology affect the environment, economy, and society. Its president, Jeremy Rifkin, has been a leading

critic of biotechnology and GM foods.

Homeland Security Institute (HSI)
URL: http://www.homeland
security.org
E-mail: homelandsecurity@
anser.org
2900 South Quincy Street
Suite 800
Arlington, VA 22206
A research and development center funded by the Department of Homeland Security, it edits an electronic journal and weekly newsletter on homeland security issues, including those related to biosecurity and agriculture.

International Association for Food Protection (IAFP)
URL: http://www.food
protection.org
E-mail: info@foodprotection.org
Phone: (800) 369-6337
6200 Aurora Avenue
Suite 200W
Des Moines, IA 50322-2864
An association of food-safety professionals that publishes a journal on food protection, helps its members keep abreast of the latest developments in the field, and provides a forum for exchange of ideas on food safety.

International Food Information Council (IFIC)
URL: http://www.ific.org
E-mail: foodinfo@ific.org
Phone: (202) 296-6540

1100 Connecticut Avenue, NW
Suite 430
Washington, DC 20036
Aims to communicate science-based information on food safety and nutrition to experts and consumers. Focused primarily on research, it is supported by the food, beverage, and agricultural industries.

National Center for Food Protection and Defense (NCFPD)
URL: http://www.fpd.umn.edu
E-mail: ncfpd@umn.edu
Phone: (612) 624-2458
University of Minnesota–Twin Cities Campus
925 Delaware Street, SE
Suite 200
Minneapolis, MN 55455
A Department of Homeland Security Center of Excellence, it links academics, government agencies, and private businesses in a consortium devoted to research and education on the safety of the nation's food supply. Its mission focuses on preventing and responding to deliberate contamination of food.

National Center for Food Safety and Technology (NCFST)
URL: http://www.iit.edu/~ncfs
Phone: (708) 563-1576
6502 South Archer Road
Summit, IL 60501
A research consortium associated with the Illinois Institute of Technology. Composed of scientists from academia, the Food and Drug Administration, and food related industries,

239

it allows members to pool their scientific expertise and perspectives on food-safety issues.

National Research Council (NRC)
URL: http://www.nationalacademies.org/nrc
E-mail: web form
Phone: (202) 334-2000
500 Fifth Street, NW
Washington, DC 20001
A unit of the National Academies that provides science, technology, and health policy advice. In publishing studies on food-safety topics, it has made objective and scientifically based recommendations for improving meat-inspection methods.

Partnership for Food Safety Education (PFSE)
URL: http://www.fightbac.org
Phone: (202) 220-0651
655 15th Street, NW
7th Floor
Washington, DC 20005
A public-private partnership created to reduce the incidence of foodborne illness by educating Americans about safe food-handling practices. It is funded by industry trade associations with technical assistance and support from government agencies and consumer organizations.

Pew Charitable Trusts
URL: http://pewtrusts.org
E-mail: info@pewtrusts.org
Phone: (202) 347-9044
1331 H Street, NW
Suite 900
Washington, DC 20005
A charitable organization that aims to inform the public about important issues and to advance policy solution to social problems. It has funded the Initiative on Food and Biotechnology to offer accurate and unbiased information on agricultural biotechnology and GM foods.

RAND Corporation
URL: http://www.rand.org
E-mail: web form
Phone: (310) 393-0411
1776 Main Street
P.O. Box 2138
Santa Monica, CA 90407-2138
A nonprofit research organization focused on using data to make decisions in the private and public sector that has sponsored several studies of agricultural terrorism.

Society of Toxicology (SOT)
URL: http://www.toxicology.org
E-mail: sothq@toxicology.org
Phone: (703) 438-3115
1821 Michael Faraday Drive
Suite 300
Reston, VA 20190
The nation's largest professional organization of toxicologists, those who study the adverse effects of drugs, chemicals, and other agents such as pesticides and natural chemicals in food.

PART III

APPENDICES

APPENDIX A

FOOD ADDITIVES (1992)

Those opposed to the use of additives in food have harshly criticized the Food and Drug Administration (FDA), the agency responsible for approving preservatives, flavor enhancers, and other chemicals added to food during the manufacturing process. This document from the FDA describes the benefits of using additives and the procedures in place for approving them. Although critics will dispute many of its claims, the document offers a guide to how government regulators have for several decades evaluated the safety of food additives.

Food additives play a vital role in today's bountiful and nutritious food supply. They allow our growing urban population to enjoy a variety of safe, wholesome and tasty foods year-round. And, they make possible an array of convenience foods without the inconvenience of daily shopping.

Although salt, baking soda, vanilla and yeast are commonly used in foods today, many people tend to think of any additive added to foods as complex chemical compounds. All food additives are carefully regulated by federal authorities and various international organizations to ensure that foods are safe to eat and are accurately labeled. The purpose of this brochure is to provide helpful background information about food additives, why they are used in foods and how regulations govern their safe use in the food supply.

WHY ARE ADDITIVES USED IN FOODS?

Additives perform a variety of useful functions in foods that are often taken for granted. Since most people no longer live on farms, additives help keep food wholesome and appealing while en route to markets sometimes thousands of miles away from where it is grown or manufactured. Additives also improve the nutritional value of certain foods and can make them more appealing by improving their taste, texture, consistency or color.

243

Threats to Food Safety

Some additives could be eliminated if we were willing to grow our own food, harvest and grind it, spend many hours cooking and canning, or accept increased risks of food spoilage. But most people today have come to rely on the many technological, aesthetic and convenience benefits that additives provide in food.

Additives are used in foods for five main reasons:

- To maintain product consistency. Emulsifiers give products a consistent texture and prevent them from separating. Stabilizers and thickeners give smooth uniform texture. Anti-caking agents help substances such as salt to flow freely.
- To improve or maintain nutritional value. Vitamins and minerals are added to many common foods such as milk, flour, cereal and margarine to make up for those likely to be lacking in a person's diet or lost in processing. Such fortification and enrichment has helped reduce malnutrition among the U.S. population. All products containing added nutrients must be appropriately labeled.
- To maintain palatability and wholesomeness. Preservatives retard product spoilage caused by mold, air, bacteria, fungi or yeast. Bacterial contamination can cause foodborne illness, including life-threatening botulism. Antioxidants are preservatives that prevent fats and oils in baked goods and other foods from becoming rancid or developing an off-flavor. They also prevent cut fresh fruits such as apples from turning brown when exposed to air.
- To provide leavening or control acidity/alkalinity. Leavening agents that release acids when heated can react with baking soda to help cakes, biscuits and other baked goods to rise during baking. Other additives help modify the acidity and alkalinity of foods for proper flavor, taste and color.
- To enhance flavor or impart desired color. Many spices and natural and synthetic flavors enhance the taste of foods. Colors, likewise, enhance the appearance of certain foods to meet consumer expectations. Examples of substances that perform each of these functions are provided in the chart "Common Uses of Additives."

Many substances added to food may seem foreign when listed on the ingredient label, but are actually quite familiar. For example, ascorbic acid is another name for Vitamin C; alphatocopherol is another name for Vitamin E; and beta-carotene is a source of Vitamin A. Although there are no easy synonyms for all additives, it is helpful to remember that all food is made up of chemicals. Carbon, hydrogen and other chemical elements provide the basic building blocks for everything in life.

WHAT IS A FOOD ADDITIVE?

In its broadest sense, a food additive is any substance added to food. Legally, the term refers to "any substance the intended use which results or may reasonably be expected to result—directly or indirectly—in its becoming a component or otherwise affecting the characteristics of any food." This definition includes any substance used in the production, processing, treatment, packaging, transportation or storage of food.

If a substance is added to a food for a specific purpose in that food, it is referred to as a direct additive. For example, the low-calorie sweetener aspartame, which is used in beverages, puddings, yogurt, chewing gum and other foods, is considered a direct additive. Many direct additives are identified on the ingredient label of foods.

Indirect food additives are those that become part of the food in trace amounts due to its packaging, storage or other handling. For instance, minute amounts of packaging substances may find their way into foods during storage. Food packaging manufacturers must prove to the U.S. Food and Drug Administration (FDA) that all materials coming in contact with food are safe, before they are permitted for use in such a manner.

WHAT IS A COLOR ADDITIVE?

A color additive is any dye, pigment or substance that can impart color when added or applied to a food, drug, or cosmetic, or to the human body. Color additives may be used in foods, drugs, cosmetics, and certain medical devices such as contact lenses. Color additives are used in foods for many reasons, including to offset color loss due to storage or processing of foods and to correct natural variations in food color.

Colors permitted for use in foods are classified as certified or exempt from certification. Certified colors are man-made, with each batch being tested by the manufacturer and FDA to ensure that they meet strict specifications for purity. There are nine certified colors approved for use in the United States. One example is FD&C Yellow No. 6, which is used in cereals, bakery goods, snack foods and other foods.

Color additives that are exempt from certification include pigments derived from natural sources such as vegetables, minerals or animals.

For example, caramel color is produced commercially by heating sugar and other carbohydrates under strictly controlled conditions for use in sauces, gravies, soft drinks, baked goods and other foods. Most colors exempt from certification also must meet certain legal criteria for specifications and purity.

HOW ARE ADDITIVES REGULATED?

Additives are not always byproducts of 20th-century technology or modern know-how. Our ancestors used salt to preserve meats and fish; added herbs and spices to improve the flavor of foods; preserved fruit with sugar; and pickled cucumbers in a vinegar solution.

Over the years, however, improvements have been made in increasing the efficiency and ensuring the safety of all additives. Today food and color additives are more strictly regulated than at any other time in history. The basis of modern food law is the Federal Food, Drug, and Cosmetic (FD&C) Act of 1938, which gives the Food and Drug Administration (FDA) authority over food and food ingredients and defines requirements for truthful labeling of ingredients.

The Food Additives Amendment to the FD&C Act, passed in 1958, requires FDA approval for the use of an additive prior to its inclusion in food. It also requires the manufacturer to prove an additive's safety for the ways it will be used.

The Food Additives Amendment exempted two groups of substances from the food additive regulation process. All substances that FDA or the U.S. Department of Agriculture (USDA) had determined were safe for use in specific food prior to the 1958 amendment were designated as prior-sanctioned substances. Examples of prior-sanctioned substances are sodium nitrite and potassium nitrite used to preserve luncheon meats.

A second category of substances excluded from the food additive regulation process are generally recognized as safe or GRAS substances. GRAS substances are those whose use is generally recognized by experts as safe, based on their extensive history of use in food before 1958 or based on published scientific evidence. Salt, sugar, spices, vitamins and monosodium glutamate are classified as GRAS substances, along with several hundred other substances. Manufacturers may also request FDA to review the use of a substance to determine if it is GRAS.

Since 1958, FDA and USDA have continued to monitor all prior sanctioned and GRAS substances in light of new scientific information. If new evidence suggests that a GRAS or prior sanctioned substance may be unsafe, federal authorities can prohibit its use or require further studies to determine its safety.

Appendix A

In 1960, Congress passed similar legislation governing color additives. The Color Additives Amendments to the FD&C Act require dyes used in foods, drugs, cosmetics and certain medical devices to be approved by FDA prior to their marketing.

In contrast to food additives, colors in use before the legislation were allowed continued use only if they underwent further testing to confirm their safety. Of the original 200 provisionally listed color additives, 90 have been listed as safe and the remainder have either been removed from use by FDA or withdrawn by industry.

Both the Food Additives and Color Additives Amendments include a provision which prohibits the approval of an additive if it is found to cause cancer in humans or animals. This clause is often referred to as the Delaney Clause, named for its Congressional sponsor, Rep. James Delaney (D-N.Y.).

Regulations known as Good Manufacturing Practices (GMP) limit the amount of food and color additives used in foods. Manufacturers use only the amount of an additive necessary to achieve the desired effect.

HOW ARE ADDITIVES APPROVED FOR USE IN FOODS?

To market a new food or color additive, a manufacturer must first petition FDA for its approval. Approximately 100 new food and color additives petitions are submitted to FDA annually. Most of these petitions are for indirect additives such as packaging materials.

A food or color additive petition must provide convincing evidence that the proposed additive performs as it is intended. Animal studies using large doses of the additive for long periods are often necessary to show that the substance would not cause harmful effects at expected levels of human consumption. Studies of the additive in humans also may be submitted to FDA.

In deciding whether an additive should be approved, the agency considers the composition and properties of the substance, the amount likely to be consumed, its probable long-term effects and various safety factors. Absolute safety of any substance can never be proven. Therefore, FDA must determine if the additive is safe under the proposed conditions of use, based on the best scientific knowledge available.

If an additive is approved, FDA issues regulations that may include the types of foods in which it can be used, the maximum amounts to be used, and how it should be identified on food labels. Additives proposed for use in meat and poultry products also must receive specific authorization by USDA. Federal officials then carefully monitor the extent of Americans'

247

consumption of the new additive and results of any new research on its safety to assure its use continues to be within safe limits.

In addition, FDA operates an Adverse Reaction Monitoring System (ARMS) to help serve as an ongoing safety check of all additives. The system monitors and investigates all complaints by individuals or their physicians that are believed to be related to specific foods; food and color additives; or vitamin and mineral supplements. The ARMS computerized database helps officials decide whether reported adverse reactions represent a real public health hazard associated with food, so that appropriate action can be taken.

SUMMARY

Additives have been used for many years to preserve, flavor, blend, thicken and color foods, and have played an important role in reducing serious nutritional deficiencies among Americans. Additives help assure the availability of wholesome, appetizing and affordable foods that meet consumer demands from season to season.

Today, food and color additives are more strictly regulated than at any time in history. Federal regulations require evidence that each substance is safe at its intended levels of use before it may be added to foods. All additives are subject to ongoing safety review as scientific understanding and methods of testing continue to improve.

Source: Selections from U.S. Food and Drug Administration, January 1992 (URL: http://www.cfsan.fda.gov/~lrd/foodaddi.html)

APPENDIX B

FOOD ALLERGIES: RARE BUT RISKY (1994)

Only a small part of the population has food allergies, but the threat to life and well-being of those with the allergies is serious. This summary from the Food and Drug Administration highlights what risks the various types of food allergies present and how victims can help protect themselves.

Do you start itching whenever you eat peanuts? Does seafood cause your stomach to churn? Symptoms like these cause millions of Americans to suspect they have a food allergy.

But true food allergies affect a relatively small percentage of people: Experts estimate that only 2 percent of adults, and from 2 to 8 percent of children, are truly allergic to certain foods. Food allergy is different from food intolerance, and the term is sometimes used in a vague, all-encompassing way, muddying the waters for people who want to understand what a real food allergy is.

"Many people who have a complaint, an illness, or some discomfort attribute it to something they have eaten. Because in this country we eat almost all the time, people tend to draw false associations between food and illness," says Dean Metcalfe, M.D., head of the Mast Cell and Physiology Section at the National Institute of Allergy and Infectious Diseases.

ALLERGY AND INTOLERANCE— DIFFERENT PROBLEMS

The difference between an allergy and an intolerance is how the body handles the offending food. In a true food allergy, the body's immune system recognizes a reaction-provoking substance, or allergen, in the food—usually a protein—as foreign and produces antibodies to halt the "invasion." As the battle rages, symptoms appear throughout the body. The most common sites are the mouth (swelling of the lips), digestive tract (stomach cramps, vomiting, diarrhea), skin (hives, rashes or eczema), and the airways (wheezing or breathing problems). People with allergies must avoid the offending foods altogether.

Cow's milk, eggs, wheat, and soy are the most common sources of food allergies in children. Allergists believe that infant allergies are the result of immunologic immaturity and, to some extent, intestinal immaturity. Children sometimes outgrow the allergies they had as infants, but an early peanut allergy may be lifelong. Adults are usually most affected by tree nuts, fish, shellfish, and peanuts.

Food intolerance is a much more common problem than allergy. Here, the problem is not with the body's immune system, but, rather, with its metabolism. The body cannot adequately digest a portion of the offending food, usually because of some chemical deficiency. For example, persons who have difficulty digesting milk (lactose intolerance) often are deficient in the intestinal enzyme lactase, which is needed to digest milk sugar (lactose). The deficiency can cause cramps and diarrhea if milk is consumed. Estimates are that about 80 percent of African-Americans have lactose intolerance, as do many people of Mediterranean or Hispanic origin. It is quite different from the true allergic reaction some have to the proteins in milk. Unlike allergies, intolerances generally intensify with age.

DANGEROUS DISHES

For people with true food allergies, the simple pleasure of eating can turn into an uncomfortable—and sometimes even dangerous—situation. For some, food allergies cause only hives or an upset stomach; for others, one bite of the wrong food can lead to serious illness or even death.

Food intolerance may produce symptoms similar to food allergies, such as abdominal cramping. But while people with true food allergies must avoid offending foods altogether, people with food intolerance can often eat some of the offending food without suffering symptoms. The amount that may be eaten before symptoms appear is usually very small and varies with each individual.

WHEN FOOD ADDITIVES ARE A PROBLEM

Over the years, people have reported to FDA adverse reactions to certain food additives, including aspartame (a sweetener), monosodium glutamate (a flavor enhancer), sulfur-based preservatives, and tartrazine, also known as FD&C Yellow No. 5 (a food color). The federal Food, Drug, and Cosmetic Act requires that FDA ensure the safety of all substances added to foods, but individual health conditions sometimes cause problems with certain additives.

- **Aspartame**

  After reviewing scientific studies, FDA determined in 1981 that aspartame was safe for use in foods. In 1987, the General Accounting Office investigated the process surrounding FDA's approval of aspartame and confirmed the agency had acted properly. However, FDA has continued to review complaints alleging adverse reactions to products containing aspartame. To date, FDA has not determined any consistent pattern of symptoms that can be attributed to the use of aspartame, nor is the agency aware of any recent studies that clearly show safety problems.

  Carefully controlled clinical studies show that aspartame is not an allergen. However, certain people with the genetic disease phenylketonuria (PKU), and pregnant women with hyperphenylalanine (high levels of phenylalanine in blood) have a problem with aspartame because they do not effectively metabolize the amino acid phenylalanine, one of aspartame's components. High levels of this amino acid in body fluids can cause brain damage. Therefore, FDA has ruled that all products containing aspartame must include a warning to phenylketonurics that the sweetener contains phenylalanine.

- **Monosodium glutamate**

  Monosodium glutamate (MSG) has been used for many years in home and restaurant foods, and in processed foods. People sensitive to MSG may have mild and transitory reactions when they eat foods that contain large amounts of MSG (such as would be found in heavily flavor-enhanced foods). Because MSG is commonly used in Chinese cuisine, these reactions were initially referred to as "Chinese restaurant syndrome."

  FDA believes that MSG is a safe food ingredient for the general population. It is regarded by the agency as among food ingredients that are "generally recognized as safe." FDA has studied adverse reaction reports and other data concerning MSG's safety. The agency also has an ongoing contract with the Federation of American Societies for Experimental Biology to re-examine the scientific data on possible adverse reactions to glutamate in general. MSG must be declared on the label of any food to which it is added.

- **Sulfites**

  Of all the food additives for which FDA has received adverse reaction reports, the ones that most closely resemble true allergens are sulfur-based preservatives. Sulfites are used primarily as antioxidants to prevent or reduce discoloration of light-colored fruits and vegetables, such as dried apples and potatoes, and to inhibit the growth of microorganisms in fermented foods such as wine.

Though most people don't have a problem with sulfites, they are a hazard of unpredictable severity to people, particularly asthmatics, who are sensitive to these substances. FDA uses the term "allergic-type responses" to describe the range of symptoms suffered by these individuals after eating sulfite-treated foods. Responses range from mild to life-threatening.

FDA's sulfite specialists say scientists, at this time, are not sure how the body reacts to sulfites. To help sulfite-sensitive people avoid problems, FDA requires the presence of sulfites in processed foods to be declared on the label, and prohibits the use of sulfites on fresh produce intended to be sold or served raw to consumers (see "A Fresh Look at Food Preservative" in the October 1993 *FDA Consumer*).

- **FD&C Yellow No. 5**

  Color additives must go through the same safety approval process as food additives. But one color, FD&C Yellow No. 5 (listed as tartrazine on medicine labels), may prompt itching or hives in a small number of people.

  Since 1980 (for drugs taken orally) and 1981 (for foods), FDA has required all products containing Yellow No. 5 to list it on the labels so sensitive consumers could avoid it. (As of May 8, 1993, food labels must list all certified colors as part of the requirements of the Nutrition Labeling and Education Act of 1990. See "From Shampoo to Cereal, Seeing to the Safety of Color Additives" in the December 1993 *FDA Consumer*.)

TRUE ALLERGIES

Heredity may cause a predisposition to have allergies of any type, and repeated exposure to allergens starts sensitizing those who are susceptible. Some experts believe that, rarely, a specific allergy can be passed on from parent to child. Several studies have indicated that exclusive breast-feeding, especially with maternal avoidance of major food allergens, may deter some food allergies in infants and young children. (Smoking during pregnancy can also result in the increased possibility that the baby will have allergies.) Most patients who have true food allergies have other types of allergies, such as dust or pollen, and children with both food allergies and asthma are at increased risk for more severe reactions.

LIFE-THREATENING REACTIONS

The greatest danger in food allergy comes from anaphylaxis, a violent allergic reaction involving a number of parts of the body simultaneously. Like less serious allergic reactions, anaphylaxis usually occurs after a person is exposed to an allergen to which he or she was sensitized by previous exposure (that is, it does not usually occur the first time a person eats a particular food). Although any food can trigger anaphylaxis (also known as anaphylactic shock), peanuts, tree nuts, shellfish, milk, eggs, and fish are the most common culprits. As little as one-fifth to one-five-thousandth of a teaspoon of the offending food has caused death.

Anaphylaxis can produce severe symptoms in as little as 5 to 15 minutes, although life-threatening reactions may progress over hours. Signs of such a reaction include: difficulty breathing, feeling of impending doom, swelling of the mouth and throat, a drop in blood pressure, and loss of consciousness. The sooner that anaphylaxis is treated, the greater the person's chance of surviving. The person should be taken to a hospital emergency room, even if symptoms seem to subside on their own.

There is no specific test to predict the likelihood of anaphylaxis, although allergy testing may help determine what a person may be allergic to and provide some guidance as to the severity of the allergy. Experts advise people who are susceptible to anaphylaxis to carry medication, such as injectable epinephrine, with them at all times, and to check the medicine's expiration date regularly. Doctors can instruct patients with allergies on how to self-administer epinephrine. Such prompt treatment can be crucial to survival.

Injectable epinephrine is a synthetic version of a naturally occurring hormone also known as adrenaline. For treatment of an anaphylactic reaction, it is injected directly into a thigh muscle or vein. It works directly on the cardiovascular and respiratory systems, causing rapid constriction of blood vessels, reversing throat swelling, relaxing lung muscles to improve breathing, and stimulating the heartbeat.

Epinephrine designed for emergency home use comes in two forms: a traditional needle and syringe kit known as Ana-Kit, or an automatic injector system known as Epi-Pen. Epi-Pen's automatic injector design, originally developed for use by military personnel to deliver antidotes for nerve gas, is described by some as "a fat pen." The patient removes the safety cap and pushes the automatic injector tip against the outer thigh until the unit activates. The patient holds the "pen" in place for several seconds, then throws it away.

While Epi-Pen delivers one premeasured dosage, the Ana-Kit provides two doses. Which system a patient uses is a decision to be made by the doctor and patient, taking into account the doctor's assessment of the patient's individual needs. . .

FOOD ALLERGIES AND BIOTECHNOLOGY

People with food allergies have expressed the concern that new varieties of food, developed through the new techniques of biotechnology (such as gene splicing), may introduce allergens not found in the food before it was altered.

FDA addressed this concern in its 1992 biotechnology policy statement and said it will regulate whole foods developed through biotechnology by applying the same rigorous safety standards as for all other foods. The agency is taking steps to ensure that foods developed through biotechnology do not pose any new risks for consumers.

Under the new policy guidelines, a protein copied by genetic engineering from a food commonly known to cause an allergic reaction is presumed to be allergenic unless clearly proven otherwise. Any food product of biotechnology that contains such proteins must list the allergen on the label.

Labeling would not be required if the manufacturer could demonstrate that the allergen was not transferred. For example, if a food company were to breed potatoes containing a genetically engineered soy protein (to which some people might be allergic), the labeling on the potatoes would have to disclose the presence of the soy protein. But labeling would not be required if scientific data clearly showed that the protein had been changed and no longer contained the soy allergen.

To ensure that FDA has state-of-the-art information for its food biotechnology policy, the agency will sponsor a scientific conference in the spring of 1994 to discuss what makes a substance a food allergen. . .

Source: Selections from U.S. Food and Drug Administration, May 1994 (URL: http://www.cfsan.fda.gov/~dms/wh-alrg1.html)

APPENDIX C

ASSESSING HEALTH RISKS FROM PESTICIDES (1999)

Although beneficial for producing healthy crops, the use of pesticides in farming has the less desirable consequence of leaving chemical residue on food consumed by humans. The Environmental Protection Agency (EPA), which has responsibility for regulating pesticide use, has been in the center of controversy over the harm of this chemical residue for human health. This fact sheet put out by the agency attempts to explain government procedures for assessing pesticide risks.

The Federal Government, in cooperation with the States, carefully regulates pesticides to ensure that they do not pose unreasonable risks to human health or the environment. As part of that effort, the Environmental Protection Agency (EPA) requires extensive test data from pesticide producers that demonstrate pesticide products can be used without posing harm to human health and the environment. EPA scientists and analysts carefully review these data to determine whether to register (license) a pesticide product or a use and whether specific restrictions are necessary. This fact sheet is a brief overview of EPA's process for assessing potential risks to human health when evaluating pesticide products.

BACKGROUND

There are more than 865 active ingredients registered as pesticides, which are formulated into thousands of pesticide products that are available in the marketplace. About 350 pesticides are used on the foods we eat, and to protect our homes and pets.

EPA plays a critical role in evaluating these chemicals prior to registration, and in reevaluating older pesticides already on the market, to ensure that they can be used with a reasonable certainty of no harm. The process EPA uses for evaluating the health impacts of a pesticide is called risk assessment.

EPA uses the National Research Council's four-step process for human health risk assessment:

Step One: Hazard Identification
Step Two: Dose-Response Assessment
Step Three: Exposure Assessment
Step Four: Risk Characterization

STEP ONE: HAZARD IDENTIFICATION (TOXICOLOGY)

The first step in the risk assessment process is to identify potential health effects that may occur from different types of pesticide exposure. EPA considers the full spectrum of a pesticide's potential health effects.

Generally, for human health risk assessments, many toxicity studies are conducted on animals by pesticide companies in independent laboratories and evaluated for acceptability by EPA scientists. EPA evaluates pesticides for a wide range of adverse effects, from eye and skin irritation to cancer and birth defects in laboratory animals. EPA may also consult the public literature or other sources of supporting information on any aspect of the chemical.

STEP TWO: DOSE-RESPONSE ASSESSMENT

Paracelsus, the Swiss physician and alchemist, the "father" of modern toxicology (1493–1541) said,

The dose makes the poison.

In other words, **the amount of a substance a person is exposed to** is as important as **how toxic the chemical might be.** For example, small doses of aspirin can be beneficial to people, but at very high doses, this common medicine can be deadly. In some individuals, even at very low doses, aspirin may be deadly.

Dose-response assessment involves considering the dose levels at which adverse effects were observed in test animals, and using these dose levels to calculate an equal dose in humans.

Appendix C

STEP THREE: EXPOSURE ASSESSMENT

People can be exposed to pesticides in three ways:

1. Inhaling pesticides (inhalation exposure),
2. Absorbing pesticides through the skin (dermal exposure), and
3. Getting pesticides in their mouth or digestive tract (oral exposure).

Depending on the situation, pesticides could enter the body by any one or all of these routes. Typical sources of pesticide exposure include:

- **Food:** Most of the foods we eat have been grown with the use of pesticides. Therefore, pesticide residues may be present inside or on the surfaces of these foods.
- **Home and Personal Use Pesticides:** You might use pesticides in and around your home to control insects, weeds, mold, mildew, bacteria, lawn and garden pests and to protect your pets from pests such as fleas. Pesticides may also be used as insect repellants which are directly applied to the skin or clothing.
- **Pesticides in Drinking Water:** Some pesticides that are applied to farmland or other land structures can make their way in small amounts to the ground water or surface water systems that feed drinking water supplies.
- **Worker Exposure to Pesticides:** Pesticide applicators, vegetable and fruit pickers and others who work around pesticides can be exposed due to the nature of their jobs. To address the unique risks workers face from occupational exposure, EPA evaluates occupational exposure through a separate program. All pesticides registered by EPA have been shown to be safe when used properly.

STEP FOUR: RISK CHARACTERIZATION

Risk characterization is the final step in assessing human health risks from pesticides. It is the process of combining the hazard, dose-response and exposure assessments to describe the overall risk from a pesticide. It explains the assumptions used in assessing exposure as well as the uncertainties that are built into the dose-response assessment. The strength of the overall database is considered, and broad conclusions are made. EPA's role is to evaluate both toxicity and exposure and to determine the risk associated with use of the pesticide.

Simply put, RISK = TOXICITY × EXPOSURE.

This means that the risk to human health from pesticide exposure depends on both the toxicity of the pesticide and the likelihood of people coming into contact with it. At least *some* exposure and *some* toxicity are required to result in a risk. For example, if the pesticide is very poisonous, but no people are exposed, there is no risk. Likewise, if there is ample exposure but the chemical is non-toxic, there is no risk. However, usually when pesticides are used, there is some toxicity and exposure, which results in a potential risk.

EPA recognizes that effects vary between animals of different species and from person to person. To account for this variability, *uncertainty factors* are built into the risk assessment. These uncertainty factors create an additional margin of safety for protecting people who may be exposed to the pesticides. FQPA requires EPA to use an extra 10-fold safety factor, if necessary, to protect infants and children from effects of the pesticide.

TYPES OF TOXICITY TESTS EPA REQUIRES FOR HUMAN HEALTH RISK ASSESSMENTS

EPA evaluates studies conducted over different periods of time and that measure specific types of effects. These tests are evaluated to screen for potential health effects in infants, children and adults.

Acute Testing: Short-term exposure; a single exposure (dose).

- Oral, dermal (skin), and inhalation exposure
- Eye irritation
- Skin irritation
- Skin sensitization
- Neurotoxicity

Sub-chronic Testing: Intermediate exposure; repeated exposure over a longer period of time (i.e., 30–90 days).

- Oral, dermal (skin), and inhalation
- Neurotoxicity (nerve system damage)

Chronic Toxicity Testing: Long-term exposure; repeated exposure lasting for most of the test animal's life span. Intended to determine the effects of a pesticide after prolonged and repeated exposures.

- Chronic effects (non-cancer)
- Carcinogenicity (cancer)

Developmental and Reproductive Testing: Identify effects in the fetus of an exposed pregnant female (birth defects) and how pesticide exposure affects the ability of a test animal to successfully reproduce.

Mutagenicity Testing: Assess a pesticide's potential to affect the cell's genetic components.

Hormone Disruption: Measure effects for their potential to disrupt the endocrine system. The endocrine system consists of a set of glands and the hormones they produce that help guide the development, growth, reproduction, and behavior of animals including humans.

RISK MANAGEMENT

Once EPA completes the risk assessment process for a pesticide, we use this information to determine if (when used according to label directions), there is a reasonable certainty that the pesticide will not harm a person's health.

Using the conclusions of a risk assessment, EPA can then make a more informed decision regarding whether to approve a pesticide chemical or use, as proposed, or whether additional protective measures are necessary to limit occupational or non-occupational exposure to a pesticide. For example, EPA may prohibit a pesticide from being used on certain crops because consuming too much food treated with the pesticide may result in an unacceptable risk to consumers. Another example of protective measures is requiring workers to wear personal protective equipment (PPE) such as a respirator or chemical resistant gloves, or not allowing workers to enter treated crop fields until a specific period of time has passed.

If, after considering all appropriate risk reduction measures, the pesticide still does not meet EPA's safety standard, the Agency will not allow the proposed chemical or use. Regardless of the specific measures enforced, EPA's primary goal is to ensure that legal uses of the pesticide are protective of human health, especially the health of children, and the environment.

HUMAN HEALTH RISK ASSESSMENT AND THE LAW

Federal law requires detailed evaluation of pesticides to protect human health and the environment. In 1996, Congress made significant changes to strengthen pesticide laws through the Food Quality Protection Act (FQPA).

Many of these changes are key elements of the current risk assessment process. FQPA required that EPA consider:

- **A New Safety Standard:** FQPA strengthened the safety standard that pesticides must meet before being approved for use. EPA must ensure with a reasonable certainty that no harm will result from the legal uses of the pesticide.
- **Exposure from All Sources:** In evaluating a pesticide, EPA must estimate the combined risk from that pesticide from all non-occupational sources, such as: Food Sources, Drinking Water Sources, Residential Sources.
- **Cumulative Risk:** EPA is required to evaluate pesticides in light of similar toxic effects that different pesticides may share, or "a common mechanism of toxicity." At this time, EPA is developing a methodology for this type of assessment.
- **Special Sensitivity of Children to Pesticides:** EPA must ascertain whether there is an increased susceptibility from exposure to the pesticide to infants and children. EPA must build an additional 10-fold safety factor into risk assessments to ensure the protection of infants and children, unless it is determined that a lesser margin of safety will be safe for infants and children.

Source: U.S. Environmental Protection Agency, January 1999 (URL: http://www.epa.gov/pesticides/factsheets/riskassess.htm)

APPENDIX D

FOOD IRRADIATION: A SAFE MEASURE (2000)

The Food and Drug Administration views food irradiation as a safe way to kill harmful bacteria and in this document makes the case for greater use of the practice. Opponents of food irradiation would argue instead that food irradiation does more harm than good. Still, this largely positive summary represents the viewpoint of a key government agency responsible for food safety.

Food safety is a subject of growing importance to consumers. One reason is the emergence of new types of harmful bacteria or evolving forms of older ones that can cause serious illness. A relatively new strain of *E. coli*, for example, has caused severe, and in some cases life-threatening, outbreaks of food-borne illness through contaminated products such as ground beef and unpasteurized fruit juices.

Scientists, regulators and lawmakers, working to determine how best to combat food-borne illness, are encouraging the use of technologies that can enhance the safety of the nation's food supply.

Many health experts agree that using a process called irradiation can be an effective way to help reduce food-borne hazards and ensure that harmful organisms are not in the foods we buy. During irradiation, foods are exposed briefly to a radiant energy source such as gamma rays or electron beams within a shielded facility. Irradiation is not a substitute for proper food manufacturing and handling procedures. But the process, especially when used to treat meat and poultry products, can kill harmful bacteria, greatly reducing potential hazards.

The Food and Drug Administration has approved irradiation of meat and poultry and allows its use for a variety of other foods, including fresh fruits and vegetables, and spices. The agency determined that the process is safe and effective in decreasing or eliminating harmful bacteria. Irradiation

261

also reduces spoilage bacteria, insects and parasites, and in certain fruits and vegetables it inhibits sprouting and delays ripening. For example, irradiated strawberries stay unspoiled up to three weeks, versus three to five days for untreated berries.

Food irradiation is allowed in nearly 40 countries and is endorsed by the World Health Organization, the American Medical Association and many other organizations.

Irradiation does not make foods radioactive, just as an airport luggage scanner does not make luggage radioactive. Nor does it cause harmful chemical changes. The process may cause a small loss of nutrients but no more so than with other processing methods such as cooking, canning, or heat pasteurization. Federal rules require irradiated foods to be labeled as such to distinguish them from non-irradiated foods.

Studies show that consumers are becoming more interested in irradiated foods. For example, the University of Georgia created a mock supermarket setting that explained irradiation and found that 84 percent of participating consumers said irradiation is "somewhat necessary" or "very necessary." And consumer research conducted by a variety of groups, including the American Meat Institute, the International Food Information Council, the Food Marketing Institute, the Grocery Manufacturers of America, and the National Food Processors Association has found that a large majority of consumers polled would buy irradiated foods.

Some special interest groups oppose irradiation or say that more attention should be placed on food safety in the early stages of food processing such as in meat plants. Many food processors and retailers reply that irradiation can be an important tool for curbing illness and death from foodborne illness. But it is *not* a substitute for comprehensive food safety programs throughout the food distribution system. Nor is irradiation a substitute for good food-handling practices in the home.

Source: Selections from U.S. Food and Drug Administration, January 2000 (URL: http://www.fda.gov/opacom/catalog/irradbro.html)

APPENDIX E

STATEMENT BY JOSEPH A. LEVITT, DIRECTOR, CENTER FOR FOOD SAFETY AND APPLIED NUTRITION (2000)

This statement made before Congress summarizes the views of the Food and Drug Administration (FDA) on genetically modified (GM) food. The agency takes a more positive view than critics of GM food do, and this document explains how new foods created through biotechnology are regulated and why the FDA believes its regulations are sufficient to protect the safety of food. Although not the final word on the issue, the FDA statement helps explain current government policies.

INTRODUCTION

Mr. Chairman and members of the Committee, thank you for giving the Food and Drug Administration (FDA or the Agency) the opportunity to testify today on its regulatory program for foods derived from plants using the tools of modern biotechnology—also known as genetically engineered, or bioengineered, foods. I am Joseph A. Levitt, Director of FDA's Center for Food Safety and Applied Nutrition (CFSAN). Within FDA, CFSAN oversees bioengineered plant products or ingredients intended for human consumption. Our Center for Veterinary Medicine oversees bioengineered plant products used as or in animal feed, as well as bioengineered products used to improve the health or productivity of animals (including fish).

We believe it is very important for the public to understand how FDA is regulating the new bioengineered foods being introduced into the marketplace and to have confidence in that process. To that end, I appreciate this opportunity to describe our policies and procedures to the Committee and to the public.

First, let me state that FDA is confident that the bioengineered plant foods on the U.S. market today are as safe as their conventionally bred counterparts. This conclusion was echoed by a report by the National Resource Council of the National Academy of Sciences which stated, "The committee is not aware of any evidence that foods on the market are unsafe to eat as a result of genetic modification." Since FDA's 1994 evaluation of the Flavr Savr tomato, the first genetically-engineered plant food to reach the U.S. market, FDA has reviewed the data on more than 45 other products, ranging from herbicide resistant soybeans to a canola plant with modified oil content. To date, there is no evidence that these plants are significantly different in terms of food safety from crops produced through traditional breeding techniques.

The topic of bioengineering has generated much controversy, particularly about whether these foods should be labeled or not. As I discuss in more detail later in my testimony, FDA held three public meetings on bioengineered foods late last year, the second one of which I chaired. We wanted to hear the views from all, and importantly, we wanted to discuss and obtain feedback on ways in which information on bioengineered foods could be most appropriately and helpfully conveyed.

Partly in response to information gained from the public meetings and comments received by the Agency, FDA announced on May 3, 2000, that it will be taking steps to modify our current voluntary process for bioengineered foods to establish mandatory premarket notification and make the process more transparent. Further, we will be developing guidance for food manufacturers who wish voluntarily to label their products regarding whether or not they contain bioengineered ingredients. To ensure that the Agency has the best scientific advice, we also are adding experts in this field to our foods and veterinary medicine advisory committees. FDA is taking these steps to help provide consumers with continued confidence in the safety of the U.S. food supply and to ensure that the Agency's oversight procedures will meet the challenges of the future. The proposed notification rule and draft guidance are currently under development. . .

LEGAL AND REGULATORY ISSUES

FDA regulates bioengineered plant food in conjunction with the United States Department of Agriculture (USDA) and the Environmental Protection Agency (EPA). FDA has authority under the Federal Food, Drug, and Cosmetic (FD&C) Act to ensure the safety of all domestic and imported foods for man or other animals in the United States market, except meat, poultry and egg products which are regulated by USDA. (Note that the safety of animal drug residues in meat and poultry is regulated by FDA's Center for Veterinary Medicine.) Pesticides are regulated primarily by EPA, which reviews safety and sets tolerances (or establishes exemptions from tolerance) for pesticides. FDA enforces the pesticide tolerances set by EPA. USDA's Animal & Plant Health Inspection Service (APHIS) oversees the agricultural and environmental safety of planting and field testing of bioengineered plants.

Bioengineered foods and food ingredients must adhere to the same standards of safety under the FD&C Act that apply to their conventionally-bred counterparts. This means that these products must be as safe as the traditional foods in the market. FDA has broad authority to initiate regulatory action if a product fails to meet the standards of the FD&C Act.

FDA relies primarily on two sections of the FD&C Act to ensure the safety of foods and food ingredients:

(1) The adulteration provisions of section 402(a)(1). Under this postmarket authority, FDA has the power to remove a food from the market (or sanction those marketing the food) if the food poses a risk to public health. It is important to note that the FD&C Act places a legal duty on developers to ensure that the foods they market to consumers are safe and comply with all legal requirements.

(2) The food additive provisions (section 409). Under this section, a substance that is intentionally added to food is a food additive, unless the substance is generally recognized as safe (GRAS) or is otherwise exempt (e.g., a pesticide, the safety of which is overseen by EPA).

The FD&C Act requires premarket approval of any food additive—regardless of the technique used to add it to food. Thus, substances introduced into food are either (1) new food additives that require premarket approval by FDA or (2) GRAS, and are exempt from the requirement for premarket review (for example, if there is a long history of safe use in food). Generally, foods such as fruits, vegetables, and grains, are not subject to premarket approval because they have been safely consumed over many years. Other than the food additive system, there are no premarket approval requirements for foods generally.

In 1992, knowing that bioengineered products were on the horizon, FDA published a policy explaining how existing legal requirements would apply to products developed using the tools of biotechnology (57 FR 22984; May 29,1992; "Statement of Policy: Foods Derived from New Plant Varieties"). The 1992 policy was designed to answer developers' questions about these products prior to marketing to assist them in meeting their legal duty to provide safe and wholesome foods to consumers. The basic principle of the 1992 policy is that the traits and characteristics of the foods should be the focus of safety assessment for all new varieties of food crops, no matter which techniques are used to develop them.

Under FDA policy, a substance that would be a food additive if it were added during traditional food manufacturing is also treated as a food additive if it is introduced into food through bioengineering of a food crop. Our authority under section 409 permits us to require premarket approval of any food additive and thus, to require premarket review of any substance intentionally introduced via bioengineering that is not generally recognized as safe.

Generally, substances intentionally introduced into food that would be reviewed as food additives include those that have unusual chemical functions, have unknown toxicity, or would be new major dietary components of the food. For example, a novel sweetener bioengineered into food would likely require premarket approval. In our experience with bioengineered food to date, however, we have reviewed only one substance under the food additive provisions, an enzyme produced by an antibiotic resistance gene, and we approved that one. In general, substances intentionally added to food via biotechnology to date have been well-characterized proteins and fats, and are functionally very similar to other proteins and fats that are commonly and safely consumed in the diet and thus are presumptively GRAS.

In 1994, for the first bioengineered product planned for introduction into the market, FDA moved deliberately, following the 1992 policy. We conducted a comprehensive scientific review of Calgene's data on the Flavr Savr™ tomato and the use of the kanamycin resistance marker gene. FDA also held a public meeting of our Food Advisory Committee (the Committee) to examine applicability of the 1992 policy to products such as the Flavr Savr™ tomato. The Committee members agreed with FDA that the scientific approach presented in the 1992 policy was sound and that questions regarding the Flavr Savr™ had been addressed. The Committee members also suggested that we remove unnecessary reviews to provide an expedited decision process on the marketing of bioengineered foods that do not raise substantive scientific issues.

In response, that same year, FDA established a consultative process to help companies comply with the FD&C Act's requirements for any new food, including a bioengineered food, that they intend to market. Since that time, companies have used the consultative process more than 45 times as they sought to introduce genetically altered plants representing ten different crops into the U.S. market. We are not aware of any bioengineered food product on the market under FDA's jurisdiction that has not been evaluated by FDA through the current consultation process.

Typically, the consultation begins early in the product development stage, before it is ready for market. Company scientists and other officials will meet with FDA scientists to describe the product they are developing. In response, the Agency advises the company on what tests would be appropriate for the company to assess the safety of the new food.

After the studies are completed, the data and information on the safety and nutritional assessment are provided voluntarily to FDA for review. The Agency evaluates the information for all of the known hazards and also for potential unintended effects on plant composition and nutritional properties, since plants may undergo changes other than those intended by the breeders. Specifically, FDA scientists are looking to assure that the newly expressed compounds are safe for food consumption, there are no allergens new to the food, no increased levels of natural toxicants, and no reduction of important nutrients. They are also looking to see whether the food has been changed in any substantive way such that the food would need to be specially labeled to reveal the nature of the change to consumers.

Some examples of the information reviewed by FDA includes: the name of the food and the crop from which it is derived; the uses of the food, including both human food and animal feed uses; the sources, identities, and functions of introduced genetic material and its stability in the plant; the purpose or intended technical effect of the modification and its expected effect on the composition or characteristic properties of the food or feed; the identity and function of any new products encoded by the introduced genetic material, including an estimate of its concentration; comparison of the composition or characteristics of the bioengineered food to that of food derived from the parental variety or other commonly consumed varieties with special emphasis on important nutrients, anti-nutrients, and toxicants that occur naturally in the food; information on whether the genetic modification altered the potential for the bioengineered food to induce an allergic response; and, other information relevant to the safety and nutritional assessment of the bioengineered food.

It should be noted that if a plant developer used a gene from a plant whose food is commonly allergenic, FDA would presume that the modified food may be allergenic unless the developer could demonstrate that the food would not cause allergic reactions in people allergic to food from the source plant.

If FDA scientists have more questions about the safety data, the company either provides more detailed answers or conducts additional studies. Our experience has been that no bioengineered product has gone on the market until FDA's questions about the product have been answered.

LABELING

Labeling, either mandatory or voluntary, of bioengineered foods is a controversial issue. Section 403 of the FD&C Act sets labeling requirements for all foods. All foods, whether derived using bioengineering or not, are subject to these labeling requirements.

Under section 403(a)(1) of the FD&C Act, a food is misbranded if its labeling is false or misleading in any particular way. Section 201(n) of the FD&C Act provides additional guidance on how labeling may be misleading. It states that labeling is misleading if it fails to reveal all facts that are "material in light of such representations (made or suggested in the labeling) or material with respect to consequences which may result from the use of the article to which the labeling or advertising relates under the conditions of use prescribed in the labeling or advertising thereof or under such conditions of use as are customary or usual."

While the legislative history of section 201(n) contains little discussion of the word "material," there is precedent to guide the Agency in its decision regarding whether information on a food is in fact material within the meaning of 201(n). Historically, the Agency has generally limited the scope of the materiality concept to information about the attributes of the food itself. FDA has required special labeling on the basis of it being "material" information in cases where the absence of such information may: 1) pose special health or environmental risks (e.g., warning statement on certain protein diet products); 2) mislead the consumer in light of other statements made on the label (e.g., requirement for quantitative nutrient information when certain nutrient content claims are made about a product); or 3) in cases where a consumer may assume that a food, because of its similarity to another food, has nutritional, organoleptic, or functional characteristics of the food it resembles when in fact it does not (e.g., reduced fat margarine not suitable for frying).

FDA does not require labeling to indicate whether or not a food or food ingredient is a bioengineered product, just as it does not require labeling to indicate which breeding technique was used in developing a food plant. Rather, any significant differences in the food itself have to be disclosed in labeling. If genetic modifications do materially change the composition of a food product, these changes must be reflected in the food's labeling. This would include its nutritional content, (for example, more folic acid or greater iron content) or requirements for storage, preparation, or cooking, which might impact the food's safety characteristics or nutritional qualities. For example, one soybean variety was modified to alter the levels of oleic acid in the beans; because the oil from this soybean is significantly different when compared to conventional soybean oil, we advised the company to adopt a new name for that oil, a name that reflects the intended change.

If a bioengineered food were to contain an allergen not previously found in that food, information about the presence of the allergen would be material as to the potential consequences of consumption of the food. If FDA determined that labeling would be sufficient to enable the food to be safely marketed, the Agency would require that the food be labeled to indicate the presence of the allergen.

FDA has received comments suggesting that foods developed through modern biotechnology should bear a label informing consumers that the food was produced using bioengineering. While we have given careful consideration to these comments, we do not have data or other information that would form a basis for concluding under the FD&C Act that the fact that a food or its ingredients was produced using bioengineering is material within the meaning of 201(n) and thus, is a fact that must be disclosed in labeling. Hence, we believe that we have neither a scientific nor legal basis to require such labeling. We are developing, however, draft guidance for those that wish voluntarily to label either the presence or absence of bioengineered food in food products. . . .

NEW INITIATIVES

As I mentioned, FDA announced on May 3, as part of an Administration initiative, that we will be taking steps to strengthen the premarket notification program for bioengineered foods. We also intend to provide guidance to food manufacturers who wish voluntarily to label their products regarding whether or not they contain bioengineered ingredients. Our goal is to enhance public confidence in the way in which FDA is regulating bioengineered foods. We want the public to know, loud and clear, that FDA stands behind the safety of these products.

As part of this initiative, we will be proposing regulations to make it mandatory that developers of bioengineered plant varieties notify FDA at least 120 days before they intend to market such products. FDA will require that specific information be submitted to help determine whether the foods pose any safety or labeling concerns. The Agency will be providing further guidance to industry on the scientific data needed to ensure that foods developed through bioengineering are safe for human consumption. To help make the process more transparent, the Agency has made a commitment to ensuring that, consistent with information disclosure laws, consumers have access to information submitted to FDA as part of the notification process and to FDA's responses in a timely fashion.

The proposed rule on premarket notification and the draft labeling guidance are both high priorities for the Agency, and we intend to publish each of these later this fall. Both will provide a full opportunity for public comment before final policies are established. Let me assure you that when we come to a decision regarding these matters, FDA will operate in an open, transparent manner so that the public can understand our regulatory approach and continue to provide us with feedback about its impact. As a scientific organization we are comfortable with debate over complex scientific issues, and welcome the discussions that have occurred at public meetings to date. It is important that the public, including the scientific community, clearly understand FDA's policy on bioengineered foods.

Source: Selections from U.S. Food and Drug Administration, September 2000 (URL: http://www.cfsan.fda.gov/~lrd/stbioeng.html)

APPENDIX F

FOOD SAFETY IN THE KITCHEN: A "HACCP" APPROACH (2002)

The Hazard Analysis and Critical Control Point (HACCP) system has been lauded as an effective approach to reducing the contamination of meat and other foods by bacteria, viruses, and other pathogens. Although primarily used for improving the handling and packaging of food during the manufacturing process, the system applies to home kitchens as well. This document offers a useful description of the HACCP system that consumers can understand and gives practical advice that cooks can use in the kitchen.

Processing plants will be required to test meat and poultry for bacteria under new USDA rules intended to reduce disease-producing organisms known as "pathogens." The plants must implement HACCP (Hazard Analysis and Critical Control Points) systems as a means of controlling their processes to prevent microbial contamination.

Even though HACCP in the plants will significantly reduce pathogens on meat and poultry products, these foods will not be sterile. While it's not practical to do microbial testing in home kitchens, the HACCP approach is also valid to help the consumer learn and practice safe food handling and preparation of all meat and poultry at home.

The improved inspection system will not replace good sanitation and safe food handling in the home. Consumers must still share in the responsibility for safe food and safe food handling. Meat and poultry which are properly handled and cooked at home should be safe.

ABOUT THE NEW RULE

USDA's Food Safety and Inspection Service (FSIS) is pursuing a broad and long-term science-based strategy to improve the safety of meat and poultry products and to better protect the public health. Part of this strategy is a farm-to-table approach to improve the safety of meat and poultry at each step in the food production, distribution, and marketing chain.

As a result, FSIS has published new regulations to modernize USDA's meat and poultry inspection system. Part of these regulations include a HACCP system of process controls to prevent food safety hazards.

HACCP focuses on problem prevention. It involves taking a look at processes or food handling practices and identifying critical control points, or steps, where failure to take appropriate action is most likely to result in foodborne illness.

WHAT DOES HACCP MEAN TO THE CONSUMER IN THE HOME?

Recent surveys show that consumers are more aware these days of food safety issues. According to Bessie Berry, Manager of USDA's Meat and Poultry Hotline, "A recent Associated Press poll revealed that 89% of those surveyed said they follow the safety handling instructions on raw meat and poultry products. The safe handling instructions are really part of a HACCP approach which starts in the store and continues in the home." But do consumers really understand what hazards and critical control points are? As in the meat and poultry plants, potential hazards in the home can be divided into three categories:

1. biological (bacteria);
2. chemical (cleaning agents); and
3. physical (equipment).

This focus will be on the biological hazards, or foodborne bacteria, which can lead to illness if the food is mishandled, particularly for those more at risk—the very young, the elderly and the immuno-compromised.

Certain processes or handling practices by consumers in the home have been identified as being essential or critical in preventing foodborne illness. These practices, which prevent or control the "dinner plate" microbial contamination associated with foodborne illness, are under the direct control of the consumer, from food acquisition through disposal.

They are purchasing, storing, pre-preparation, cooking, serving, and handling leftovers. Failure to take appropriate action at these critical points could result in foodborne illness.

CRITICAL POINT 1: PURCHASING

- Purchase meat and poultry products last and keep packages of raw meat and poultry separate from other foods, particularly foods that will be eaten without further cooking. Consider using plastic bags to enclose individual packages of raw meat and poultry.

- Make sure meat and poultry products—whether raw, pre-packaged, or from the deli—are refrigerated when purchased.
- USDA strongly advises against purchasing fresh, pre-stuffed whole birds.
- Canned goods should be free of dents, cracks or bulging lids.
- Plan to drive directly home from the grocery store. You may want to take a cooler with ice for perishables. Always refrigerate perishable food within 2 hours. Refrigerate within 1 hour when the temperature is above 90°F.

CRITICAL POINT 2: HOME STORAGE

- Verify the temperature of your refrigerator and freezer with an appliance thermometer—refrigerators should run at 40°F or below; freezers at 0°F. Most foodborne bacteria grow slowly at 40°F, a safe refrigerator temperature. Freezer temperatures of 0°F stop bacterial growth.
- At home, refrigerate or freeze meat and poultry immediately.
- To prevent raw juices from dripping on other foods in the refrigerator, use plastic bags or place meat and poultry on a plate.
- Wash hands with soap and water for 20 seconds before and after handling any raw meat, poultry, or seafood products.
- Store canned goods in a cool, clean dry place. Avoid extreme heat or cold which can be harmful to canned goods.
- Never store any foods directly under a sink and always keep foods off the floor and separate from cleaning supplies.

CRITICAL POINT 3: PRE-PREPARATION

- The importance of hand washing cannot be overemphasized. This simple practice is the most economical, yet often forgotten way to prevent contamination or cross-contamination.
- Wash hands (gloved or not) with soap and water for 20 seconds: before beginning preparation; after handling raw meat, poultry, seafood or eggs; after touching animals; after using the bathroom; after changing diapers; or after blowing the nose.
- Don't let juices from raw meat, poultry or seafood come in contact with cooked foods or foods that will be eaten raw, such as fruits or salad ingredients.

- Wash hands, counters, equipment, utensils, and cutting boards with soap and water immediately after use. Counters, equipment, utensils and cutting boards can be sanitized with a chlorine solution of 1 teaspoon liquid household bleach per quart of water. Let the solution stand on the board after washing, or follow the instructions on sanitizing products.
- Thaw in the refrigerator, Never On the Counter. It is also safe to thaw in cold water in an airtight plastic wrapper or bag, changing the water every 30 minutes till thawed. Or, thaw in the microwave and cook the product immediately.
- Marinate foods in the refrigerator, Never On the Counter.
- USDA recommends that if you choose to stuff whole poultry, it is critical that you use a meat thermometer to check the internal temperature of the stuffing. The internal temperature in the center of the stuffing should reach 165°F before removing it from the oven. Lacking a meat thermometer, cook the stuffing outside the bird.

CRITICAL POINT 4: PRE-COOKING

- Always cook thoroughly. If harmful bacteria are present, only thorough cooking will destroy them; freezing or rinsing the foods in cold water is not sufficient to destroy bacteria.
- Use a meat thermometer to determine if your meat or poultry or casserole has reached a safe internal temperature. Check the product in several spots to assure that a safe temperature has been reached and that harmful bacteria like *Salmonella* and certain strains of *E. coli* have been destroyed.
- Avoid interrupted cooking. Never refrigerate partially cooked products to later finish cooking on the grill or in the oven. Meat and poultry products must be cooked thoroughly the first time and then they may be refrigerated and safely reheated later.
- When microwaving foods, carefully follow manufacturers instructions. Use microwave-safe containers, cover, rotate, and allow for the standing time, which contributes to thorough cooking.

CRITICAL POINT 5: SERVING

- Wash hands with soap and water before serving or eating food.
- Serve cooked products on clean plates with clean utensils and clean hands. Never put cooked foods on a dish that has held raw products unless the dish is washed with soap and hot water.

Appendix F

- Hold hot foods above 140°F and cold foods below 40°F.
- Never leave foods, raw or cooked, at room temperature longer than 2 hours. On a hot day with temperatures above 90°F, this decreases to 1 hour.

CRITICAL POINT 6: HANDLING LEFTOVERS

- Wash hands before and after handling leftovers. Use clean utensils and surfaces.
- Divide leftovers into small units and store in shallow containers for quick cooling. Refrigerate within 2 hours of cooking.
- Discard anything left out too long.
- Never taste a food to determine if it is safe.
- When reheating leftovers, reheat thoroughly to a temperature of 165°F or until hot and steamy. Bring soups, sauces and gravies to a rolling boil.
- If in doubt, throw it out.

Source: Food Safety and Inspection Service, July 2002 (URL: http://www.fsis.usda.gov/Fact_Sheets/Food_Safety_in_the_Kitchen)

APPENDIX G

HHS ISSUES NEW RULES TO ENHANCE SECURITY OF THE U.S. FOOD SUPPLY (2003)

Those concerned about terrorist attacks on the United States have highlighted the risks of contamination and poisoning of food by terrorists. The Department of Health and Human Services (HHS) has major responsibilities to prevent such events. This press release from former HHS secretary Thompson describes recent steps taken to prevent or minimize the harm of terrorist contamination of imported or domestic food.

HHS Secretary Tommy G. Thompson today [October 9, 2003] announced the issuance of two Food and Drug Administration regulations that will bolster the safety and security of America's food supply. The new regulations will enable better targeted efforts to monitor and inspect imported foods and will allow quick identification and notification of food processors and other establishments involved in any deliberate or accidental contamination of food.

"By requiring advance notice for imported food shipments and registering domestic and foreign food facilities, we are providing critical new tools for the FDA to identify potentially dangerous foods and better keep our food supply safe and secure," Secretary Thompson said. "These new requirements represent the latest steps in our ongoing efforts to respond to new threats and improve the safety of all the foods that we eat in this country."

The two new regulations will implement key provisions of the Public Health Security and Bioterrorism Preparedness and Response Act of 2002, which provided FDA new authority to protect the nation's food supply against actual or threatened terrorist acts and other food-related emergencies.

"With input from the private sector, our partners in the federal government and the governments of our trading partners, we will use these regu-

Appendix G

lations to work more effectively than ever to protect America's food supply, while maintaining the regular,free flow of commerce that is so vital to the well being of our citizens," said FDA Commissioner Mark B. McClellan, M.D., Ph.D. "Coupled with other counter-terrorism initiatives, these regulations mark a new era of international collaboration, one that strengthens the free market and free trade even as we face new threats to our security. We will keep working to build on these important regulations to fulfill our mission of helping Americans get diverse, affordable food products that are as safe and secure as possible."

The first regulation requires food importers to provide the FDA with advance notice of human and animal food shipments imported or offered for import on or after Dec. 12, 2003. This will allow FDA to know, in advance, when specific food shipments will be arriving at U.S. ports of entry and what those shipments will contain. This advance information will allow the FDA, working with U.S. Customs and Border Protection (CBP), to more effectively target inspections and ensure the safety of imported foods. The FDA expects to receive about 25,000 notifications about incoming shipments each day.

The second regulation requires domestic and foreign food facilities that manufacture, process, pack or hold food for human or animal consumption in the United States to register with the agency by Dec. 12, 2003. As a result, FDA will have for the first time a complete roster of foreign and domestic food facilities. The requirements will enable the FDA to quickly identify and locate affected food processors and other establishments in the event of deliberate or accidental contamination of food. The FDA expects about 420,000 facilities to register under this requirement.

The FDA worked closely with CBP to ensure the new regulations promote a coordinated strategy for border protection.

"Using the electronic data required under these regulations and a sophisticated automated targeting system, CBP and the FDA will be working side-by-side to make joint decisions about food shipments that could pose a potential threat to the United States," said Commissioner Robert C. Bonner, U.S. Customs and Border Protection, Department of Homeland Security. "This integrated risk-management process will increase our security and facilitate the movement of legitimate commerce—objectives shared by both agencies. We look forward to continuing our work with the FDA to implement the regulations in a manner that meets these shared objectives."

The regulations reflect comments from a broad array of law enforcement, national security, industry and other experts as the FDA worked to effectively improve food safety and security without adding unnecessary costs to domestic or international trade.

Threats to Food Safety

"We have listened carefully to what stakeholders said about the proposals, in order to develop rules that are both workable and feasible," said Dr. McClellan. "The rules we are announcing today are intended to fulfill our goal of making the food supply safer and more secure without hindering trade."

Under the prior notice regulation, prior notice of imported foods must be received and confirmed electronically by FDA no more than five days before its arrival and no fewer than:

- two hours before arrival by land via road;
- four hours before arrival by air or by land via rail; or
- eight hours before arrival by water.

In addition, for international mail shipments, notifications must be made before the shipment is mailed. Also, when an individual carries or otherwise transports foods subject to the new requirement, advance notice of two, four or eight hours is required—depending on the mode of transportation. The food must also be accompanied by confirmation of receipt for FDA review.

The regulation's timeframes reflect the FDA's work, in collaboration with other agencies, to reduce substantially the required time for advance notice to minimize unnecessary costs. For example, the proposed rule issued earlier this year would have required that importers give notice by noon the day before the arrival of a shipment of food into the United States for all modes of transportation, including by land by road. The final regulation requires only two hours notice before arrival of food by land by road and could be reduced further in the future as part of FDA-CBP plan to coordinate border-management activities more efficiently.

The advance notice to the FDA may be submitted electronically in most circumstances using Customs' existing ABI/ACS system, making it easier for importers to comply with the new law. In addition, the FDA will operate a new Prior Notice System Interface that can receive such notifications.

The second regulation requires the owner, operator, or agent in charge of a domestic or foreign food facility to register with FDA, providing information about the name and address of each facility at which, and all trade names under which, the registrant conducts business, and information about certain categories of food the facility produces. For a foreign facility, the registration must include the name of the U.S. agent for the facility.

Registration is required for domestic facilities whether or not food from the facility enters interstate commerce. Domestic facilities are also required to provide emergency contact information. All changes to such information must be reported within 60 days.

278

Appendix G

Except for specific exemptions, the registration requirements apply to all facilities that manufacture, process, pack or hold food regulated by FDA, including animal feed, dietary supplements, infant formula, beverages (including alcoholic beverages) and food additives.

Registration would not be required for private residences of individuals; certain food transport vehicles; facilities that manufacture food contact substances and pesticides; farms; restaurants; other retail food establishments; nonprofit food establishments in which food is prepared for or served directly to the consumer; non-processing fishing vessels; and facilities (such as meat and poultry slaughterhouses) that are regulated exclusively by the U.S. Department of Agriculture. Also exempt are foreign facilities if the food from the facility is to undergo further processing or packaging by another facility before it is exported to the U.S.

The registration may be submitted electronically, via the Internet, or by paper through surface mail or by fax. Registrations may also be submitted on CD-ROM by mail. The FDA will be able to accept electronic registration from anywhere in the world 24 hours a day, 7 days a week, beginning Oct. 16. Filling out registration online should take about 15 minutes if a facility has its paperwork ready. A registering facility will receive confirmation of electronic registration and its registration number instantaneously once all the required fields on the registration screen are filled in. There is no fee associated with registration.

The rules take effect Dec. 12, 2003, in accordance with the Bioterrorism Act . . .

Source: U.S. Department of Health and Human Services, October 2003 (URL: http://www.hhs.gov/news/press/2003pres/20031009.html)

APPENDIX H

EXPANDED "MAD COW" SAFEGUARDS ANNOUNCED TO STRENGTHEN EXISTING FIREWALLS AGAINST BSE TRANSMISSION (2004)

Although authorities have discovered a few U.S. cows infected with BSE or mad cow disease, no reported cases of death caused by eating infected beef have occurred here. Aiming to ensure that this record does not change, the Department of Health and Human Services (HHS) has taken several steps to keep infected beef out of the food chain. This press release from the office of former HHS secretary Thompson describes the safeguards and firewall protection put in place in response to this threat to food safety.

HHS Secretary Tommy G. Thompson today [January 26, 2004] announced several new public health measures, to be implemented by the Food and Drug Administration (FDA), to strengthen significantly the multiple existing firewalls that protect Americans from exposure to the agent thought to cause bovine spongiform encephalopathy (BSE, also known as mad cow disease) and that help prevent the spread of BSE in U.S. cattle.

The existing multiple firewalls, developed by both the U.S. Department of Agriculture (USDA) and HHS, have been extremely effective in protecting the American consumer from exposure to BSE. The first firewall is based on import controls started in 1989. A second firewall is surveillance of the U.S. cattle population for the presence of BSE, a USDA firewall that led to the finding of the BSE cow in December. The third firewall is FDA's 1997 animal feed ban, which is the critical safeguard to help prevent the spread of BSE through cattle herds by prohibiting the feeding of most mammalian protein to ruminant animals, including cattle. The fourth firewall, recently announced by USDA, makes sure that no bovine tissues known to be at high risk for carrying the agent of BSE enter the human food supply regulated by USDA. The fifth firewall is effective response planning to contain the potential for any damage from a BSE positive animal, if one is discovered. This contingency response plan, which had been developed over the past several years, was initiated immediately upon the discovery of a BSE positive cow in Washington State December 23.

The new safeguards being announced today are science-based and further bolster these already effective safeguards.

Specifically, HHS intends to ban from human food (including dietary supplements), and cosmetics a wide range of bovine-derived material so that the same safeguards that protect Americans from exposure to the agent of BSE through meat products regulated by USDA also apply to food products that FDA regulates.

FDA will also prohibit certain currently allowed feeding and manufacturing practices involving feed for cattle and other ruminant animals. These additional measures will further strengthen FDA's 1997 "animal feed" rule.

"Today's actions will make strong public health protections against BSE even stronger," Secretary Thompson said. "Although the current animal feed rule provides a strong barrier against the further spread of BSE, we must never be satisfied with the status quo where the health and safety of our animals and our population is at stake. The science and our own experience and knowledge in this area are constantly evolving. Small as the risk may already be, this is the time to make sure the public is protected to the greatest extent possible."

"Today we are bolstering our BSE firewalls to protect the public," said FDA Commissioner Mark B. McClellan, M.D., Ph.D. "We are further strengthening our animal feed rule, and we are taking additional steps to further protect the public from being exposed to any potentially risky materials from cattle. FDA's vigorous inspection and enforcement program has helped us achieve a compliance rate of more than 99 percent with the feed ban rule, and we intend to increase our enforcement efforts to assure compliance with our enhanced regulations. Finally, we are continuing to assist in the development of new technologies that will help us in the future improve even further these BSE protections. With today's actions, FDA will be doing more than ever before to protect the public against BSE by eliminating additional potential sources of BSE exposure."

To implement these new protections, FDA will publish two interim final rules that will take effect immediately upon publication, although there will be an opportunity for public comment after publication.

The first interim final rule will ban the following materials from FDA-regulated human food, (including dietary supplements) and cosmetics:

- Any material from "downer" cattle. ("Downer" cattle are animals that cannot walk.);
- Any material from "dead" cattle. ("Dead" cattle are cattle that die on the farm (i.e. before reaching the slaughter plant);
- Specified Risk Materials (SRMs) that are known to harbor the highest concentrations of the infectious agent for BSE, such as the brain, skull, eyes, and spinal cord of cattle 30 months or older, and a portion of the small intestine and tonsils from all cattle, regardless of their age or health; and
- The product known as mechanically separated beef, a product which may contain SRMs. Meat obtained by Advanced Meat Recovery (an automated system for cutting meat from bones), may be used since USDA regulations do not allow the presence of SRMs in this product.

The second interim final rule is designed to lower even further the risk that cattle will be purposefully or inadvertently fed prohibited protein. It was the feeding of such protein to cattle that was the route of disease transmission that led to the BSE epidemic in United Kingdom cattle in the 1980's and 1990's.

This interim final rule will implement four specific changes in FDA's present animal feed rule. First, the rule will eliminate the present exemption in the feed rule that allows mammalian blood and blood products to be fed to other ruminants as a protein source. Recent scientific evidence suggests that blood can carry some infectivity for BSE.

Second, the rule will also ban the use of "poultry litter" as a feed ingredient for ruminant animals. Poultry litter consists of bedding, spilled feed, feathers, and fecal matter that are collected from living quarters where poultry is raised. This material is then used in cattle feed in some areas of the country where cattle and large poultry raising operations are located near each other. Poultry feed may legally contain protein that is prohibited in ruminant feed, such as bovine meat and bone meal. The concern is that spillage of poultry feed in the chicken house occurs and that poultry feed (which may contain protein prohibited in ruminant feed) is then collected as part of the "poultry litter" and added to ruminant feed.

Third, the rule will ban the use of "plate waste" as a feed ingredient for ruminants. Plate waste consists of uneaten meat and other meat scraps that are currently collected from some large restaurant operations and rendered into meat and bone meal for animal feed. The use of "plate waste" con-

Appendix H

founds FDA's ability to analyze ruminant feeds for the presence of prohibited proteins, compromising the Agency's ability to fully enforce the animal feed rule.

Fourth, the rule will further minimize the possibility of cross-ontamination of ruminant and non-ruminant animal feed by requiring equipment, facilities or production lines to be dedicated to non-ruminant animal feeds if they use protein that is prohibited in ruminant feed. Currently, some equipment, facilities and production lines process or handle prohibited and non-prohibited materials and make both ruminant and non-ruminant feed – a practice which could lead to cross-contamination.

To accompany these new measures designed to provide a further layer of protection against BSE, FDA will in 2004 step up its inspections of feed mills and renderers. FDA will itself conduct 2,800 inspections and will make its resources go even further by continuing to work with state agencies to fund 3,100 contract inspections of feed mill and renderers and other firms that handle animal feed and feed ingredients. Through partnerships with states, FDA will also receive data on 700 additional inspections, for a total of 3,800 state contract and partnership inspections in 2004 alone, including annual inspections of 100 percent of all known renderers and feed mills that process products containing materials prohibited in ruminant feed.

"We have worked hard with the rendering and animal feed production industries to try and achieve full compliance with the animal feed rule," said Dr. McClellan, "and through strong education and a vigorous enforcement campaign, backed by additional inspections and resources, we intend to maintain a high level of compliance."

Dr. McClellan also noted that, in response to finding a BSE positive cow in Washington state December 23, FDA inspected and traced products at 22 facilities related to that positive cow or products from the cow, including feed mills, farms, dairy farms, calf feeder lots, slaughter houses, meat processors, transfer stations, and shipping terminals. Moreover, FDA has conducted inspections at the rendering facilities that handled materials from the positive cow, and they were found to be fully in compliance with FDA's feed rule.

To further strengthen protections for Americans, FDA/HHS intends to work with Congress to consider proposals to assure that these important protective measures will be implemented as effectively as possible.

FDA is also continuing its efforts to assist in the development of better BSE science, to achieve the same or greater confidence in BSE protection at a lower cost. For example, to enhance the ability of our public health system to detect prohibited materials in animal feed, FDA will continue to support the development and evaluation of diagnostic tests to identify prohibited materials. These tests would offer a quick and reliable method of testing animal feeds for prohibited materials and for testing other products for contamination with the agent thought to cause BSE.

Source: U.S. Department of Health and Human Services, January 2004 (URL: http://www.hhs.gov/news/press/2004pres/20040126.html)

INDEX

Locators in **boldface** indicate main topics. Locators followed by *c* indicate chronology entries. Locators followed by *b* indicate biographical entries. Locators followed by *g* indicate glossary entries.

Threats to Food Safety

Index

Index

Index

Index

293

Index

295

Threats to Food Safety

296

Index

297

Index

299